# Traditional South Asian Medicine

Founded by Rahul Peter Das and Ronald Eric Emmerick (†)
Edited by Rahul Peter Das

VOLUME 8
2008

DR. LUDWIG REICHERT VERLAG WIESBADEN

**Traditional South Asian Medicine** (TSAM) is a scholarly journal devoted to research into all aspects of traditional medicine in South Asia. It does not appear regularly, but only when enough contributions of high standard have been submitted. Contributions may be in English, French or German, but the use of English is preferred. Longer contributions in a language other than English should be accompanied by an English summary. Priority will be given to contributions submitted as electronic files and written with WordPerfect under MSDOS or Windows. If other wordprocessors are used, the text should be submitted in plain ASCII format. Unsolicited books cannot be returned to their senders but will be reviewed at the editor's discretion. All correspondence is to be addressed to: The Editor, Traditional South Asian Medicine, Dorotheenring 5, 25451 Quickborn, Germany (das.rp@t-online.de). For orders, subscriptions, review copies, etc. contact: Dr. Ludwig Reichert Verlag, Tauernstr. 11, 65199 Wiesbaden, Germany (info@reichert-verlag.de).

**Traditional South Asian Medicine** continues the Journal of the European Āyurvedic Society (JEĀS), which was intended to be the organ of the European Āyurvedic Society (EĀS), founded in 1983 in Groningen, Netherlands, as a forum for scholars resident in Europe who have an interest in Āyurveda; this society is no longer active. Volume 1 was published with the financial assistance of the Johanna und Fritz Buch-Gedächtnistiftung. Five volumes of JEĀS have appeared; TSAM continues the numbering of its volumes.

ISSN 1618-1522



ISBN: 978-3-89500-626-5

# CONTENTS

*Articles*



*Reviews and Notices*

## CONTENTS (Contd.)

# Arion Thomas Roşu
# (1.2.1924–4.4.2007)

EUGEN CIURTIN

Prin moartea lui Arion Thomas Roşu, în dimineaţa zilei de 4 aprilie 2007 la spitalul din Versailles, indianistica franceză şi internaţională se desparte de unul dintre savanţii cei mai rari şi mai preţuiţi. Nestor al orientaliştilor de origine română, Arion Roşu şi-a consacrat partea principală a cercetărilor sale de o viaţă medicinei indiene, iar opera sa dispune de toate trăsăturile necesare pentru a fi considerată una dintre cele mai redutabile şi mai semnificative pentru epoca în care Āyurveda şi-a căpătat, în indianistică, un drept de cetate major.

Micul Arion se naşte la Bucureşti, la 1 februarie 1924, şi avea să trăiască primii ani la Sinaia, mic oraş la poalele Carpaţilor Prahovei fondat, spre 1700, în jurul mânăstirii omonime şi amintind de pelerinajul la Muntele Sinai al spătarului muntean Mihail Cantacuzino. După 1883, când Carol I şi Regina Elisabeta – între altele corespondenţi ai lui Max Müller – inaugurează Castelul Peleş ca reşedinţă de vară a Casei Regale, Sinaia avea să devină un oraş atractiv. Arion Roşu nu va uita până târziu cum, jucându-se în împrejurimi, avea să vadă coborând dintr-o maşină frânând brusc în faţa sa un mai vârstnic, chipeş băiat, despre care va afla că e Mihai I (n. 1921), ultim rege (1940-1947) al unei Românii care, brăzdată de convulsii nenumărate, îi va marca pentru totdeauna adolescenţa şi anii de studenţie.

Nu departe de alte vechi ctitorii cantacuzine, familia sa modestă se va strămuta în capitala Regatului României Mari în 1931, şi aici Arion va relua cursuri şcolare al căror parcurs e clătinat de instabilitatea economică, de gravele incertitudini suscitate de situaţia politică locală şi, curând, de venirea războiului. Martor şi victimă a persecuţiilor rasiale şi ideologice, al dictaturilor care se vor succeda în România până târziu, în 1989, va fi protejat la început doar de solidaritatea exemplară a familiei, de rarele burse ale unor instituţii private sărace şi, în pragul şi de-a lungul războiului, în plină formare intelectuală, de prietenia luminoasă cu colegi evrei şi catolici atraşi de lumea Indiei şi de civilizaţiile Asiei. Îi va evoca astfel toată viaţa pe adolescenţii de odinioară, Anton Zigmund-Cerbu (1923-1964), Liza Zigmund-Cerbu (1924-1965), Marcel Leibovici (1924-2005), Anton, Marcel şi Arion făcând parte din aceeaşi clasă – ameninţată de legislaţia antievreiască de tip *numerus clausus* – şi împărtăşind fervoarea aceloraşi rare, dificile lecturi. Drumurile lor se vor despărţi totuşi, cei trei, spre deosebire de Arion Roşu, izbutind să emigreze în Franţa deja în 1947, unde vor urma un parcurs orientalist durabil mai ales la École Pratique des Hautes Études şi la Centre National de la Recherche Scientifique, regăsindu-se în cele din urmă distinşi cercetători (Liza Zigmund-Cerbu, în câmpul studiilor siriace), sau profesori de istorie a religiilor asiatice la Columbia University (Anton Zigmund-Cerbu), sau de asiriologie la Universitatea din Montréal (Marcel Leibovici). Îi va lega însă pentru totdeauna apartenenţa la o primă generaţie de orientalişti români, căreia i se adaugă un alt mare prieten, Sergiu Al-George (1922-1981). Aşa cum va scrie Arion Roşu despre soţii Cerbu, 'ils se partagèrent, pour ainsi dire, l'Orient, d'une part l'Asie orientale, de l'autre l'Asie antérieure, qui englobait l'Orient chrétien auquel était rattachée l'Europe de l'Est'.

Manifestată foarte timpuriu, vocaţia adâncă a lui Arion Roşu pentru studiul Indiei nu a fost concurată de nimic, precum nimic nu i-a putut înfrânge dorinţa de a i se consacra, sprijinindu-se şi pe formaţia sa solidă în domeniile filologiei clasice, ilustrată convingător pe atunci de Universitatea din Bucureşti. Asemeni colegilor săi, s-a putut bucura în prima tinereţe de existenţa, la Bucureşti, a unui indianist şi istoric al religiilor care va deveni pretutindeni cunoscut: Mircea Eliade (1907-1986). Stimulat de intensa lui pledoarie în favoarea studiului Indiei, Arion Roşu va descoperi, asimila şi continua teza sa de doctorat despre Yoga susţinută la Bucureşti în 1933 şi publicată în 1936 (*Yoga. Essai sur les origines de la mystique indienne*[1]). Nicăieri altundeva nu e atât de profund şi personal exprimat parcursul lui Arion Roşu – între 'cet indianisme sans école' care a fost şi avea să rămână până azi cel românesc, şi incomparabila indianistică franceză şi europeană – decât aşa cum se regăseşte el într-un articol rămas inedit, pe care îl dedica 'Profesorului Mircea Eliade la împlinirea a 70 de ani':[2]

---

[1] Bucureşti: Fundaţiile Regale / Paris: Librairie orientaliste Paul Geuthner.

[2] Manuscris din anii 1970 dăruit nouă de autor; a doua redactare, pp. 4f.

> Les premiers travaux d'indianisme de Mircea Eliade, notamment sa thèse sur le *Yoga*, préparée en Inde sous la direction de S.N. Dasgupta, ont suscité à Bucarest un vif intérêt et allumé chez de jeunes philologues classiques tels que Zigmund-Cerbu et moi-même la flamme du sanskrit et de la pensée indienne. La direction féconde de son analyse des techniques corporelles et spirituelles du Yoga est rejointe par mes travaux philologiques entrepris à Paris depuis 1965 sur la médecine indienne traditionnelle, spécialement sur la psychosomatique de l'Āyurveda. Attiré dans les années 1940 par l'orientalisme sous l'impulsion des recherches de Mircea Eliade, dont je n'ai fait la connaissance qu'un quart de siècle plus tard en Occident, un long détour m'a ramené en fait à son inspiration. Ma rencontre, attendue quatre lustres, avec les maîtres français en indianisme m'a en effet reconduit en quelque sorte au point de départ, à savoir l'analyse donnée par Mircea Eliade des pratiques psychosomatiques du Yoga. C'est elle qui a été déterminante pour ma démarche intellectuelle. Comme dans la légende hassidique interprétée par Heinrich Zimmer, où un pieux rabbin de Cracovie a dû faire un voyage à Prague pour découvrir finalement son propre trésor caché derrière le poêle de sa maison, de même j'ai dû personnellement faire un long voyage d'initiation pour pouvoir retrouver l'idée qui m'avait poussé, encore collégien à Bucarest, à me consacrer aux études sanskrites. D'autre part, j'ai renoué avec la tradition savante de mon devancier Constantin Georgian. Il y a un siècle celui-ci avait en effet été auditeur de la conférence de sanskrit que donnait Abel Bergaigne à l'École des Hautes Études, et ce génial védisant a marqué la destinée de Sylvain Lévi, le maître de mes maîtres, Louis Renou et Jean Filliozat.

Opera lui Arion Roşu cuprinde aproape o centurie de studii monografice, articole, bibliografii, precum şi peste şaizeci de recenzii critice, note şi notiţe bibliografice. Un studiu despre 'La musicothérapie en perspective historique et transculturelle', redactat în ultimii ani, ar fi trebuit să înceapă astfel: 'Tout arrive pour celui qui sait attendre'. Arion Roşu ştia bine ce însemnase să aştepte. Impregnat de cultura franceză şi stimulat de existenţa unui Institut français la Bucureşti, dirijat pe atunci de Alphonse Dupront (viitor Rector al Sorbonei) sau a unui Liceul francez Bossuet, a încercat să se apropie de timpuriu de numele venerate care l-au ghidat de-a lungul întregii opere. S-a înscris astfel la finele anilor '40 la École Pratique des Hautes Études, însă a trebuit într-adevăr să aştepte douăzeci de ani pentru a se integra astfel – şi numai după stabilirea la Paris, în 1965 – mediului indianist parizian.

Arion Roşu a debutat în 1956, cu un articol despre diferitele 'nume ale pupilei în sanscrită', publicat în franceză la Berlin. Data nu trebuie să înşele: ea reflectă mai degrabă condiţiile mai mult decât precare care sugrumau, în Europa orientală captivă a acelor ani, orice studiu umanist. Dar Prof.Dr. Raghu Vira, pe atunci Director al International Academy of Indian Culture (New Delhi), îi va scrie la 10 iunie 1958, înainte de a veni la Bucureşti: 'You have devoted your time and energy to the study of India and that makes you a bridge between India and Romania.' Împreună cu bunul său prieten şi coleg Al-George (cu care avea să păstreze o lungă corespondenţă) îşi clădeşte pregătirea filologică şi istorică temeinică în condiţii de izolare, precaritate şi risc, despre care povestea anevoie, privilegiind totuşi amintirea înseninată, aşa cum a făcut, alături de fiica sa Myriam, în 2001, când s-a aflat pentru ultima oară în România.

Întâlnirea cu şcoala lui Louis Renou (pe care îl venera din adolescenţă) şi mai cu seamă a lui Jean Filliozat, adoptarea sa la biblioteca muzeului Guimet (1965-1967) şi mai apoi în Centre National de la Recherche Scientifique (1967-1990), i-au permis vocaţiei să se împlinească. Recunoştinţa şi ataşamentul său pentru Franţa, limba şi cultura sa au fost întotdeauna desăvârşite. În opera extraordinar de solidă şi diversă şi în personalitatea umanistă a lui Jean Filliozat Arion Roşu a regăsit, direct şi indirect, stimulul cel mai preţios, chiar dacă descoperirea scrierilor medicului sas al lui Ranjit Singh, Honigberger, sau cărţile lui Reinhold F.G. Müller l-au atras deja în anii 1950 tocmai spre medicina tradiţională a Asiei de Sud. Sub direcţia maestrului său va sintetiza, în teza clasică susţinută în 1974 şi publicată în 1978 – *Les conceptions psychologiques dans les textes médicaux indiens* – întreaga problematică şi literatură a Indiei antice şi medievale referitoare la unitatea psihosomatică, recitind şi rescriind neîncetat, cu o extremă densitate şi concizie ('te cunosc bine, eşti un "perfecţionist" pătimaş', îi va scrie Eliade la 29 septembrie 1977). Probleme esenţiale în gândirea medicală indiană nu au mai fost studiate cu aceeaşi acurateţe şi acuitate din 1978 şi până azi. Multe studii din anii 1970-2000 aveau să aprofundeze traiectoria dicipolului devenit maestru într-un canton al indianisticii clasice multă vreme prea puţin frecventat şi asumat în chip de prioritate umanistă. Coerenţa şi rigoarea tuturor studiilor sale organizează de la sine câteva volume în care, reluate în chip de *Kleine Schriften*, ar putea lesne amplifica tematica şi metoda unei cercetări de o viaţă, novatoare şi solidă, iar acesta şi fusese gândul lui Arion Roşu în ultimii ani.

Dorind să construiască o operă demnă de vigoarea aceleia a lui Jean Filliozat, Arion Roşu s-a orientat astfel, cu metodă şi scrupulozitate, spre chestiunile fundamentale, căutând totdeauna să lumineze particularităţi din cultura medicală şi religioasă indiană rămase obscure, câteva din ele niciodată lămurite până la el. A scris astfel despre unele tratate esenţiale precum *Mādhavanidāna* (1977) sau *Rasendracūḍāmaṇi*, din care a excerptat, precum odinioară P.C. Ray, editat, tradus şi adnotat un dificil fragment (1997), în cadrul celui mai laborios şi novator efort inedit al său. A studiat deontologia medicală în India (1981, 1985), tradiţia şi revirimentul modern al Āyurvedei (1981, 1982, 1984, 1987, 1991) şi evoluţia tradiţiilor medicale din subcontinent (2002), acordând prioritate studiilor despre *rasāyana* şi *rasaśāstra* (1975, 1976, 1984, 1986, 1988, 1997, în pregătire), despre medicină, alchimie şi Yoga (1982) sau despre careurile magice (1987, 1989) în Āyurveda. Studiile sale despre *trivarga* (1978), *marman* (1981), *mantra* şi *yantra* (1986) ori *vajrolī mudrā* (2002) sunt dotate cu o fiabilitate care concede foarte puţin timpului scurs de la publicarea lor. O ultimă ilustrare amplă a îmbinării ştiinţelor filologice şi istorice cu o curiozitate nesecată e monografia despre apă în India (cuprinzând studii apărute între 1999 şi 2007). Apariţia ediţiei şi traducerii tratatului *Rasendracūḍāmaṇi* (*Le joyau de diadème pour le mercure*) au fost anunţate încă din 1985 (*IASTAM Newsletter* 5). Arion Roşu a realizat întâiul survol complet al acestui tratat într-o epocă în care, dincolo de rădăcinile diverse ale unui interes crescând pentru medicinile tradiţionale, nu exista nici o ediţie şi traducere completă a vreunui text alchimic sau iatrochimic indian. Ataşamentul său pentru *realia*, de pildă, e observabil deja din adnotările unei traduceri româneşti din Kālidāsa (1964). Păstrate de familie, trei mici *Carnets de mission* păstrează sute de pagini cu observaţii directe şi lecturi rare făcute pe parcursul călătoriilor sale în India (1978-1982), atingând practic zeci de teme clasice în Āyurveda şi majoritatea zonelor subcontinentu lui. Cunoscând toate calităţile cercetărilor lui Arion Roşu, e de sperat că apariţia acestei cărţi (aflată în grija prietenilor săi Pierre-

Sylvain Filliozat, Dominik Wujastyk şi David Gordon White) nu va întârzia, şi va răsplăti astfel stăruinţele autorului fie şi postum.

Se cuvine menţionat că printre axele lor principale se află şi prezenţa Indiei în cultura română şi în Europa de Est, plecând de la studiile sale despre medicul Johann Martin Honigberger (1959-1960, 1962, 1963, 2004 şi în pregătire), Constantin Georgian (1966), Mihai Eminescu (1970) şi până la paginile despre Al-George (1982), Zigmund-Cerbu (1999-2000) şi Eliade, cu care se va afla în corespondenţă din 1965, întâlnindu-se abia începând din septembrie 1968, când fac în sfârşit cunoştinţă la Neuilly. Totodată, trebuie amintit că Arion Roşu a studiat cu acribie şi rolul învăţaţilor francezi sau al misionarilor europeni în istoria ştiinţelor şi tehnicii în India (1991; 1993, 2003), scriind şi despre savanţi indianişti, precursori sau contemporani, precum Marcelin Berthelot (1983, 1986, 1990), Chandragiri Dwarakanath (1980), Jeannine Auboyer (1990) – cea care avea să joace un rol esenţial în emigrarea sa în Franţa, după ce îi publicase primele articole –, Albert Le Bonheur (1993-1994), Priya Vrat Sharma (1997), şi mai cu seamă despre istoria medicinei indiene în spaţiul francez, de la Gustave Liétard et Palmyr Cordier (1989) la Jean Filliozat (1984, 1993-1994).

Majoritatea acestor contribuţii au apărut în periodice franceze consacrate Indiei, precum *Arts Asiatiques* (1957-1967), *Journal Asiatique* (din 1968, când devine membru al Société Asiatique, până în 2005, fiind unul dintre cei mai prezenţi indianişti şi chiar orientalişti provenind din Europa de Est, din întreaga istorie a celui mai vechi periodic asiatic european), *Bulletin de l'École française d'Extrême-Orient* (1969-1982, 2001) şi mai ales, încă de la fondarea lui în 1983 şi până la moartea sa, *Bulletin d'Études Indiennes*. Avea să publice, în periodicul fondat de Nalini Balbir şi Georges-Jean Pinault, editat de Nalini Balbir, peste 200 de pagini, incluzând 9 articole şi nu mai puţin de 55 de recenzii critice şi note bibliografice, cea mai mare parte a lor consacrând-o publicaţiilor indiene atingătoare de Āyurveda. Alături de contribuţiile sale în periodice germane, indiene şi româneşti de indianistică şi studii asiatice, Arion Roşu a reprezentat Franţa în acel comitet de redacţie al seriei iniţiale a acestui periodic (1990-2001), contribuind în *Journal of the European Āyurvedic Society / Traditional South Asian Medicine* pentru volumele 2-7 (1992-2003). Institut d'Études

Indiennes al Collège de France păstrează, alături de cele ale lui Louis Renou, o bibliotecă impresionantă de *separata* închinate medicinei indiene şi indianisticii clasice, provenind din toate colţurile lumii. Lor li se adaugă acum o bibliotecăde specialitate, astfel că acest Fond Arion Roşu poate fi considerat cel mai semnificativ pentru istoria medicinei şi alchimiei indiene din întreaga lume francofonă.

Ultimele evenimente publice la care avea să ia parte au fost legate, *comme pour boucler la boucle*, de maestrul său francez şi de ţara natală. La 17 noiembrie 2006 participa la colocviul 'Sciences et médecine en Asie' închinat centenarului Jean Filliozat de Académie des Inscriptions et Belles-Lettres – al cărei laureat Arion Roşu fusese în 1979, iar la 8 decembrie 2006, în cadrul unei recepţii la Ambasada României de la Paris, i se decerna ordinul 'Meritul cultural' în grad de Comandor conferit de Preşedintele României la Bucureşti în septembrie 2006. Foarte puţin timp apoi, suferinţe mai vechi, unele purtate încă din adolescenţă, l-au încolţit: lunile petrecute în spital aveau să fie ultimele.

Funeraliile au avut loc la 7 aprilie 2007, în sâmbăta dinaintea Paştilor, la Biserica Saint Symphorien din Versailles. Soţia sa Claude Roşu, cea care l-a veghеat şi care i-a fost alături vreme de aproape patruzeci de ani, nu avea să-i supravieţuiască decât până în decembrie. Odihnesc unul alături de celălalt în cimitirul normand din Sées.

În urma sa rămâne o operă fundamentală pentru istoria medicinei şi a religiilor indiene. Ea e cu atât mai rară cu cât Arion Roşu a clădit-o, cum reamintea Profesorul Pierre-Sylvain Filliozat în faţa Societăţii Asiatice din Paris, în împrejurări eroice, în care numai puterea vocaţiei şi un destin ieşit din comun puteau împlini. Cei cărora le-a fost, pe rând sau împreună, prieten, coleg, maestru nu-l pot uita, cum nici Arion Roşu nu-i uita pe aceia de odinioară. Rigoarea şi demnitatea, modestia şi discreţia, bunătatea lui – inconfundabile toate pentru cei care l-au cunoscut îndeaproape, cărora li se încredinţa 'cu veche prietenie' – ne angajează recunoştinţa care îi supravieţuieşte.

## Notă

O bibliografie completă a scrierilor lui Arion Roşu (până în 2004) a apărut în *Du corps humain, au carrefour de plusieurs savoirs en Inde. Mélanges offerts à Arion Roşu par ses collègues et ses amis à l'occasion de son 80e anniversaire. The Human Body, at the Crossroads of Multiple Indian Ways of Knowing. Papers Presented to Arion Roşu by His Colleagues and Friends on the Occasion of his Eightieth Birthday*, Bucarest: Université de Bucarest/Paris: De Boccard 2004 (= *Studia Asiatica* 4-5 ⟨2003-2004⟩), pp. 23-39, volum care se deschide cu o evocare a Doamnei Colette Caillat (1921-2007), Membre de l'Institut de France, îmbogăţită în *Comptes rendus de l'Académie des Inscriptions et Belles-Lettres*, avril-juin 2005: 539-541. Au apărut între timp 'En marge des pratiques tantriques du *JA* 290.1.2002, p. 293-313', *Journal Asiatique* 293,1 (2005): 379-381, nota despre David Gordon White, *Kiss of the Yoginī. 'Tantric Sex' in Its South Asian Context*, Chicago/London: University of Chicago Press 2003 (în *Archives de sciences sociales des religions* 132 ⟨2005⟩: 72), precum şi necrologia în amintirea lui 'David Pingree (1933-2005)', 'Chronique de l'eau (suite) [IV]', notele bibliografice despre David Pingree (*Catalogue of* Jyotiṣa *Manuscripts in the Wellcome Library: Sanskrit Astral and Mathematical Literature*, Leiden/Boston: Brill 2004) şi Priya Vrat Sharma (*Six Decades of Āyurveda ⟨1941-2000⟩. A Collection of Selected Articles and Lectures*, Delhi: Chaukhamba Sanskrit Pratisthan 2005), toate în *Bulletin d'Études Indiennes* 22-23 (2004-2005): 13f., 585, 642f. şi 644. 'Le *kuṇḍalinīyoga* et les charmeurs des serpents' se află sub tipar în Nalini Balbir şi Georges-Jean Pinault (eds.), *Penser, dire et représenter l'animal dans le monde indien, Colloque international, Paris, 25-28 mars 2002*, Paris 2008 (Bibliothèque de l'École des Hautes Études 345). A doua parte a studiului despre *rasāyana* (cf. *Indo-Iranian Journal* 17 ⟨1975⟩: 1-29 şi 395), precum şi lucrări despre craniolatrie sau medicul transilvan J.M. Honigberger, redactatate în colaborare în ultimii ani, îşi aşteaptă apariţia. Altele însă, redactate în stadiu incipient sau doar schiţate, vor rămâne probabil în stadiu embrionar. Cea mai însemnată contribuţie încă inedită rămâne cu certitudine ediţia şi traducerea franceză din *Rasendracūḍāmaṇi*.

Necrologul citit de Pierre-Sylvain Filliozat, Membre de l'Institut de France, la şedinţa din 11 mai 2007 a Société Asiatique (Paris), va fi publicat în *Journal Asiatique* 295,2 (2007). Alte mărturii despre Arion Roşu vor apărea în *Bulletin d'Études Indiennes*, *Indologica Taurinensia* şi *Studia Asiatica*.

## Translation*

With the death of Arion Thomas Roşu in the morning of April 4, 2007 at Versailles hospital centre, both French and international Indian studies lose one of their most exceptional and valuable scholars. Nestor of Romanian scholars of Asia, Arion Roşu devoted the major part of his lifetime research to Indian medicine. His work can be considered as among the most significant and venerated in an age of Indian studies in which Āyurveda gained primary status.

Little Arion was born in Bucharest on February 1, 1924, and spent his first years in Sinaia, a small town in the Prahova valley in the Carpathians founded about 1700 around the monastery of the same name, which refers to the Vallachian *Spathaire* Michael Cantacuzino's pilgrimage to Mount Sinai. After 1883, when Charles I of Romania and his Queen Elizabeth (the two being, furthermore, correspondents of Max Müller) inaugurated the Peleş Castle as the summer residence of the Royal House, Sinaia developed into an attractive small town. Arion Roşu would remember late in life how, playing as a small child in Sinaia, he once saw, alighting from his car with a sudden braking, an older, handsome young man. He would later find out that the young man was Michael I (born 1921), last King (1940-1947) of a country which would indelibly imprint its countless historical upheavals on Arion's adolescence and college years.

Not far from other architectural monuments founded by the Cantacuzins, his modest Roşu family moved to the capital of the kingdom of Greater Romania in 1931. Here, Arion continued his school years under high economic instability, an uncertain political setting and, soon enough, war. A witness and a victim of racist and ideological persecutions, of succeeding dictatorships governing over Romania until very recently in 1989, Arion was protected at first solely by the exemplary solidarity of his family. Later, he obtained rare fellowships given by ill-funded private institutions, and, right before and during the war, during the years of his intellectual formation, he enjoyed the enlightening friendship of some Jewish and Catholic colleagues attracted by the Indian world and Asian civilisations. He would remember all his life the erstwhile adolescents Anton Zigmund-Cerbu (1923-1964), Liza Zigmund-Cerbu (1924-1965), Marcel Leibovici (1924-2005). Anton, Marcel and Arion were in the same class menaced by anti-Jewish *numerus clausus* and sharing the fervour of their rare, difficult common readings. Their paths would, however, separate, the three young men, unlike Arion Ro-

* Translated by Lucian Petrescu. The verbal tenses have been brought into line with common English usage.

şu, being able to emigrate to France already in 1947, where they would follow a solid course in Asian Studies at the École Pratique des Hautes Études and at the Centre National de la Recherche Scientifique, and become finally distinguished researchers (Liza Zigmund-Cerbu, in the field of Syriac studies), or professors of the history of Asian religions at Columbia University (Anton Zigmund-Cerbu) and of the Ancient Near East at the University of Montreal (Marcel Leibovici). Their belonging to a first generation of Romanian Asian scholars, to which another great friend, Sergiu Al-George (1922-1981), belongs, will always connect them. As later Arion Roşu wrote on the Cerbu couple, 'ils se partagèrent, pour ainsi dire, l'Orient, d' une part l'Asie orientale, de l'autre l'Asie antérieure, qui englobait l'Orient chrétien auquel était rattachée l'Europe de l'Est'.

Arion Roşu's ardent calling for the study of India, aroused very early, had not been rivalled by anything, and nothing could hold back his desire to dedicate himself to it. He was supported in his endeavour by his solid education in classical philology, an education which could be very efficaciously completed at that time at the University of Bucharest. Together with his colleagues, he could enjoy in his first youth the presence in Bucharest of an Indologist and historian of religions who would later be acclaimed everywhere: Mircea Eliade (1907-1986). Stimulated by its intense advocacy for the study of India, Arion Roşu discovered, assimilated and continued Eliade's PhD thesis on Yoga defended at Bucharest in 1933 and published in 1936 (*Yoga. Essai sur les origines de la mystique indienne*[1]). We will not find anywhere else the intellectual journey of Arion Roşu – conducted between 'cet indianisme sans école', which was and still remains the Romanian one, and the incomparable tradition of French and European Indology – expressed as we find it in an unpublished article which he dedicated to 'Professor Mircea Eliade on his 70th birthday':[2]

> Les premiers travaux d'indianisme de Mircea Eliade, notamment sa thèse sur le *Yoga*, préparée en Inde sous la direction de S.N. Dasgupta, ont suscité à Bucarest un vif intérêt et allumé chez de jeunes philologues classiques tels que Zigmund-Cerbu et moi-même la flamme du sanskrit et de la pensée indienne. La direction féconde de son analyse des techniques corporelles et spirituelles du Yoga est rejointe par mes travaux philologiques entrepris à Paris depuis 1965 sur la médicine indienne traditionnelle, spécialement sur la psychosomatique de l'Āyurveda. Attiré dans les années 1940 par l'orientalisme sous l'impulsion des recherches de Mircea Eliade,

---

[1] Bucureşti: Fundaţiile Regale / Paris: Librairie orientaliste Paul Geuthner.

[2] Manuscript dating from the 1970s, relinquished to us by the author; revised version, pp. 4f.

dont je n'ai fait la connaissance qu'un quart de siècle plus tard en Occident, un long détour m'a ramené en fait à son inspiration. Ma rencontre, attendue quatre lustres, avec les maîtres français en indianisme m'a en effet reconduit en quelque sorte au point de départ, à savoir l'analyse donnée par Mircea Eliade des pratiques psychosomatiques du Yoga. C'est elle qui a été déterminante pour ma démarche intellectuelle. Comme dans la légende hassidique interprétée par Heinrich Zimmer, où un pieux rabbin de Cracovie a dû faire un voyage à Prague pour découvrir finalement son propre trésor caché derrière le poêle de sa maison, de même j'ai dû personnellement faire un long voyage d'initiation pour pouvoir retrouver l'idée qui m'avait poussé, encore collégien à Bucarest, à me consacrer aux études sanskrites. D'autre part, j'ai renoué avec la tradition savante de mon devancier Constantin Georgian. Il y a un siècle celui-ci avait en effet été auditeur de la conférence de sanskrit que donnait Abel Bergaigne à l'École des Hautes Études, et ce génial védisant a marqué la destinée de Sylvain Lévi, le maître de mes maîtres, Louis Renou et Jean Filliozat.

The work of Arion Roşu contains almost a hundred monographic studies, articles, and bibliographies, together with over sixty book reviews, notes and short notices. A study on 'La musicothérapie en perspective historique et transculturelle', written in the last years of his life, begins with the phrase: 'Tout arrive pour celui qui sait attendre'. Arion Roşu knew very well what it meant to wait. Permeated by French culture and stimulated by the existence of a French Institute in Bucharest, directed back then by Alphonse Dupront (the future president of the Sorbonne), and of a French upper secondary school, the Lycée Bossuet, Arion Roşu tried very early to approach the famous names which had guided him along his career. He enrolled himself in a programme at the École Pratique des Hautes Études at the end of the 1940s, but he really had to wait twenty years before feeling integrated via this means – and only after his arrival in France in 1965 – in the Parisian Indologist milieu.

Arion Roşu debuted in 1956, with an article on 'the different names of the pupil [of the eye] in Sanskrit', published in French in Berlin. The date of publication must not delude us: it reflects, in fact, the precariousness suffocating any study in the humanities in the occupied Eastern Europe of those years. But Prof.Dr. Raghu Vira, who was, back then, the Director of the International Academy of Indian Culture in New Delhi, would write to him on June 10, 1958, just before coming to Bucharest: 'You have devoted your time and energy to the study of India and that makes you a bridge between India and Romania.' Together with his good friend and colleague Al-George (with whom he kept up a long correspondence) Arion Roşu built a strong philological and historical education – in those poor, risky and isolating conditions which he rarely recalled, preferring a serene evoking, like the recollection he gave with his daughter Myriam in 2001 while visiting Romania for the last time.

His encounter with the school of Louis Renou (whom he deeply admired since his adolescence), and foremost with Jean Filliozat, his inclusion in the library of the Musée Guimet (1965-1967), and then in the Centre National de la Recherche Scientifique (1967-1990), allowed him to carry out his vocation. His gratefulness and attachment towards France, towards its culture and language, were always intact. In Jean Filliozat's solid and extraordinarily diverse work, as well as in his humanist personality, Arion Roşu found, directly and indirectly, a priceless inspiration. However, the discovery of the writings of Ranjit Singh's Transylvanian Saxon doctor, Honigberger, or of the writings of Reinhold F.G. Müller, had drawn him already in the 1950s towards South Asian traditional medicine. Under the direction of his teacher he would synthesise the entire problematics of ancient India literature regarding the psychosomatic unity of the human body in his classic PhD thesis defended in 1974 and published in 1978 – *Les conceptions psychologiques dans les textes médicaux indiens* –, rereading and rewriting it constantly, in an extremely close and concise manner ('I know you very well, you are a passionate "perfectionist",' Eliade wrote to him in September 29, 1977). Essential issues in Indian medical thought have not been studied so accurately since his thesis. Many studies from the period 1970-2000 shaped this trajectory of a disciple become master in a sphere of classical Indology less frequented and rarely assumed to be a humanist priority. The coherence and rigour of all of his studies would effortlessly encompass a few volumes, which, republished as *Kleine Schriften*, could easily amplify the theme and the method of an innovative and solid lifetime research – and this had been Arion Roşu's desire in his last years.

Wishing to build a work worthy of the vigour of that of Jean Filliozat, Arion Roşu thus oriented himself, methodically and scrupulously, towards fundamental questions, searching always to clarify obscure details from South Asian medical and religious culture, some of which had never been brought to light until his endeavour. He has thus written on some essential treatises such as the *Mādhavanidāna* (1977) or the *Rasendracūḍāmaṇi*, of which he extracted (as erstwhile P.C. Ray), edited, translated and annotated a difficult fragment in 1997, as part of his most innovative and laborious unpublished effort. He studied the Indian medical deontology (1981, 1985), the tradition of the modern revival of Āyurveda (1981, 1982, 1984, 1987, 1991) and the evolution of the medical traditions of the Subcontinent (2002), giving priority to studies on *rasāyana* and *rasaśāstra* (1975, 1976, 1984, 1986, 1988, 1997, forthcoming), on the relationships between medicine, alchemy and Yoga (1982), or on the magic squares (1987, 1989) in Āyurveda. His studies on *trivarga* (1978), *marman* (1981), *mantra* and *yantra*

(1986) or the *vajrolī mudrā* (2002) are endowed with such reliability that they concede but little to the time which has passed since their publication. One last ample example of his combining philological and historical instruments with undivided curiosity is his monograph on water in India (comprising studies published between 1999 and 2007). The appearance of the edition and translation of the *Rasendracūḍāmaṇi* (*Le joyau de diadème pour le mercure*) has been announced since 1985 (*IASTAM Newsletter* 5). Arion Roşu accomplished the first complete survey of this treatise in an era when, despite the diverse strands of developing interest in traditional medicine and alchemy, there was no complete translation of any alchemical or iatrochemical Indian text. His attachment towards realia can, for instance, be observed already in his annotations of a Romanian translation of Kālidāsa (1964). Preserved by his family, three little *Carnets de mission* hold hundreds of pages with direct observations and rare lectures from his travels in India (1978-1982), covering, in fact, dozens of classic subjects of Āyurveda and many areas of the Subcontinent. Knowing all the qualities of Arion Roşu's research, one can but hope that the appearance of this volume (now under the care of his friends Pierre-Sylvain Filliozat, Dominik Wujastyk and David Gordon White) will not be delayed, and will thus posthumously reward the painstaking efforts of the author.

One must mention that among his main areas of study is also the presence of India in Romanian culture and in Eastern Europe – starting with his studies on Dr Johann Martin Honigberger (1959-1960, 1962, 1963, 2004 and forthcoming), on Constantin Georgian (1966), Mihai Eminescu (1970) up to his pages on Al-George (1982), Zigmund-Cerbu (1999-2000) and Eliade, with whom he corresponded since 1965, but whom he did not meet until September 1968, in Neuilly. Also, one needs to note that Arion Roşu studied keenly the role played by French scholars and by European missionaries in the history of science and technology in India (1991, 1993, 2003), writing also on forerunners or contemporary scholars like Marcelin Berthelot (1983, 1986, 1990), Chandragiri Dwarakanath (1980), Jeannine Auboyer (1990) – who played an essential role in his emigration to France, after publishing his first articles –, Albert Le Bonheur (1993-1994), and Priya Vrat Sharma (1997), but particularly on the history of Indian medicine in France, from Gustave Liétard and Palmyr Cordier (1989) until Jean Filliozat (1984, 1993-1994).

The largest part of these researches was published in French journals dedicated to the study of India, like *Arts Asiatiques* (1957-1967), *Journal Asiatique* (starting from 1968, when he becomes a member of the Société Asiatique, until 2005, he was one of the most present Indologists and Asian scholars coming from Eastern Europe during the entire history of the oldest Asian journal in Europe), *Bulletin de l'École française d'Extrême-Orient* (1969-1982, 2001) and especially, since its founding in 1983 until his death, in the *Bulletin d'Études Indiennes*. He published over 200 pages in the journal founded by Nalini Balbir and Georges-Jean Pinault, edited by Nalini Balbir, including nine articles and no less than 55 critical reviews and short notices, most of which were dedicated to Indian publications concerning Āyurveda. Together with his contributions in German, Indian and Romanian journals of Indian and Asian studies, Arion Roşu represented France on the editorial board (1990-2001) of the initial series of this very journal, contributing to volumes 2-7 (1992-2003) of the *Journal of the European Āyurvedic Society / Traditional South Asian Medicine*. In Paris, the *Institut d'Études Indiennes* of the Collège de France now holds, together with the library of Louis Renou, his impressive library of offprints dedicated to the study of Indian medicine and classical Indology, with items coming from all over the world. His special library has now been added, so that the Arion Roşu Collection seems now to be the most important one for the history of medicine and Indian alchemy from the entire Francophone world.

His last public events have been devoted, *comme pour boucler la boucle*, to his French teacher and to his native country. On November 17, 2006 he participated in the colloquium 'Sciences et médecine en Asie', dedicated to the centenary of Jean Filliozat, of the Académie des Inscriptions et Belles-Lettres, which honoured Arion Roşu in 1979, and on December 8, 2006 he took part in a reception by the Romanian Embassy in Paris, celebrating his being awarded the 'Cultural Merit' order in the rank of Commander by the President of Romania in September 2006 at Bucharest. Shortly afterwards, his old afflictions, some of which he bore since his adolescence, caught up with him; the months he spent in the hospital would be his last ones.

The funeral took place on April 7, 2007, the Saturday before Easter at the Saint Symphorien Church in Versailles. His wife Claude Roşu, who cared for and was with him for almost forty years, did not survive him for more than a few months. She died in December. They both rest near each other in the Normand cemetery of Sées.

He leaves behind a fundamental opus on the history of medicine and of Indian religions. It is a most rare work, for he built it, as Professor Pierre-Sylvain Filliozat said before the Asiatic Society in Paris, in heroic circumstances, which only the strength of his mission and an extraordinary destiny could overcome. Those to whom he has been a friend, a colleague, a teacher, or more than one of these, cannot forget him, as he himself did not forget his old teachers, colleagues, and friends. His rigour and dignity, his modesty and discretion, his kindness – all of which are unmistakable for those who knew him closely, in whom he confided 'in old friendship' – engender our gratefulness, which survives him.

**Note**

A complete bibliography of Arion Roşu's writings (until 2004) has appeared in *Du corps humain, au carrefour de plusieurs savoirs en Inde. Mélanges offerts à Arion Roşu par ses collègues et ses amis à l'occasion de son 80e anniversaire. The Human Body, at the Crossroads of Multiple Indian Ways of Knowing. Papers Presented to Arion Roşu by His Colleagues and Friends on the Occasion of his Eightieth Birthday*, Bucarest: Université de Bucarest/Paris: De Boccard 2004 (= *Studia Asiatica* 4-5 ⟨2003-2004⟩), pp. 23-39, a volume opening with the tribute of Madame Colette Caillat (1921-2007), Membre de l'Institut de France, further in *Comptes rendus de l'Académie des Inscriptions et Belles-Lettres*, avril-juin 2005: 539-541. Since then there have appeared 'En marge des pratiques tantriques du *JA* 290.1.2002, p. 293-313', *Journal Asiatique* 293,1 (2005): 379-381, a note on David Gordon White, *Kiss of the Yoginī. 'Tantric Sex' in Its South Asian Context*, Chicago/London: University of Chicago Press 2003 (in *Archives de sciences sociales des religions* 132 ⟨2005⟩: 72), as well as an obituary remembering 'David Pingree (1933-2005)', 'Chronique de l'eau (suite) [IV]', and short bibliographical notices on David Pingree (*Catalogue of* Jyotiṣa *Manuscripts in the Wellcome Library: Sanskrit Astral and Mathematical Literature*, Leiden/Boston: Brill 2004) and Priya Vrat Sharma (*Six Decades of Āyurveda ⟨1941-2000⟩. A Collection of Selected Articles and Lectures*, Delhi: Chaukhamba Sanskrit Pratisthan 2005), all in *Bulletin d'Études Indiennes* 22-23 (2004-2005): 13f., 585, 642f. and 644. 'Le *kuṇḍalinīyoga* et les charmeurs des serpents' is forthcoming in Nalini Balbir and Georges-Jean Pinault (eds.), *Penser, dire et représenter l'animal dans le monde indien, Colloque international, Paris, 25-28 mars 2002*, Paris 2008 (Bibliothèque de l'École des Hautes Études 345). The second part of his study on *rasāyana* (cf. *Indo-Iranian Journal* 17 ⟨1975⟩: 1-29 and 395), together with works on craniolatry and on the Transylvanian doctor J.M. Honigberger, written in collaboration these past few years, are waiting to be printed. Other works, only started or sketched, will probably remain in an embryo status. His most remarkable unpublished contribution certainly remains his edition and French translation of the *Rasendracūḍāmaṇi*.

The obituary read by Pierre-Sylvain Filliozat, Membre de l'Institut de France, on May 11, 2007 at the Société Asiatique (Paris) will be published in *Journal Asiatique* 295,2 (2007). Other tributes to Arion Roşu will appear in *Bulletin d'Études Indiennes*, *Indologica Taurinensia* and *Studia Asiatica*.

# Some Neglected Aspects of Āyurveda
# or
# The Illusion of a Consistent Theory
## *II: The* Suśrutasaṃhitā

GERRIT JAN MEULENBELD

The first part of this investigation[1] dealt with the relationship between *agni*[2] and *pitta* in the *Carakasaṃhitā* and, to a minor extent, the *Bhelasaṃhitā*. The conclusion reached was that *agni* is often different from *pitta*; as a separate agent, it is able to corrupt other bodily constituents and to cause disorders, while it is also a constituent liable to corruption by the *doṣa*s. The *Carakasaṃhitā* thus shows traces of a not yet completed elaboration of the *tridoṣa* doctrine. The commentators strive to make these vestiges subservient to the prevailing classical theory which makes the *doṣa*s into the only truly corrupting entities.

The relationship between *agni* and *pitta* is explicitly discussed in a prose passage of the *vraṇapraśna* chapter of the Sūtrasthāna (21,9). This well-known chapter is about the *doṣa*s, blood, and the *kriyākāla*.[3]

The relevant passage appears abruptly and unexpectedly after a summarising verse,[4] expressing that *kapha*, *pitta* and *vāta* sustain the body in the same way as moon (*soma*), sun (*sūrya*) and wind (*vāta*) sustain the world by their respective actions, consisting of emission (*visarga*), taking away (*ādāna*) and dispersion (*vikṣepa*). The parallelism of macro- and microcosm is at issue again here, as it was in the *vātakalākalīya* chapter of the *Carakasaṃhitā*.

---

[1] MEULENBELD *forthcoming*. At the time of going to press, this first part had not yet been published.

[2] The stem forms of the Sanskrit terms are not marked (i.e. *agni* instead of *agni-*), as this proved too cumbersome.

[3] *Kriyākāla* means the proper time for particular therapeutic measures, dependent on the evolutive stage of a disease process.

[4] *Suśrutasaṃhitā*, Sūtrasthāna 21,8:
*visargādānavikṣepaiḥ somasūryānilā yathā*
*dhārayanti jagad dehaṃ kaphapittānilās tathā.*

The subject matter of the prose passage that follows upon this verse surprises and catches the eye, in the same way as Marīci's words in the *vātakalākalīya* chapter. Again, one is tempted to consider the possibility of an interpolation.

The passage runs as follows:

*tatra jijñāsyaṃ kiṃ pittavyatirekād anyo 'gnir āhosvit pittam evāgnir iti. atrocyate – na khalu pittavyatirekād anyo 'gnir upalabhyate, āgneyatvāt pitte dahanapacanādiṣv abhipravartamāne 'gnivad upacāraḥ kriyate 'ntaragnir iti; kṣīṇe hy agniguṇe tatsamānadravyopayogād ativṛddhe śītakriyopayogād āgamāc ca paśyāmo na khalu pittavyatirekād anyo 'gnir iti.*

With respect to this (*tatra*) one would like to know if there exists another fire (*agni*) than *pitta* or if *pitta* and fire are identical. The answer to this question is: certainly no other fire than *pitta* is known. The reason is that *pitta*, due to its fiery nature, and being engaged in (*abhipravartamāna*) burning (*dahana*), cooking (*pacana*) and the like, is, metaphorically speaking, like *agni* and therefore called the internal fire (*antaragni*). Verily, there is no other fire than *pitta*, as can be learnt from the use of similar substances when its fiery quality (*agniguṇa*) has diminished (*kṣīṇa*)[5] and from the employment of cooling measures (*śītakriyā*) when it has increased too much; this can be learnt as well from trustworthy authorities (*āgama*).

The translation of this passage is not without some contentious points. The word *tatra*, with which it begins, has no referent in the preceding verse. The commentator Ḍalhaṇa notices this and feels obliged to list three different interpretations of *tatra*.[6]

This detail, small though it is, strengthens the thought that the passage may

---

[5] The interpretation of *tatsamānadravya* is disputed. Ḍalhaṇa is of the opinion that substances similar to *agni* are meant; others, referred to by him, are convinced that *agniguṇa* denotes *ūṣman* and that substances similar to *pitta* are intended.

[6] (1) *Tatra* refers to the problem whether or not *pitta* and *agni* are identical; (2) *tatra* means *teṣu madhye* 'amongst these things'; (3) *tatra* points back to the *ādāna* of the preceding verse. A fourth group asks why the wish to know about the relationship between *pitta* and *agni* is relevant after mentioning *ādāna* in the set *visargādānavikṣepa*.

be an addition to a more original text. The second problem is the precise meaning of the expression *agnivad upacāraḥ kriyate*, which I rendered as '(*pitta*) is, metaphorically speaking, like *agni*'. SHARMA 1999 concurs with me in translating 'it is metaphorically identified with *agni*'.[7] DUTT 1883 translated: 'it acts like fire', while SINGHAL/TRIPATHI/CHATURVEDI 1981 translate: 'it performs functions like *agni*'.[8] These differences indicate that it is not completely clear whether *upacāra* is employed in a technical or in a more general sense. Ḍalhaṇa opts for the latter alternative, as some later commentators do; the resulting translation of *agnivad upacāraḥ kriyate* as 'it performs functions like those of *agni*' is permissible and does not give a wrong sense to the expression. In my opinion, however, most probably a metaphor comes into play, as attested by the suffix *-vat* in *agnivat* and because of the ambiguity of the train of thought.[9]

As to be expected, Cakrapāṇidatta and Ḍalhaṇa present elaborate comments on the passage.

Ḍalhaṇa begins with remarking that the passage demonstrates that the identity of *agni* and *pitta* can be proved by direct observation (*pratyakṣa*), inference (*anumāna*) and reliance on trustworthy authorities (*āgama*). He proceeds by introducing an imaginary opponent, who adduces proofs contradicting the identity. This evidence to the contrary consists of the existence of substances with effects on *pitta* that differ from those on *agni*[10] and some passages from

---

[7] As will be observed later, Śrīkaṇṭhadatta also supports this interpretation.

[8] The English translation of BHISHAGRATNA 1963 has no clear equivalent of *upacāra*. Hārāṇacandra's nineteenth-century Sanskrit commentatry gives *vyavahāra* as the equivalent of *upacāra* (see BHAṬṬĀCĀRYYA et al. 1832), which means that it performs functions like those of *agni*. GHANEKAR 1952 also explains *upacāra* as *vyavahār* in his Hindī commentary.

[9] The conclusion 'it is therefore called the internal fire' does not follow from the similarities between *pitta* and *agni*.

[10] Examples adduced are: (1) ghee, which pacifies *pitta* while stimulating the fire (see *Suśrutasaṃhitā*, Sūtrasthāna 45,96); Cakrapāṇidatta gives an elaborate exposition on the actions of ghee in his comments on *Carakasaṃhitā*, Sūtrasthāna 13,13; (2) goat's milk, which has the same effects (see Sūtrasthāna 45,51cd-53ab); (3) fish, which make *pitta* increase without stimulating the fire (Sūtrasthāna 46,114 only mentions that fresh water fish stimulate *pitta*, but is

the *Suśrutasaṃhitā* itself;[11] a quotation from an unmentioned source[12] completes the evidence to the contrary. I shall return to these objections later.

This opposition is superfluous in Ḍalhaṇa's eyes, for Suśruta, as well as others, acknowledge that in reality (*paramārthataḥ*) *pitta* and *agni* are distinct. A stanza from the Nidānasthāna (13,37), to be discussed later, is cited as evidence. Ḍalhaṇa goes on by intimating that he could provide more quotations in support, but that he abstains from doing so for fear of prolixity.[13] He is apparently convinced that *agni* and *pitta* are not identical, but fails to specify of which type the difference may be. The most significant remarks occur at the end of his comments, where he declares that the statement of the *Suśrutasaṃhitā* about the absence of a difference between *agni* and *pitta* serves to show that *agni* can only be treated by means of therapeutic measures appropriate to *pitta*, because *pitta* is endowed with attributes such as taste (*rasa*), potency (*vīrya*), and the like, which *agni* does not possess;[14] otherwise, disorders of *agni* would not be amenable to treatment.

The essence of Ḍalhaṇa's train of thought is that *agni* and *pitta* are actually distinct, but that this difference is neglected for practical purposes.

Completely absent from Ḍalhaṇa's deliberations is any reference to the verse (Sūtrasthāna 21,11) enumerating the qualities (*guṇa*) of *pitta* and closing the section on this *doṣa*, even though this stanza establishes beyond the shad-

---

silent about the effect on the fire; Sūtrasthāna 21,21 mentions fish in general as one of the items making *pitta* excited; I could not find a statement in the *Suśrutasaṃhitā* corroborating that of Ḍalhaṇa); (4) sleeping by day (Sūtrasthāna 21,23 mentions *divāsvapna* as one of the factors causing excitement of *kapha*, Śārīrasthāna} 4,38 regards sleeping by day as provoking all the *doṣa*s).

11 From Sūtrasthāna 35,24 and 15,41, and Nidānasthāna 13,37 on *palita*.

12 *dravaṃ snigdham adhogaṃ ca pittaṃ vahnir ato 'nyathā.*

13 He could have referred to Uttaratantra 39,16cd-19ab on the onset of fever, where it is said that the *doṣa*s (one of which is *pitta*) make the (digestive) fire sluggish and expel the heat (*ūṣman*) from the seat of digestion, making it reach the surface of the body.

14 Substances (*dravya*) possess *guṇa*s. Obviously, *agni* is not a substance; it is a *guṇa* of *pitta* according to Ḍalhaṇa ad Sūtrasthāna 21,9: *agner guṇo yasya tad agniguṇaṃ pittam.*

ow of a doubt clear-cut differences between *pitta* and *agni*.[15]

Cakrapāṇidatta's comments on the same passage bear witness to more theoretical subtlety and less concern for practice. This author does not pay attention to the word *tatra* and begins, tying in with what has been expressed in the preceding verse, by also making an objector appear, who argues: 'Well, but how does *pitta* perform, in the same way as the sun, the action called *ādāna*?' Cakrapāṇidatta replies to his opponent that the words of Suśruta aim at dispelling the doubt that there may be a difference between *agni* and *pitta*. Valid means of acquiring knowledge (*pramāṇa*) that could attest to such a difference are simply absent. Seeming (*avabhāsaka*) statements to the contrary, such as '*pitta* makes the fire *tīkṣṇa*' (Sūtrasthāna 35,24), should not be taken literally. That is why Suśruta says '*pitta* is the same as fire on account of its fiery nature'. After establishing this point, the text of the *Suśrutasaṃhitā* makes use of inference in order to underpin its thesis (*pakṣa*) by referring to therapeutic measures which are recommended in disorders. The property (*guṇa*) of fire that has the ability to cook (*pācakatva*) as its characteristic, is its heat (*ūṣman*).[16] When this heat has diminished, substances with properties similar to fire and similar to *pitta*[17] can increase it, and conversely when the heat has increased. These effects are possible because *tejas* forms part (*avayavarūpa*) of *pitta* and acts by means of its fiery nature (*agnitva*). The substances mentioned cannot but possess this same *tejas* just because they are suitable to the purpose.

This having been settled, the thesis is also proved by having recourse to authority. Cakrapāṇidatta quotes as evidence in support Sūtrasthāna 26,20 and

---

[15] The verse runs:
*pittaṃ tīkṣṇaṃ dravaṃ pūti nīlaṃ pītaṃ tathaiva ca*
*uṣṇaṃ kaṭurasaṃ caiva vidagdhaṃ cāmlam eva ca.*
It implies that substances with opposite qualities subdue *pitta* without impairing the fire.

[16] Cakrapāṇidatta, who does not distinguish between *pitta* and *agni*, ascribes *guṇa*s to *agni*, unlike Ḍalhaṇa; evidently, Cakrapāṇidatta is one of those, referred to in Ḍalhaṇa's commentary, who regard *ūṣman* as an *agniguṇa*.

[17] This is remarkable in view of Ḍalhaṇa's statement that, depending on the interpretation of *agniguṇa*, either substances similar to fire or substances similar to *pitta* are intended.

Śārīrasthāna 4,18, two passages still to be dealt with, and a verse of Bhoja running: 'The agent bringing about cooking (*paktimat*) is therefore *pitta*, which consists of *tejas*, which is the heat (*ūṣman*) of *pitta*.'[18]

Cakrapāṇidatta, so far apparently defending that *agni* and *pitta* are identical, begins to put his opinion in perspective in the subsequent part of his comments.

He opens this part by remarking: If there were actually no distinction between the two, there could not exist between them the same connection as that between cause and effect, as exemplified in the statement: 'a *tīkṣṇa* fire is brought about by *pitta*' (Sūtrasthāna 35,24). Absence of any distinction would also contradict other statements, such as found in a verse on *grahaṇīdoṣa* from the *Carakasaṃhitā* (Cikitsāsthāna 15,65) stating that *pitta* may, like hot water, extinguish the fire by flooding it.[19] Two more passages from the *Suśrutasaṃhitā* would neither be acceptable in that case. The first of these quotations (Sūtrasthāna 45,96) lists the properties and actions of ghee, the second one (Sūtrasthāna 15,41) distinguishes a balanced state of the *doṣa*s from a balanced state of the fire.

Though statements clearly demonstrating the absence of any difference do occur, such as '(foreign objects in the body) made of gold, silver, copper, brass, tin or lead, are, after a long stay there, dissolved by the heating action (*pratāpana*) of the *tejas* of *pitta*' (Sūtrasthāna 26.20), yet words like those of Bhoja: 'The heat (*ūṣman*) of *pitta* has the capacity to cook (*paktimat*)', point to the fiery nature (*agnitva*) of *tejas* as being different from its substrate, *pitta*.

The inference (that *agni* and *pitta* are identical), based on the assertion that

---

[18] The following sentence does not form part of the text in all the manuscripts: 'This detailed exposition (*prapañca*) proves that *agni* is not distinct from *pitta*, since it exists in the form of the heat of *pitta*, and a difference between a property (*dharma*) and the substrate of that property (*dharmin*) does not exist.' The use of the terms *dharma* and *dharmin* point to this sentence as being interpolated.

[19] GAUTAM/UPĀDIIYĀY/GAUTAM 2005 refer in their article to an author called Nirañjan Dev, who determined the *pāñcabhautika* composition of *pitta* as follows: *vāyu* and *ākāśa* 10%, *pr̥thivī* 20%, *ap* 30%, *agni* 40%.

substances increasing *pitta* can also usefully be employed when the fire has grown weak, is not valid, since it is well known that some substances make the one increase while not stimulating but even hurting the other.[20]

At this point Cakrapāṇidatta reaches his conclusion. He decides that Suśruta's words about the absence of a difference between *agni* and *pitta* mean that their only difference is the same as that between an attribute and the bearer of that attribute. A verse from the *Suśrutasaṃhitā* is cited with the aim of supporting this conclusion. This verse (Sūtrasthāna 35,27) runs: "The venerable (*bhagavat*) lord (*īśvara*), the abdominal fire (*jāṭharāgni*), who cooks the food and takes up (*ādadāna*) the tastes, can, on account of its subtlety (*saukṣmya*), not be perceived (*vi√vic*)'. Subtleness is, according to Cakrapāṇidatta, a characteristic that cannot be applied to *pitta*, whereas it does suit heat (*ūṣman*). In the expression 'the sixth *kalā* is that one called *pittadharā*' (Śārīrasthāna 4, 18), the word *pitta* is employed metaphorically[21] and actually designates *agni*. The statement that substances increasing or decreasing *pitta* usually make *agni* increase or decrease as well, ought to be interpreted in a similar vein; it is to be understood in a metaphorical sense, because it does not distinguish between a property (*dharma*) and the bearer of that property (*dharmin*).

The acceptance of a distinction between the two, namely that *agni* exists in the form of the *tejas* of *pitta*, makes it intelligible that particular substances which increase the liquid part of *pitta*, but not the part consisting of *tejas*, may extinguish the fire by generating a kind of *pitta* that is *vyamla*, abnormally acid in taste.

Cakrapāṇidatta presents in this long discourse the same view as that found in his comments on Marīci's intervention in the *vātakalākalīya* chapter of the *Carakasaṃhitā*, where he is less prolix and indulges to a much lesser degree in theoretical considerations.

---

[20] In this Cakrapāṇidatta agrees with Ḍalhaṇa. Substances which are either *dīpana* or *pācana* or both simultaneously are distinguished in lists of drug actions in works like the *Śārṅgadharasaṃhitā* (1,4,1-2ab). The *Suśrutasaṃhitā* itself also has groups of drugs which are either *pācana* or *dīpana* (Sūtrasthāna 38).

[21] The term used is *aupacārikapittaśabdaprayoga*.

In short, he is convinced that the relation between *agni* and *pitta* is of the same kind as that between a property (*dharma*) and the bearer of that property (*dharmin*). Heat (*ūṣman* or *tejas*) is the *dharma* and *pitta* the *dharmin*. Cakrapāṇidatta's conclusion implies that, wherever *pitta* is present, *agni* will be present too.

This conclusion is not free from blemishes. It is questionable whether *agni* is always dependent on *pitta* in the *Carakasaṃhitā* and *Suśrutasaṃhitā*. Minor flaws are that he does not distinguish between *ūṣman* and *tejas* (these are distinct in *Suśrutasaṃhitā*, Sūtrasthāna 15,4,2) and that he considers *agni* and *ūṣman* to be identical. He obviously aims, more so than Ḍalhaṇa, at the construction of a coherent theory, in which *agni* is not allowed to have a position that makes it, even partially, independent of the *doṣa*s.

The prose passage that follows upon Sūtrasthāna 21,9 of the *Suśrutasaṃhitā* describes the five kinds of *pitta*, calling them not *pācakapitta* etc., but *pācakāgni* etc.

In this context an interesting verse from the *Suśrutasaṃhitā* which throws light on the relation between *pitta* and *ūṣman* has to be discussed. This verse was so conspicuous and problematic in the eyes of the commentators that it prompted them to expound and defend their views on *agni* and *pitta* in sometimes long discourses.

The pertinent verse is found in the chapter on *kṣudraroga*s of the Nidānasthāna (13,37) and forms also part of the chapter on the same subject of the *Mādhavanidāna* (55,32). Four comments are therefore available, those of Gayadāsa and Ḍalhaṇa on the *Suśrutasaṃhitā* and those of Śrīkaṇṭhadatta and Vācaspati on the *Mādhavanidāna*.[22]

The verse runs:

*krodhaśokaśramakṛtaḥ śarīroṣmā śirogataḥ*
*pittaṃ ca keśān pacati palitaṃ tena jāyate*

The bodily heat (*śarīroṣman*), brought about by anger (*krodha*), grief (*śoka*), or

[22] Hārāṇacandra's commentary on the Nidānasthāna of the *Suśrutasaṃhitā* is not available to me.

> fatigue (*śrama*), and having moved to the head, cooks (*pacati*), together with *pitta*, the hair of the head; this generates greyness (*palita*).

It is important to see how the commentators reflect upon the juxtaposition of bodily heat and *pitta* in this stanza.

Gayadāsa, the oldest of the four, begins with remarking that, according to some, this is a case where two agents (*kartr̥*) are put together, namely bodily heat and *pitta*. That is not proper in his opinion. Obviously, Gayadāsa does not admit that two distinct types of agent produce, in collaboration, one and the same disorder. That makes him go on as follows: However, there does exist a difference, because pathological (*vaikr̥ta*) greyness is brought about by the heat of *pācakapitta*, and naturally occurring (*svābhāvika*) greyness by the *pitta* of one's constitution. In this interpretation, Gayadāsa identifies the bodily heat with the heat of *pācakapitta*. He proceeds by presenting an imaginary opponent who objects that, if things are thus, we have here a case (*prasaṅga*) of greyness that arises without a *doṣa*. The reply to this argument is: That is not correct, for greyness arises from a property (*dharma*) of *pitta*. This reasoning is evidently of the same type as that of Cakrapāṇidatta.

After a lacuna in the manuscript, Gayadāsa says: The situation is as follows: pathological greyness finds its origin in *pitta*, whereas natural greyness occurs in persons with a balanced constitution (*samadoṣaprakr̥ti*). For that reason it is not right to accept that two agents are mentioned in the verse; natural greyness is found in persons with a constitution dominated by *pitta*, and, as has repeatedly been explained, a constitution does not lead to pathological changes (*vikāra*), on account of the small amount of the *doṣa* (*alpadoṣatva*) in a particular constitution.[23]

Gayadāsa thus subsumes bodily heat under the concept of *pitta* and refuses to recognise it as a separate agent. He solves the problem by distinguishing a pathological and a natural type of greyness of the hair. An imperfection in his reasoning is that he attributes natural greyness first to persons with a balanced constitution and later to those with a constitution dominated by *pitta*.

---

[23] Cf. *Suśrutasaṃhitā*, Śārīrasthāna 5,79.

Ḍalhaṇa also dislikes the two agents mentioned in the verse. He argues that bodily heat generates pathological greyness and *pitta* the naturally occurring type. Otherwise, since *pitta* and heat are the same, we would have here a case of useless repetition (*punaruktidoṣa*). He quotes the author of the commentary called *Pañjikā*, who says: 'Bodily heat is the fire (*pāvaka*) and *pitta* is its substrate (*āśaya*); these two, having become one, perform the action of cooking.' Ḍalhaṇa remarks that in this way the option of a pathological type of greyness, brought about by heat only, has been removed, for that would have been a disorder coming about without a *doṣa*.

Ḍalhaṇa's line of thought thus resembles that of Gayadāsa, but without having recourse to the concept of constitution. Remarkable is that he here disowns his opinion, expressed on a former occasion, that *agni* and *pitta* are actually distinct.

Both Gayadāsa and Ḍalhaṇa do not want to acknowledge that two agents are found in the verse, keen as they are on dispelling any danger to the *tridoṣavāda*.

Śrīkaṇṭhadatta's comments are very long and replete with quotations, which makes it expedient to present a condensed rendering.

He begins by saying: The bodily heat is the bodily fire; *pitta* is mentioned as having moved to the head too, in the same way as the bodily heat. An opponent may object that *pitta* is identical with fire because, at several instances, it is said to be endowed with the action of cooking (*pācakatva*); what may therefore be the reason that *pitta* and the fire are mentioned separately?

Śrīkaṇṭhadatta replies that this objection can be refuted. The internal fire (*antaragni*) and *pitta* are not identical to such an extent. This has been established more than once in authoritative statements. A reference to *Suśrutasaṃhitā*, Sūtrasthāna15,41 (*samadoṣaḥ samāgniś ca*), together with an unidentified quotation (*samaprakopau sarveṣāṃ doṣāṇām agnisaṃśrayau*), make Śrīkaṇṭhadatta declare that *agni* and *pitta* differ from each other, both being separately mentioned. He adds that the statement '*agni* becomes *tīkṣṇa* through the action of *pitta*' is an example of a contradiction in terms (*svātmani kriyāvirodhaḥ*). The difference between *agni* and *pitta* is, moreover, established by the use of the term *upacāra* in the *Suśrutasaṃhitā* (Sūtrasthāna 21,9): a metaphor is not applicable in cases of identity. He also disagrees with the view that the identity of the two is established by the fact that substances with qualities similar to those of *pitta* make the fire increase; he adduces as a counter-example that, though substances with properties similar to those of *kapha* make semen increase, this does not prove at all that *kapha* and semen are identical. At the end of this part of his discourse, he mentions, as other commentators do, that ghee, which pacifies *pitta*, stimulates the fire; some new examples of the same phenomenon are provided: accumulation of *pitta* does not result in increase of the fire, and *peyā* (a thin kind of gruel) makes the fire increase without increasing *pitta*.[24]

He proceeds by bringing forward that *pitta* is an aggregate (*samudāya*) of a fluid (*drava*) and a fiery part (*tejas*). The *tejas* part of *pitta* cannot, as fire does, reduce something to ashes (*aṅgārākāra*), since a whole differs from its component parts. The *tejas* part of *pitta* is the agent responsible for the cooking action.

Quotations serve to settle that assertions about the identity of *agni* and *pitta* should be interpreted metaphorically. A second question is then raised: Well, how can, if *pitta* makes the fire *tīkṣṇa*, this same *pitta* extinguish (*praśamana*) the fire, as has been said in the *Carakasaṃhitā* (Cikitsāsthāna 15,65) with the words: 'an abundant amount of *pitta* inundates the fire, in the same way as hot water'?

Śrīkaṇṭhadatta replies: When, by the intake of particular substances, *pitta* has increased, the fire becomes *tīkṣṇa* due to the abundantly present *tejas* part of *pitta*; when, by the intake of other substances, *pitta*, accompanied by *kapha*, has increased, the fire is extinguished due to the prevalence of the liquid part of *pitta*.

Jatūkarṇa is quoted in support; this authority says: 'The fire is, like a lamp, extinguished by excited *vāta*; it is extinguished by excited *pitta* as by hot water, and by excited *kapha* as by water.' Śrīkaṇṭhadatta concludes that it is there-

[24] See *Suśrutasaṃhitā*, Sūtrasthāna 46,341cd-342ab.

fore proper to mention the fire separately.

Having reached this point, he is ready to interpret the verse of the *Mādhavanidāna* that occasioned this digression.

The fire, being part of *pitta*, is brought about by anger, for anger arises from excitement of *pitta*. The bodily heat has moved to the head by the dispersive action (*vikṣepaṇa*) of *vāta*, which originates from grief and fatigue. In this way *vāta* also plays its role; *pitta* is mentioned explicitly. The word *ca* in *pittaṃ ca* adds *kapha*, which whitens the hair.

Thus interpreted, the verse expresses that greyness of the hair is caused by bodily heat, together with the three *doṣa*s. This is in conformity with what the *Carakasaṃhitā* says (Cikitsāsthāna 26,132): '(*Tejas*), together with *vāta* and the other *doṣa*s, having burnt the scalp, gives rise to baldness (*khalati*); when this burning is slight, greyness results or a reddish (*harit*) colour of the hair.'

Our author proceeds: These are the characteristics (*lakṣaṇa*) of all types of greyness that occur at an improper time (*akāla*), that is to say before the age in which it is naturally found; the type occurring in old age (*kāla*) is, though not mentioned, included (*upalakṣaṇa*). This type also originates from heat, together with the three *doṣa*s; the latter are roused by the changes (*pariṇāma*) due to the stage of life (*vayas*); otherwise, it would be a missing item. Or, it may be that the type found in old age has been left unmentioned as a naturally occurring (*svābhāvika*) change.

Others, however, have expressed the opinion that bodily heat and *pitta* designate two agents, which boils down to an accumulation of agents with the same range of action (*viṣaya*). Actually, the range of action is twofold. The bodily heat is at the origin of pathological (*vaikr̥ta*) greyness, while *pitta* is at the origin of natural greyness, found in persons with a constitution dominated by *pitta*. This agrees with what has been said: 'A *pittaprakr̥ti* goes together with premature wrinkles and greyness' (no source mentioned).

Thus, the natural greyness of old age has also *pitta* as its cause (*hetu*). The fact that greyness is brought about by heat is therefore not a case in which the *doṣa*s are absent, because heat forms part of *pitta* as one of its attributes.

Śrīkaṇṭhadatta's elaborate discussion is not clear in all respects. He strives at incorporating everything found in his predecessors' works. On the one hand he expresses as his opinion that *ūṣman* is the fiery part of *pitta*, while, on the other, he gives some scope to the view that greyness of the hair arises from the bodily heat, together with the three *doṣa*s.

The verse discussed appears, however, to recognise bodily heat as an agent distinct from *pitta*.

Vācaspati's short remarks do not provide new material. He regards *śarīroṣman* and *pitta* as identical. The view that *agni* and *pitta* are distinct is referred to, as well as the opinion that *palita* is brought about by the three *doṣa*s.

Another verse from the *Suśrutasaṃhitā* may also establish that *agni* is distinct from the *doṣa*s. As to be expected, it is therefore often quoted and made to mean that this is not the case. This verse (Sūtrasthāna 15,41) runs: 'A person is called healthy (*svastha*) when the *doṣa*s and the fire are in a balanced state, when the functions (*kriyā*) of the *dhātu*s and the *mala*s are balanced, and when the *ātman*, the senses and *manas* are in a tranquil (*prasanna*) condition.'[25]

Ḍalhaṇa's comments are conspicuous in being in conformity with what he expressed on an earlier occasion. First, he raises the question why the *ācārya*, i.e., Suśruta, refers to the *doṣa*s and *agni* separately, since a balanced state of *agni* and of the other constituents mentioned is brought about by a balanced state of the *doṣa*s. His answer is: It is not obligatory that a balanced state of *agni* and of other constituents of the body is dependent on the *doṣa*s. The argument he adduces is that the *doṣa*s and *agni* are distinct as to treatment, for ghee and goat's milk remove *pitta* and increase *agni*. In this way Ḍalhaṇa repeats his conviction that *agni* and *pitta* are not identical.

Cakrapāṇidatta also sticks to his opinion. He solves the difficulties raised by the verse by interpreting it as expressing that a person with balanced *doṣa*s is characterised by a balanced fire and by balanced functions of the *dhātu*s and *mala*s. This reasoning implies that *agni* and *pitta* are identical.

A prose passage of the *Suśrutasaṃhitā* also gives the impression that *agni*

---

[25] *samadoṣaḥ samāgniś ca samadhātumalakriyaḥ*
*prasannātmendriyamanāḥ svastha ity abhidhīyate.*

and the *doṣa*s are distinct. This passage (from Sūtrasthāna 35,24) says: '*Agni* is the agent that cooks the food (*annasya pācakaḥ*). … When subject to a disorder (*vikriyām āpannaḥ*) it is of three types: … [it becomes] *tīkṣṇa* by *pitta*.'[26] This passage is well known to the commentators, who quote it when discoursing on the status of *agni*, but neither Cakrapāṇidatta nor Ḍalhaṇa makes any remark on this topic in their comments on this occasion.

The *Suśrutasaṃhitā* contains, moreover, a verse that may not only confirm that *agni* is distinct from the *doṣa*s, but also that it is a separate corrupting agent. This verse, from the chapter of the Uttaratantra on diarrhoea (*atīsāra*) and the chronic diarrhoea called *grahaṇīroga* (Uttaratantra 40,167), runs: 'When, in cases of diarrhoea, or even when this has ceased, the patient whose digestive fire is weak (*mandāgni*) indulges in unwholesome food, the fire becomes more corrupted; thereupon this fire corrupts (*abhidūṣayati*) the *grahaṇī*.'[27]

This verse expresses that the digestive fire is corrupted in diarrhoea; this is a corruption caused by the *doṣa*s. The already corrupted fire gets more corrupted, not by the *doṣa*s, but by the intake of unwholesome food; then, in its turn, it corrupts its seat, the grahaṇī.

Ḍalhaṇa does not pay much attention to this verse, which makes *agni* into a separate agent, able to corrupt the *grahaṇī*. As a corrupting agent, however, it is not independent in this case and its corrupting action may, in Āyurvedic theory, be derived from the *doṣa*s. This would agree with a tenet of Āyurvedic theory declaring that constituents of the body, in particular those called *dhātu*, may transmit their corruption, caused by the *doṣa*s, to other constituents, in this case the *grahaṇī*. A corrupting capacity of the fire that is independent from the *doṣa*s cannot be proved by the help of this verse.

Provisionally, it can be concluded that the *Suśrutasaṃhitā* contains, as does the *Carakasaṃhitā*, verses and passages in prose about *agni* and the *doṣa*s, in particular about the connection between *agni* and *pitta*, attesting that the elab-

---

[26] *agnir annasya pācakaḥ. … vikriyām āpannas trividho bhavati. … tīkṣṇaḥ pittena.*

[27] *atisāre nivṛtte 'pi mandāgner ahitāśinaḥ*
*bhūyaḥ sandūṣito vahnir grahaṇīm abhidūṣayet.*

oration of the *tridoṣa* doctrine was still a process in flux. Remnants of competing theories can be discovered, next to a tendency to encapsulate disagreeing concepts within the system that gradually succeeded in dominating medical thought.[28]

Statements that appeared to jeopardise the *tridoṣavāda* caught the eye of the commentators and gave them much food for thought in their efforts to avert any danger to the prevailing theory. The obvious meaning of some discordant utterances was twisted until concurring with the system. Passages that were ambiguous and susceptible to various interpretations were made to conform. A conspicuous aspect of the reasonings met with is the tendency to avoid the acceptance of any bodily constituent as a factor capable, independently of the *doṣa*s, of initiating physiological and, more especially, pathogenetic processes. The champion in this field is Cakrapāṇidatta, while Ḍalhaṇa is prone to give most weight to considerations relating to medical practice.

## Bibliography

BHAṬṬĀCĀRYYA, Candrakānta et al. (ed.) 1832: *Suśrutasaṃhitā – prathamakhaṇḍam – sūtrasthānātmakam. Rāmapuraboyāliyā-pravāsi-śrīHārāṇacandracakravartikavirāja-viracita-suśrutārthasandīpanabhāṣya-sametam.* Kalikātā: Satyayantra Śaka era 1832.

BHISHAGRATNA, Kunjalal (trans. and ed.) 1963: *An English Translation of the Sushruta Samhita based on Original Sanskrit Text, with a Full and Comprehensive introduction, Additional Texts, Different Readings, Notes, Comparative Views, Index, Glossary and Plates. Vol. I. Sutra-sthāna.* Second editon. Varanasi: Chowkhamba Sanskrit Series Office. The Chowkhamba Sanskrit Studies 30.

DUTT, Udoy Chand (trans.) 1883: *The Sus'ruta-samhitá. The Hindu System of Medicine according to Sus'ruta.* Calcutta: Baptist Mission Press. Bibliotheca Indica, New Series 500.

GAUTAM, Māṇḍ'vī; UPĀDHYĀY, Om Prakāś; GAUTAM, Vinod Kumār 2005: 'Pitt evaṃ agni vivecan', *Sachitra Ayurved* 58,6: 424-427.

GHANEKAR, Bhaskar Govind (comm.) 1952: *Sushruta Saṃhitā with Hindi Commentary named "Āyurveda Rahasyadīpikā". Volume one (Sūtra-Nidān-Sthān).* Second edition.

[28] GAUTAM/UPĀDHYĀY/GAUTAM 2005, an article on the relationship between *pitta* and *agni*, concludes that they are similar (*sādharmya*) as to their actions (*karmātmak*) and treatment (*upacārātmak*), but different (*vaidharmya*) as to their own nature (*svarūp*). This makes them members of the same group (*varg*), able to cooperate.

Delhi: Meharchand Lachhmandas.

*Mādhavanidāna*: *Mâdhavanidâna by Mâdhavakara with the Commentary Madhukosha by Vijayarakshita and Shrîkaṇthadatta and Commentary Âtankadarpaṇa by Vâchaspati Vaidya*. Edited by Vaidya Jâdowjī Tricumjī Âchârya. Bombay: Nirnaya-Sâgar Press 1920.

MEULENBELD, G. JAN *forthcoming*: 'Some Neglected Aspects of Āyurveda or The Illusion of a Consistent Theory', in: Dominik Wujastyk and Michio Yano (eds.), *Mathematics and Medicine. Proceedings of the 12th World Sanskrit Conference, Helsinki 2003* (working title).

SHARMA, Priya Vrat (ed. and trans.) 1999: *Suśruta-saṃhitā with English Translation of Text and Ḍalhaṇa's Commentary along with Critical Notes. Vol. I (Sūtrasthāna)*. Varanasi: Chaukhambha Visvabharati. Haridas Ayurveda Series 9.

SINGHAL, G.D.; TRIPATHI, S.N.; CHATURVEDI, G.N. 1981: *Fundamental and Plastic Surgery Considerations in Ancient Indian Surgery (based on chapters 1-27 of Sūtra-sthāna of Suśruta Saṃhitā)*. Varanasi: Institute of Medical Sciences, Banaras Hindu University. Ancient Indian Surgery 1.

*Suśrutasaṃhitā*: *Sushrut-Sañhitā (Sūtra Sthān) With Bhānumatī Commentary by Chakrapāṇi Datta*. ... Edited by Vaidya Jādavajī Trikamajī Āchārya and Pt. Nandkishor Sharmā Bhishagāchārya. Agra: Swāmī Lakshmī Rām Trust 1939. Shrī Swāmī Lakshmī Rām Trust Series 1.

—: *The Suśrutasaṃhitā of Suśruta With the Nibandhasañgraha Commentary of Śrī Dalhaṇāchārya* [sic] *and the Nyāyachandrikā Pañjikā of Śrī Gayadāsāchārya on Nidānasthāna*. Edited ... by Vaidya Jādavji Trikamji Āchārya and ... Nārāyaṇ Rām Āchārya. Revised third edition. Bombay: Nirṇaya Sāgar Press 1938.

# *Rasāyana* und die āyurvedische Krankheitskunde[*]

OLIVER HELLWIG

Das *rasāyana*, eine āyurvedische Therapie zur Wiederherstellung von körperlicher und geistiger Fitness, ist in mehreren Publikationen untersucht worden (z.B. ROŞU 1975, MAHDIHASSAN 1979, ROŞU 1982, WHITE 1996). Der Fokus dieser Darstellungen liegt auf kulturgeschichtlichen oder religionswissenschaftlichen Themen, so auf der körperlichen Transformation des Therapierten in ROŞU 1975 und WHITE 1996 oder den Verbindungen zwischen *rasāyana* und Askese in MAHDIHASSAN 1979. Die medizinischen Wirkmechanismen der Therapie werden in diesen Darstellungen dagegen oft nur skizziert.

Die meisten Autoren gehen dazu von CA, Ci 1,1,8 aus, wo das *rasāyana* als *lābhopāyo ... śastānāṃ rasādīnām* definiert wird, also ein 'Mittel, um guten *rasa* usw. zu erhalten'. Der Terminus *rasa* wird dann, z.B. unter Bezug auf Aruṇadattas Kommentar zu AH, Ut 39,2, mit dem ersten der 'Körperelemente' (*dhātus*) gleichgesetzt, die aus verdauter Nahrung aufgebaut werden und deren feinstes, der Samen (*śukra*), die Zeugungsfähigkeit eines Manns garantiert. Die Einwirkung der Zeit stört diesen Verdauungsprozeß, der dann mithilfe der *rasāyana*-Therapie repariert werden muß. Durch die neu gewonnene Verdauungskraft wird der Körper des Patienten schließlich in einen jugendlichen Zustand zurückversetzt. Die Wirkungsweise der Therapie orientiert sich damit am geläufigen āyurvedischen Krankheitsmodell, das die Bedeutung der Verdauung und des *tridoṣa*-Komplexes betont.[1] Diese moderne Interpretation der *rasāyana*-Therapie, die sich vor allem auf Aussagen der CA stützt, wird im folgenden

---

[*] Zu den im Aufsatz verwendeten Abkürzungen siehe das Verzeichnis am Ende. – Sanskritwörter, die in der Stammform angegeben werden, werden nicht besonders gekennzeichnet (z.B. *dhātu* statt *dhātu-*).

[1] Der dargestellte Argumentationsgang findet sich z.B. bei ROŞU 1975: 3ff. WHITE 1996: 25ff. folgt dieser Interpretation und verknüpft sie mit verschiedenen Zeitmodellen der āyurvedischen Texte. Eine ähnliche Erklärung des Begriffs setzt der von Roşu zitierte Müller an, der *rasāyana* holprig als 'den Saft (*rasa*) [ursprünglich der Nahrung] hingehen-lassend [zur Verjüngung]' erklärt (MÜLLER 1960: 411, Anm. 76). MAHDIHASSAN 1979: 60ff. bietet weitere, sehr gewagte Etymologien.

als *Standarddefinition* bezeichnet.

Eine genauere Untersuchung theoretischer Aussagen zeigt allerdings, daß die *Standarddefinition* die *rasāyana*-Therapie in drei Punkten nicht angemessen beschreibt. Dabei handelt es sich um das Zusammenspiel des *rasāyana*s mit dem Verdauungsprozeß, um die Rolle der Zeit im *rasāyana*-Konzept und schließlich um die Annahme konzeptioneller Homogeneität āyurvedischer Texte.

Der gravierendste Mangel der *Standarddefinition* ist ihre Beschränkung auf die verlockend einfache 'etymologische' Erklärung, nach der *rasāyana* 'den *rasa* zum Laufen bringt' (*rasāyanam = rasasyāyanam*). Eine genauere Untersuchung der theoretischen Aussagen zeigt nämlich, daß das *rasāyana* in vielen Fällen nicht mit Störungen des Verdauungsprozesses, sondern mit der Klasse der *svābhāvika*-Krankheiten assoziiert wird. Diese Verbindung wird von ROŞU 1975: 5 zwar erwähnt, aber nicht weiter verfolgt. Nun ist die Stellung der *svābhāvika*-Krankheiten innerhalb des Āyurvedas alles andere als gefestigt. Teilweise lassen sie sich so schlecht mit anderen Theorien der Pathologie verbinden, daß JOLLY 1901: 47 ihren Status als eigenständige Krankheitsklasse anzweifelt und damit die bis heute weit verbreitete Meinung wiedergibt, daß in der āyurvedischen Pathologie nur drei Krankheitsklassen (*śārīra*, *mānasa* und *āgantu*) eine bedeutende Rolle spielen. Die wichtigste dieser Klassen ist die der 'körperlichen Krankheiten' (*śārīra*, *nija*), deren prominentester Vertreter das Fieber (*jvara*) ist. Hier wird das 'Gleichgewicht' (*sāmya*) der drei *doṣa*s durch eine genau definierte Menge externer oder mentaler Faktoren gestört. Die 'erzürnten' (√*kup*) *doṣa*s beeinflussen dann die Verdauung, was schließlich zum Ausbruch der Krankheit führt. Als zweite Krankheitsklasse werden mentale Krankheiten (*mānasa*) angesetzt, die aus Fehlverhalten wie Zorn, nach anderen Theorien aber auch aus einer Störung des *doṣa*-Systems entstehen können. Diese Klasse wurde u.a. von Arion Roşu detailliert untersucht (ROŞU 1978). Die dritte Klasse der *āgantu*-Krankheiten umfaßt hauptsächlich Verletzungen; eine Interaktion mit dem *tridoṣa* ist hier nicht immer eindeutig erkennbar.

Die Klassifizierung der Krankheiten wird durch drei Variablen gesteuert:

(1) durch die 'erste Ursache' (*nidāna*), die die krankhaften Veränderungen in Gang setzt (z.B. falsche Ernährung, der Wechsel der Jahreszeiten oder Ver-

letzungen),

(2) durch den innerkörperlichen Prozeß, der den Ausbruch der Krankheit bewirkt; zumindest bei den *śārīra*-Krankheiten treten hier neben einer Veränderung im *doṣa*-Gleichgewicht (*doṣavaiṣamya*) häufig Störungen im Verdauungsprozeß auf,

(3) durch den Erscheinungsort der Krankheit (*adhiṣṭhāna*), der wenigstens *śārīra*- und *mānasa*-Klassen differenziert.

*Svābhāvika*-Krankheiten fallen sowohl hinsichtlich der ersten Ursache als auch der innerkörperlichen Vorgänge aus dem Schema heraus, das durch die drei typischen Krankheitsklassen festgelegt ist. So sind sowohl *doṣavaiṣamya* als auch Störungen im Verdauungsprozeß bei dieser Krankheitsklasse irrelevant. Aus seiner Rolle als spezialisiertes Heilmittel für diese wenig beachtete Krankheitsklasse lassen sich daher interessante Rückschlüsse auf die therapeutische Bewertung des *rasāyana*s im Āyurveda ziehen.

Auch die Ursachen für die Störungen im Verdauungsprozeß werden in der *Standarddefinition* nicht klar definiert. WHITE 1996: 23-25 sieht einen Zusammenhang zwischen dem Schwund von *rasa* und *śukra*, der eine *rasāyana*-Therapie nötig mache, und zyklischen Zeitphänomenen wie dem Mondzyklus und der Wiederkehr der heißen Jahreszeit. Gleichzeitig wird – wie auch bei ROṢU 1975: 4 – die Verbindung der Therapie mit der Geriatrie betont. Diese Annahmen verbinden das zyklische Zeitmodell der Jahre(szeiten) mit demjenigen der Lebenszeit (*vayas*) und widersprechen damit den Aussagen āyurvedischer Texte, die das zyklische Modell mit *śārīra*- bzw. *nija*-Krankheiten, das lineare Lebenszeit-Modell dagegen eindeutig mit *svābhāvika*-Krankheiten verbinden.

Der dritte Kritikpunkt an den bisher vorliegenden Darstellungen ist die Vermischung von Passagen verschiedener āyurvedischer Texte, der das oft unausgesprochene Axiom zugrundeliegt, daß diese Texte eine einheitliche medizinische Tradition repräsentieren, obwohl, wie DAS 2003: 32 anmerkt, die vorliegenden Editionen nicht problemlos als homogene Texte von fixierbaren Autoren angesehen werden können. Daher werden im folgenden SU und CA als separate Basiseinheiten angesetzt, die, wie sich im Laufe der Untersuchung herausstellen wird, unterschiedliche Lehrmeinungen zum *rasāyana* und zur Pathogenese vortragen.

Die Untersuchung beschränkt sich auf die 'theoretischen' Passagen von SU und CA, die sich am besten durch Ausschluß der zahlreichen āyurvedischen Rezepte und Therapiebeschreibungen eingrenzen lassen. Die Auswertung der Rezepte mit statistischen Methoden und der Vergleich dieser Ergebnisse mit den theoretischen Aussagen bleibt eine lohnende Aufgabe, die hier aus Platzgründen aber nicht durchgeführt werden kann.

## 1. *Suśrutasaṃhitā*

In der SU und ihren Kommentaren finden sich vier verschiedene Einschätzungen der *rasāyana*-Therapie. Den breitesten Raum nimmt der Einsatz bei *svābhāvika*-Krankheiten ein (unten, §1.1). Mit einer Variante der *Standarddefinition* erklärt Ḍalhaṇa die Wirkung des *rasāyana*s bei *ojas*-Schwund (unten, S. 46). Daneben besitzt die Therapie in den theoretischen Passagen der SU den Status eines 'Wunderheilmittels', das bei unheilbaren Krankheiten eingesetzt wird (S. 47). Eine kurze Notiz bei Ḍalhaṇa deutet schließlich darauf hin, daß zumindest diesem Kommentator auch die *Standarddefinition* geläufig war (S. 49).

### 1.1. *Rasāyana* als Mittel gegen *svābhāvika*-Krankheiten

In SU, Sū 1,8 wird *rasāyana* als siebtes von acht *aṅga*s des Āyurveda definiert. Der Text spricht ihm drei Wirkungen zu:

1. Konsolidierung und Verlängerung der Lebensspanne (*vayaḥsthāpana*, *āyuṣkara*). – Der Begriff *vayaḥsthāpana* bezeichnet nach Ḍalhaṇa die Fähigkeit des *rasāyana*s, dem Patienten zu der vollen Lebensspanne von 100 Jahren zu verhelfen. *āyuṣkara* bezieht sich dagegen auf eine Lebensverlängerung über diese hundert Jahre hinaus (vgl. ROȘU 1982: 364ff.).
2. Verbesserung von körperlicher und geistiger Fitness (*medhābalakara*).
3. Beseitigung von Krankheiten (*rogāpaharaṇa*).

Daß es sich bei diesen Krankheiten um die Klasse der *svābhāvika*-Krankheiten handelt, hat schon ROȘU 1975: 5 angedeutet. Zur Unterstützung kann man SU, Sū 3,22 anführen, einen Vers aus dem metrischen Inhaltsverzeichnis der SU, dem gemäß sich das Kapitel SU, Ci 29 mit der Abwehr von *svābhāvika*-Krankheiten beschäftigt. Der Name von SU, Ci 29 (*Svabhāvavyādhipratiṣedhanīya*) bestätigt diese Aussage. Welche Position die *svābhāvika*-Krankheiten in der Pathologie der SU einnehmen und wie sich die medizinische Wirkung des *rasāyanas* mit diesem Krankheitskonzept erklären läßt, wird im folgenden anhand von zwei Textstellen besprochen.

### 1.1.1. Sūtrasthāna 1,24-25

In SU, Sū 1,24-25 werden vier Krankheitstypen (*vyādhi*) aufgezählt. Neben dem Typus der *āgantu*-Krankheiten ('Verletzungen') kennt der Text *śārīra*-Krankheiten, die durch eine Störung des *tridoṣas* entstehen, und mentale Leiden, die *mānasa*-Krankheiten. Den vierten Typus bilden die *svābhāvika*-Krankheiten, die mit folgenden Worten definiert werden: *svābhāvikās tu kṣutpipāsājarāmṛtyunidrāprakṛtayaḥ* (Variante: °*prabhṛtayaḥ*).

Betrachten wir zunächst die Lesart °*prakṛtayaḥ*, der Ḍalhaṇa in seinem Kommentar den Vorzug gibt. Die Interpretation des gesamten Kompositums hängt von der Bedeutung ab, die man seinem Endglied *prakṛti* zuweist. Die im āyurvedischen Kontext oft übliche Übersetzung als 'körperliche Konstitution' auf Basis des *tridoṣas* ist im vorliegenden semantischen Kontext nicht anwendbar. Ḍalhaṇa scheint auf eine Bedeutung wie 'Natur' zurückzugreifen, wenn er schreibt: *prakṛtigrahaṇāt prakṛtibhavā rogā gṛhyante*. Eine naheliegende Übersetzung dieses Satzes könnte lauten: 'Durch Benutzung [des Begriffs] *prakṛti* werden [von] Natur [aus im Menschen existente] Krankheiten erfaßt.'

Gemäß dieser Übersetzung entstehen *svābhāvika*-Krankheiten ohne einen speziellen pathogenen Einfluß wie die Verdauung bei den *śārīra*- oder Verletzungen bei den *āgantu*-Krankheiten. Es handelt sich um Anlagen, die dem menschlichen Körper inhärent sind und – das ist zu ergänzen – im Laufe des Lebens von selbst aktiviert werden. Im weiteren Verlauf des Kommentars kommen aber Zweifel an dieser Interpretation auf. Ḍalhaṇa teilt den Krankheitstypus nämlich weiter in zwei Unterklassen auf, von denen die erste durch *doṣas* hervorgerufen wird (*kadācid doṣajāḥ*), während die zweite wiederum den Namen *svābhāvika* erhält.

Um einer Begriffsverwirrung vorzubeugen, wird der Krankheitstypus *svābhāvika*mit $S_1$, seine Unterklasse *svābhāvika* mit $S_2$, seine Unterklasse *doṣaja* dagegen mit D bezeichnet. Nach Ḍalhaṇa lassen sich $S_2$ und D hauptsächlich anhand ihrer Entstehungszeit auseinanderhalten. Treten die Symptome wie

Hunger, Altern usw. an passenden Momenten im Lauf des Lebens auf, liegt die Variante $S_2$ vor, die selbst mit einer *rasāyana*-Therapie nicht geheilt werden kann. Hier handelt es sich also um Phänomene wie normalen Hunger, ein angemessenes Schlafbedürfnis oder altersgemäße Abnutzungserscheinungen. Bei unzeitgemäßem (*akālaja*) Auftreten kann man dagegen von einer *doṣa*-basierten Krankheit ausgehen, die dann mit dem *rasāyana* behandelt werden kann:

> *tatra yadaite sarve doṣebhyo jāyante tadā śārīrāḥ pratīkāryāś ca. yadā tu svabhāvatas tadā niṣpratīkārā rasāyanato'pi na pratīkāryāḥ*
> Wenn alle diese [Krankheiten] aus *doṣa*s entstehen, sind sie *śārīra*-[Krankheiten] und [damit] behandelbar. Wenn [sie] aber von selbst (*svabhāvataḥ*) [entstehen], dann sind sie unbehandelbar, [dann sind sie] selbst mit dem *rasāyana* nicht behandelbar.

Eine eindeutige Unterscheidung in $S_2$ und D ist nach Ḍalhaṇa allerdings unmöglich, da keine der beiden Klassen jemals in Reinform auftritt, sondern immer auch Züge der anderen Klasse zeigt. Die Bezeichnung (*vyapadeśa*) und damit Diagnose richtet sich daher nach dem dominierenden Faktor und – in einem gewissen Umfang – auch nach sprachlichen Konventionen.

Wie ist der Begriff *prakṛti* in Ḍalhaṇas Kommentar also zu interpretieren? Das Wort kann an dieser Stelle nicht bedeuten, daß die *svābhāvika*-Krankheiten 'von Natur aus' im Menschen angelegt sind, da in diesem Fall die Unterklasse D nicht von der Definition erfaßt wäre. Eher können die *prakṛtibhavā rogāḥ* als krankhafte *Phänomene* beschrieben werden, die bei jedem Menschen 'von Natur aus' auftreten. Der Begriff *prakṛti* sagt damit nichts über die Ursache, sondern etwas über den Phänotyp dieser Krankheiten aus. Ihre Entstehung und ihre Wirkung im Körper werden von Ḍalhaṇa nur für die Unterklasse D, die mit den *śārīra*-Krankheiten zusammenfällt, schlüssig erklärt. Wie die Unterklasse $S_2$ aktiviert wird und ob sie ihre pathogene Wirkung wie *śārīra*-Krankheiten durch eine Störung des *doṣa*-Gleichgewichts erzielt, führt er nicht weiter aus.

Ein Indiz für die Vermutung, daß Ḍalhaṇa bei der *gesamten* Klasse der *svābhāvika*s ($S_1$) andere Wirkungsmechanismen am Werk sieht als bei den restlichen *vyādhi*s, liefert allerdings sein Kommentar zu SU, Sū 1,24 (*te caturvidhā* *āgantavaḥ śārīrā mānasāḥ svābhāvikāś ceti*). Hier interpretiert er die harmlose Partikel *ca* als einen Indikator für die Sonderstellung von $S_1$: *cakāraḥ svābhāvikasya vyādher āgantuprabhr̥tibhiḥ sahātulyabalatām sūcayati* 'Das Wort *ca* zeigt an, daß die *svābhāvika*-Krankheitsklasse nicht dieselbe Kraft besitzt wie *āgantu*-[Krankheiten] usw.'

Ob der Terminus *atulya* im Sinn einer größeren oder geringeren Kraft gedeutet werden muß, verrät Ḍalhaṇa leider nicht.

Unter Einbeziehung von Ḍalhaṇas Kommentar läßt sich die Krankheitsklassifikation in Su, Sū 1,24-25 so darstellen:

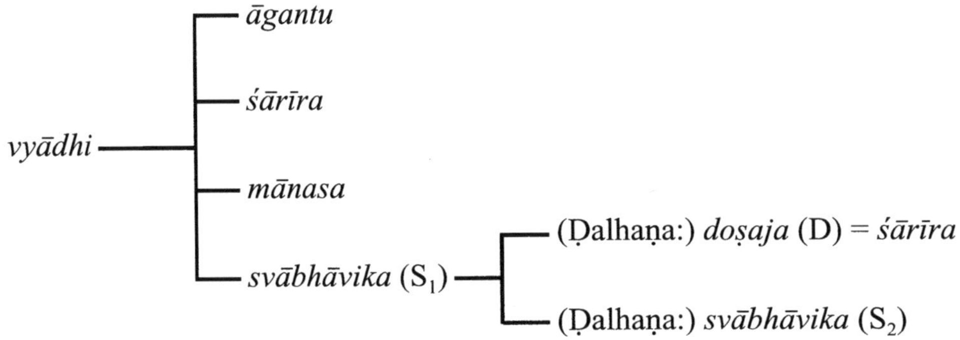


Überträgt man Ḍalhaṇas Ausführungen auf den Haupttext der Su, müßte für *prakr̥ti* in Su, Sū 1,25 eine Bedeutung wie 'natürliche/typische Erscheinung' angesetzt werden. Die *svābhāvika*-Krankheiten wären dann typische körperliche Erscheinungen wie Hunger, Durst usw. Zu einer ähnlichen Auffassung gelangt Roşu 1978: 107; hier wird der Begriff *svābhāvika* mit '[maladies] naturelles ..., c'est-à-dire inhérentes à la nature humaine' paraphrasiert.

Vernachlässigt man Ḍalhaṇas Überlegungen, könnte für *prakr̥ti* auch eine Übersetzung wie 'Ursprung' = 'Ursache' gewählt werden, was den Inhalt des Textes aber deutlich veränderte, denn Su, Sū 1,25 beschriebe nicht mehr Symptome, sondern Ursachen der *svābhāvika*-Krankheiten. Dieser Krankheitstypus würde dann aufgrund von Hunger, Durst usw. entstehen – über seine Symptomatik wäre nichts gesagt. Die Erwähnung von *mr̥tyu* spricht nicht gegen diese zweite Interpretation; daß sich āyurvedische Texte durchaus etwas unter Krankheiten vorstellen konnten, 'deren Ursache der Tod ist', zeigen z.B. Cakrapāṇidattas Ausführungen zu einem ähnlichen Thema (siehe S. 55).

Angesichts der Probleme, die bei der Interpretation von *prakṛti* auftreten, könnte man die auf S. 36 erwähnte Lesart °*prabhṛtayaḥ* in Betracht ziehen. Ḍalhaṇa erwähnt sie nur kurz am Ende seines Kommentars. Inhaltlich bietet diese Textvariante allerdings nur einen geringen Unterschied zu der von Ḍalhaṇa angesetzten Bedeutung von *prakṛti*, da der Text einfach verschiedene *svābhāvika*-Krankheiten aufzählt.

Was sagen diese Informationen aus SU und Ḍalhaṇas Kommentar über das Verhältnis von *rasāyana* und *svābhāvika*-Krankheiten aus? Als erstes ist zu betonen, daß SU, Sū 1,24-25 das *rasāyana* nicht als Therapie gegen *svābhāvika*-Krankheiten erwähnt. Die eingangs angeführten Indizien (S. 35) deuten aber darauf hin, daß die Verbindung von *rasāyana* und *svābhāvika*-Krankheiten der Intention der SU entspricht. Betrachtet man allein SU, Sū 1,25 ohne den Kommentar, zählt der Text verschiedene Krankheiten (°*prabhṛtayaḥ*) bzw. Krankheitsursachen (°*prakṛtayaḥ*) auf, die teilweise mit den in SU, Sū 1,8 angegebenen Wirkungsfeldern des *rasāyana*s übereinstimmen. Ohne weitergehende Information wirken die Aussagen im SU-Text wie die Erfüllung eines Menschheitstraums: Das *rasāyana* kann Abnutzungs- und Ermüdungserscheinungen bis hin zum Tod beseitigen. Ḍalhaṇa unternimmt dagegen den Versuch, den Begriff der *svābhāvika*-Krankheiten und die Wirkungsweise des *rasāyana*s in das dominante āyurvedische Krankheitsmodell zu integrieren, indem er die behandelbaren *svābhāvika*-Fälle auf Variante D beschränkt, die einen Standardfall im Repertoire des Āyurveda darstellt. Das *rasāyana* unterscheidet sich damit im Prinzip nicht mehr von anderen Heilmitteln gegen *śārīra*-Krankheiten.

Ḍalhaṇas Bestreben, *rasāyana* in den Kreis der āyurvedischen Heilmittel einzugliedern, zeigt sich auch in seinem Kommentar zu den Grundklassen der Heilmethoden in SU, Sū 1,27. Das *rasāyana* – wie übrigens auch die Aphrodisiaka (*vājīkaraṇa*) – läßt sich danach über den Pfad *saṃśamana* → *ābhyantara* → *rasāyana* definieren und ist somit nur eines unter vielen Mitteln zum Ausgleich ‘erzürnter’ *doṣa*s.

### 1.1.2. Sūtrasthāna 24,4-7

In Kapitel SU, Sū 24 wird ein weiteres Klassifikationsschema für Krankheiten präsentiert, das die in SU, Sū 1,24-25 erwähnten vier Krankheiten als Unterklassen umfaßt (vgl. Roşu 1978: 102). Der Text nimmt in Su, Sū 24,4 durch ein Zitat Bezug auf Su, Sū 1,23 (*tadduḥkhasaṃyogā vyādhayaḥ*) und erklärt dann, daß mit dem Terminus *duḥkha* drei Grundklassen von 'Leiden' gemeint seien, die wiederum in sieben Krankheitsklassen (*vyādhi*) unterteilt werden. Mit Ḍalhaṇas Kommentar zu Su, Sū 24,4 lassen sich die *duḥkhas* so beschreiben:

1. Die *ādhyātmika*-Leiden beruhen auf Störungen im *doṣa-dūṣya*-Komplex oder im Verdauungsprozeß. Sie umfassen u.a. *śārīra*- und *mānasa*-Krankheiten.
2. Die *ādhibhautika*-Leiden sind mit der Klasse der *āgantu*-Krankheiten identisch.
3. Die *ādhidaivika*-Leiden werden von Faktoren initiiert, die außerhalb des menschlichen Zugriffs liegen.

Jede der drei Grundklassen wird in weitere Unterklassen gegliedert, so daß sich das folgende Bild ergibt:

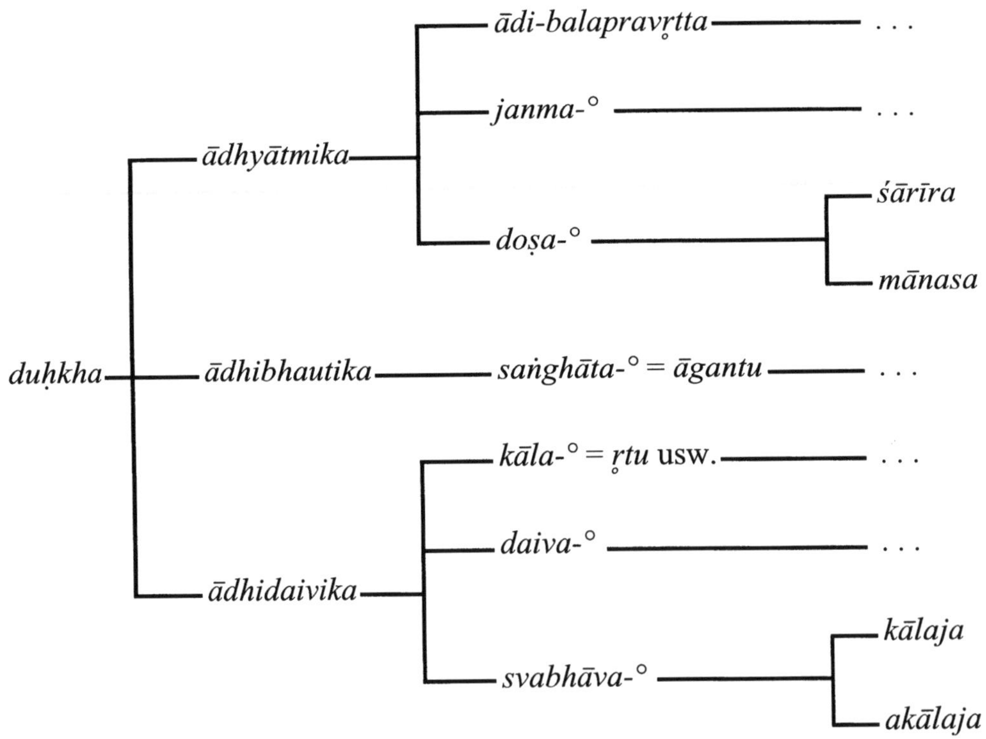

SU, Sū 24,4-7 stellt nicht nur ein Klassifikationsschema für Krankheiten auf, sondern macht auch Angaben zur Entstehung der Unterklassen, die in der folgenden Tabelle zusammengefaßt sind:

| Klasse | Unterklasse | Ursache |
|---|---|---|
| *ādhyātmika* | *ādibalapravr̥tta* | Fehler in Samen und 'Menstrualblut' (*ārtava*)[2] |
| | *janmabalapravr̥tta* | fehlerhafte Lebensführung und Ernährung der Mutter[3] |
| | *doṣabalapravr̥tta* | Folge einer anderen Erkrankung,[4] Ernährung |
| *ādhibhautika* | | Verletzungen |
| *ādhidaivika* | *kālabalapravr̥tta* | Wechsel der Jahreszeiten |
| | *daivabalapravr̥tta* | 'Götter', Verfluchung |
| | *svabhāvabalapravr̥tta* | Verstreichen der Lebenszeit |

Im Zusammenhang mit dem *rasāyana* ist die Unterklasse *ādhidaivika* → *svabhāvabalapravr̥tta* von Interesse, die anhand der aufgezählten Symptome[5] mit den *svābhāvika*-Krankheiten aus SU, Sū 1,24-25 (siehe S. 36) gleichgesetzt werden kann. Diese Identifizierung wird natürlich auch vom Namen der Krankheitsklasse nahegelegt. Der Name *svabhāvabalapravr̥tta* findet sich übrigens auch in SU, Sū 27,5, wo Körperprozesse wie Weinen, Husten oder die Urinausscheidung, durch die Fremdkörper (*śalya*) von selbst aus dem Körper entfernt werden, mit diesem Wort beschrieben werden.[6] Nimmt man einen inhaltlichen

---

[2] *śukraśoṇitadoṣānvayāḥ*; Ḍalhaṇa bezieht den Begriff *doṣa* auf den *tridoṣa*.

[3] *mātur apacārāt ... jāyante*. – Der Kommentar liefert weitere Informationen.

[4] Aus Text und Kommentar geht nicht hervor, ob es sich hier um *upasarga*-Erkrankungen handelt. Ḍalhaṇa führt nur einige Beispiele an, so z.B., daß aus Erkältung Husten entstehe (*pratiśyāyāt kāsaḥ*).

[5] *svabhāvabalapravr̥ttā ye kṣutpipāsājarāmr̥tyunidrāprabhr̥tayaḥ ...* .

[6] *tatrāśrukṣavathūdgārakāsamūtrapurīṣānilaiḥ svabhāvabalapravr̥ttair nayanādibhyaḥ patati ...* .

Zusammenhang zwischen den beiden Passagen an, sind *svabhāvabalapravṛtta*-Krankheiten – genau wie die aufgezählten Reflexe – schwer steuerbare Körpervorgänge, die nicht unbedingt von regulären pathogenen Faktoren hervorgerufen sein müssen.

Die Klasse *svabhāvabalapravṛtta* zerfällt nach SU, Sū 24,7 in zwei Unterklassen. Während die *kālaja*-Variante trotz medizinischer Vorsorge (*parirakṣaṇa*; vgl. SU, Sū 35,34) im Lauf des Lebens auftritt, entstehen *akālaja*-Krankheiten aufgrund von mangelnder Vorsorge (*aparirakṣaṇa*) zum falschen Zeitpunkt. Diese Klassifikation könnte hervorragend zur Erklärung von Ḍalhaṇas Unterteilung der *svābhāvika*-Krankheiten in $S_2$ und D herangezogen werden (*kālaja* = $S_2$, *akālaja* = D), wenn der Kommentator seinen vorher getroffenen Aussagen zum Einsatz des *rasāyana*s im Kommentar zur aktuellen Textstelle nicht widerspräche:

> *ata eva kālakṛtānāṃ nopacāro 'sti. yāpyataivāsti bhojanapānarasāyanādibhiḥ. ātyantikapratīkāro vā svabhāvavyādhicikitsitoktarasāyanavidhinā*
> Für die von der Zeit verursachten [Krankheiten] gibt es keine Behandlungsmöglichkeit. Sie lassen sich aber lindern durch [passende] Speisen, Getränke, *rasāyana* usw. Daneben gibt es ein endgültiges Gegenmittel durch die *rasāyana*-Behandlung, die im Kapitel SU, Ci 29 beschrieben wird.

Während Ḍalhaṇa im Kommentar zu SU, Sū 1,27 das *rasāyana* also gegen D = *akālaja*, die *doṣa*-basierte, zur Unzeit auftretende Variante der *svābhāvika*-Krankheiten, einsetzen will, sieht er den Einsatzbereich jetzt bei der *kālaja*-Variante = $S_2$, die sogar vollkommen geheilt werden könne.

In zwei Punkten unterscheiden sich die *svabhāvabalapravṛtta*-Krankheiten deutlich von dem Einsatzgebiet, das dem *rasāyana* in der *Standarddefinition* zugeschrieben wird. Der erste Unterschied ist das lineare Zeitmodell, das die Ursache der *svabhāvabalapravṛtta*-Krankheiten bildet. Unter den *ādhidaivika*-Krankheiten werden zwei zeitbasierte Krankheitsklassen eingeordnet. Während den *kālabalapravṛtta*-Krankheiten ein Jahreszeitenmodell zugrundeliegt, das z.B. auch in der *ṛtucaryā* benutzt wird, bezeichnet der Terminus *kāla* im Zusammenhang mit den *svabhāvabalapravṛtta*-Krankheiten die Lebenszeit. Für den 'Verfasser' des Textes war der konzeptionelle Unterschied zwischen diesen beiden Zeitskalen anscheinend groß genug, um aus ihm zwei verschiedene Krankheitsmodelle abzuleiten.[7]

Der zweite Unterschied ist, daß die Verdauung und damit verbunden die *doṣas* nach SU, Sū 24,7 bei der Entstehung von *svabhāvabalapravṛtta*-Krankheiten keine Rolle spielen. Die eben dargestellte Klassifizierung erwähnt Verdauungsprobleme und das *doṣavaiṣamya* als innerkörperliche Krankheitsursache nur bei der Klasse der *ādhyātmikas*. Die Klassen *ādhibhautika* und *ādhidaivika* müßten ihre krankhafte Wirkung im menschlichen Körper danach ohne eine Veränderung im *doṣa*-System hervorbringen. In diesem Zusammenhang sollte man berücksichtigen, daß in SU, Sū 24,8, also im direkt folgenden Satz, die *doṣas* emphatisch als Ursachen (*mūla*) *aller* Krankheiten bezeichnet werden.

Man kann diese Aussage als Rationalisierungsversuch interpretieren, durch den Krankheitsklassen wie *ādhidaivika* → *svabhāvabalapravṛtta* in die Pathologie des Āyurveda integriert werden sollen. In Anlehnung an Theorien der Pathogenese, die z.B. in SU, Sū 1,34 vorgetragen werden, könnte man die *duḥkhas* aber auch als *nidānas*, also primäre Krankheitsursachen interpretieren. Sobald eine krankhafte Störung (*roga*) im Körper entstanden ist, beruht diese wirklich allein auf dem Ungleichgewicht der *doṣas*. In dieser Funktion ist der *tridoṣa* die Ursache (*mūla*) aller Krankheiten. Vor Auftreten der Krankheit muß der *tridoṣa* allerdings zuerst ins Ungleichgewicht gebracht werden, und diese Aufgabe fällt bei der Klasse *ādhyātmika* → *doṣabalapravṛtta* u.a. der Verdauung, bei der Klasse *ādhidaivika* → *svabhāvabalapravṛtta* dagegen der Zeit zu. Diese Auffassung läßt sich so darstellen:

---

[7] Auf die Existenz verschiedener Zeitmodelle in āyurvedischen Texten hat u.a. ZIMMERMANN 1975 hingewiesen. Neben dem zyklischen Zeitmodell der Jahreszeiten, auf die der Āyurveda mit dem (*kāla-*)*sātmya* reagiert, erkennt Zimmermann in Anschluß an CA, Vi 8,125-128 ein therapeutisches Zeitmodell der *avasthās*, das die Entwicklungsstadien einer Krankheit berücksichtigt. Der Arzt muß nach Zimmermann das Leben des Patienten so organisieren, daß die 'gelebte Zeit' (*temps vécu*) des Patienten und vor allem die Phasen seiner Krankheit mit der externen zyklischen Zeit harmonieren. – Das *avasthā*-Modell der CA steht zwar im Kontrast zum zyklischen Zeitmodell, hat aber sonst wenig mit dem hier betrachteten Lebenszeit-Modell zu tun, das eher durch die Ausführungen über das *vayas* in CA, Vi 8,122 ergänzt werden kann.

SU, Sū 24,4-7: *nidāna* ≡ 3 *duḥkhas* ⊃ 7 *vyādhis*

↓

SU, Sū 24,8: *doṣavaiṣamya*

↓

*roga*

Für die Klasse der *svabhāvabalapravṛtta-* (= *svābhāvika-*)Krankheiten ergäbe sich aus dieser Überlegung, daß Krankheiten wie Alter und Tod zwar vom Verstreichen der Lebenszeit initiiert werden, dann aber ganz wie reguläre *śārīra*-Krankheiten auf ins Ungleichgewicht gebrachten *doṣa*s beruhen. Zwar harmonisiert diese Darstellung die Aussagen von SU, Sū 24,7 und SU, Sū 24,8. Ob dem 'Verfasser' der SU für die Wirkung der *svābhāvika*-Krankheiten aber wirklich die Ursachenkette *kāla* (= *vayas*) → *tridoṣa* → *roga* vorschwebte, läßt sich nicht eindeutig klären, da verschiedene Passagen der SU unterschiedliche Aussagen zu diesem Thema machen:

1. In SU, Sū 1,33-34 werden zeitliche Phänomene beschrieben, die eine Veränderung im *doṣa*-Haushalt bewirken.[8] Der Text beschränkt sich dabei wie bei den *kālabalapravṛtta*-Krankheiten auf zyklische Phänomene von der Maximaldauer eines *ayana*s. Eine direkte pathogene Wirkung der linearen Lebenszeit und damit auch der *svābhāvika*-Krankheiten ohne Zwischenschaltung von Verdauung oder *doṣa*s wird von SU, Sū 1,33 zumindest nicht widerlegt.
2. SU, Sū 35,31 verbindet dagegen die drei Lebensabschnitte von Kindheit, Erwachsensein und Alter mit der Dominanz von *kapha*, *pitta* und *vāta*.[9] Der in SU, Sū 35,29 beschriebene Schwund der Körperkraft (*bala*) ist wie die Bildung von Falten und grauen Haaren ein häufig genannter Grund, eine *rasāyana*-Behandlung zu beginnen. Gemäß SU, Sū 35,29 werden diese Phänomene durch den *vātadoṣa* hervogerufen, was der Arzt bei der Behandlung

[8] *kālakṛtāḥ pravātanivātātapacchāyājyotsnātamaḥśītoṣṇavarṣāhorātrapakṣamāsartvayanādayaḥ saṃvatsaraviśeṣāḥ ... doṣāṇāṃ sañcayaprakopapraśamapratīkārahetavaḥ.*

[9] *bāle vivardhate śleṣmā madhyame pittam eva tu*
*bhūyiṣṭhaṃ vardhate vāyur vṛddhe tad vīkṣya yojayet.*

berücksichtigen muß. Es ist zwar nicht klar, ob diese Textstelle überhaupt zur Interpretation des *rasāyana*s herangezogen werden kann, da nach SU, Ci 27,3-4 Menschen im letzten Lebensabschnitt von der *rasāyana*-Therapie ausgeschlossen sind. Trotzdem werden die Alterungserscheinungen, die Ähnlichkeiten mit den Symptomen der *svābhāvika*-Krankheiten zeigen, von einer Störung im *doṣa*-Gleichgewicht hervorgerufen, was dem Befund aus SU, Sū 24,7 widerspricht.

3. In SU, Sū 35,35 erfährt das Verhältnis der Begriffe *svabhāva*, *doṣa* und Lebenszeit eine weitere Interpretation. Inhalt der Passage ist die Diagnose von körperlicher Stärke (*bala*; siehe S. 46) und Schwäche: ... *daurbalyaṃ ca svabhāvadoṣajarādibhir avekṣitavyam* '... und [körperliche] Schwäche sollte man anhand der "Natur", der *doṣa*s, des Lebensalters usw. diagnostizieren.'

Von den drei Ursachen für die Schwächung eines Patienten sind *doṣa* und *jarā* eindeutig erklärbar. Schwieriger ist die Interpretation des Begriffs *svabhāva*. Das Wort kann an dieser Stelle nicht die im Alter einsetzende automatische Verschlechterung des Körperzustands beschreiben, da diese Funktion vom Terminus *jarā* abgedeckt ist. Ḍalhaṇa greift zur Erklärung offenbar auf das Konzept der *ādibalapravr̥tta*-Krankheiten zurück: *svabhāvān mātr̥pitr̥śoṇitaśukrasvabhāvād ity arthaḥ* 'Aus der "Natur" [bedeutet]: aus der Natur von Blut und Samen von Mutter und Vater.'

Ob Ḍalhaṇas Interpretation mit der Intention des 'Verfassers' der SU übereinstimmt, läßt sich nicht mehr nachvollziehen. Trotzdem erlaubt die Passage zwei interessante Schlußfolgerungen. Da die drei Faktoren nebeneinandergestellt sind, können Phänomene wie die Schwächung des Körpers von *doṣa*s *oder* dem Alter verursacht werden. *Doṣa*s sind also kein integraler Faktor bei jeder Verschlechterung des körperlichen Zustands; die von SU, Sū 24,8 betonte zentrale Position der *doṣa*s bei allen Erkrankungen muß sich nicht auf die *svabhāvabalapravr̥tta*- = *svābhāvika*-Krankheiten beziehen. Andererseits weckt SU, Sū 35,35 Zweifel an der inhaltlichen Gleichsetzung von *svabhāva* und Lebenszeit, die z.B. von Ḍalhaṇa bei der Interpretation von SU, Sū 1,24-25 vertreten wurde (S. 36). Offenbar existieren neben der Lebenszeit noch andere körperliche Faktoren, die als *svabhāva* bezeichnet werden und eine Schwächung des Menschen hervorrufen.

Die Aussagen von SU, Sū 24,4-7 und assoziierten Textstellen lassen sich in folgenden drei Punkten zusammenfassen:

1. *Svābhāvika-* und *svabhāvabalapravṛtta*-Krankheiten sind wahrscheinlich identisch.
2. *Svābhāvika*-Krankheiten werden von der linearen Lebenszeit hervorgerufen.
3. Bei der Entstehung von Krankheiten dieser Klasse spielen trotz der Aussagen in SU, Sū 24,8 Verdauung und *doṣa*s wohl keine Rolle.

### 1.2. *Rasāyana* als Mittel gegen Schwund von *bala* und *ojas*

Eine Variante der *Standarddefinition* findet sich im Kapitel SU, Sū 15, das sich mit den Auswirkungen einer krankhaften Vermehrung/Verminderung von *doṣa*s, *dhātu*s und *mala*s befaßt. In SU, Sū 15,19 werden die Termini *ojas* und *bala* als 'perfekte' (*para*) Form des *tejas*[10] der *dhātu*s definiert. Folgt man Ḍalhaṇas Kommentar, können die beiden Begriffe hier nicht synonym gebraucht werden; vielmehr bezeichne *ojas* einen Stoff, während *bala* eher als Eigenschaft des Körpers zu erklären, auf jeden Fall aber nicht stofflich sei. Daß tatsächlich ein Unterschied zwischen den Begriffen besteht, bestätigen die folgenden Sätze:

1. *Bala* ist hauptsächlich für die korrekte Funktion der Sinne und die menschliche Handlungsfähigkeit (*sarvaceṣṭāsvapratighāta*) verantwortlich, bewirkt aber auch eine klare Stimme, eine reine Haut (*svaravarṇaprasāda*) und festigt das Körperfleisch (*sthiropacitamāṃsatā*) (SU, Sū 15,20). Auf Grundlage der hier dargestellten Wirkungen kann man davon ausgehen, daß der in vielen *rasāyana*-Rezepten erwähnte Begriff *bala* mit dem Terminus technicus aus SU, Sū 15,19 identisch ist.
2. Das stoffliche *ojas* besitzt die 'Natur von Soma' und durchdringt lebensspendend den gesamten Körper, der nach Schwund des *ojas* folgerichtig auch verfällt (*śīryante śarīrāṇi*; SU, Sū 15,21-22).[11]

Das Verschwinden von *ojas*/*bala* – und hier kommen wir zum *rasāyana* –

---

[10] Ḍalhaṇa erwähnt eine Lehrmeinung, der gemäß *tejas* 'Essenz' (*sāra*) ist *(yat paraṃ teja iti yad utkṛṣṭaṃ sāraḥ*). Zu *para* als Bestimmung von *ojas* und *tejas* siehe DAS 2003: 530ff.

[11] Siehe auch DAS 2003: 530ff.

wird nach SU, Sū 15,23 durch Verletzungen, Anstrengungen aller Art, Kummer, aber auch Grübeln (*dhyāna*) und Hunger hervorgerufen und in typisch āyurvedischer Manier in drei Klassen (*doṣa*s) unterteilt (SU, Sū 15,25-27). Die ersten beiden, minderschweren dieser drei Klassen (*vyāpad*, *visraṃsa*) können nach SU, Sū 15,28 durch geeignete Therapien (*kriyāviśeṣa*) behandelt werden, die das *bala* wiederherstellen (*āpyāyayet*). Nach Ḍalhaṇa handelt es sich bei diesen Therapieformen u.a. um *rasāyana* und *vājīkaraṇa*.

Welchen Krankheitstyp soll das *rasāyana* nach Ḍalhaṇas Meinung an dieser Stelle bekämpfen? Einerseits sind *ojas* und *bala* Endprodukte des Verdauungsprozesses (vgl. SU, Sū 1,28). Ihr Schwund deutet auf eine Störung dieses Ablaufs hin, der Einsatz des *rasāyana*s daher auf die *Standarddefinition* der Therapie. Andererseits greifen nach SU, Sū 15,23 die äußeren Faktoren das *ojas* direkt an und treiben es aus dem Herzen (*hṛdaya*) bzw. den 'Gefäßen' (*srotas*).[12] Der Schwund von *ojas*/*bala* ist daher nicht die Folge einer krankhaften Veränderung der Verdauung. Vielmehr wird das *ojas*/*bala* in fast mechanischer Weise von seinem natürlichen Platz im Körper vertrieben. Zwar stellt das *rasāyana* an dieser Stelle die Funktion des Verdauungsprozesses wieder her – gestört wurde dieser aber nicht durch eine Form der Zeit, sondern durch externe Störungen, die den Auslösern von *āgantu*-Krankheiten ähneln.

### 1.3. *Rasāyana* als Medizin für hoffnungslose Fälle

Während *rasāyana* in den bisher besprochenen Fällen bei einem bestimmten Krankheitsbild eingesetzt wird, läßt sich eine weitere Funktion als 'Notfallmedikament' für hoffnungslos Erkrankte erkennen. Zwei dieser Fälle werden im folgenden besprochen.

Kapitel SU, Sū 33 beschäftigt sich mit Erkrankungen, die von *upadrava*s, also zur Haupterkrankung hinzutretenden Zusatzerkrankungen, begleitet sind (vgl. MEULENBELD 1974: 447f.). Das einzige Mittel gegen die in SU, Sū 33 be-

[12] Der Text der SU lautet: *ojaḥ ... ebhyo dhātugrahaṇaniḥsṛtam* Der Begriff *dhātugrahaṇa* wird von den Kommentatoren als *srotas* (Ḍalhaṇa, Cakrapāṇidatta, Hārāṇacandra) bzw. *hṛdaya* (Ḍalhaṇa) paraphrasiert. Zum Komplex *ojas*/*hṛdaya* siehe z.B. DAS 2003: 530ff., 590 – Die Übersetzung 'Gefäß' für *srotas* hat eher verdeutlichenden Charakter.

schriebenen, sonst unheilbaren Krankheiten stellt nach SU, Sū 33,3 das *rasāyana* dar. Ḍalhaṇa schreibt dazu in seinem Kommentar: *rasāyanād vineti rasāyanena hy asādhyo vyādhir api prāyaḥ sādhyate* '"Außer durch *rasāyana*" heißt: Durch *rasāyana* wird selbst eine unheilbare Krankheit meist geheilt.'

Obwohl der Text nichts über die Entstehung der Krankheiten aussagt, kann man anhand der in SU, Sū 33 aufgeführten Fälle davon ausgehen, daß es sich hauptsächlich um die *śārīra*-Variante, also die dominante āyurvedische Krankheitsklasse handelt. Der besondere Charakter des *rasāyana*s leitet sich hier nicht aus dem Krankheitstypus, sondern aus der Schwere der Erkrankung ab.

Ähnlich liegt der Fall in SU, Sū 28,5. Selbst der unmittelbar bevorstehende Tod, diagnostiziert mithilfe von *(a)riṣṭas* (körperlichen Vorzeichen des Todes, vgl. MEULENBELD 1974: 442), läßt sich mit geeigneten Methoden vermeiden: *... maraṇaṃ ... brāhmaṇais tat kilāmalaiḥ | rasāyanatapojapyatatparair vā nivāryate* 'Der Tod wird von reinen Brahmanen oder [von Leuten], die ganz auf *rasāyana*, Askese oder *japa* konzentriert sind, verhindert.'

Ḍalhaṇa verknüpft in seinem Kommentar die *rasāyana*-Therapie, das Konzept der *svābhāvika*-Krankheiten und pharmakologische Ansätze:

> *rasāyanaparā iti svabhāvavyādhinivāraṇaviśiṣṭauṣadhacintakās te rasavīryauṣadhaprabhāveṇa maraṇaṃ nivārayanti*
> 'Ganz auf *rasāyana* konzentriert' heißt: Sie machen sich Gedanken über Heilmittel, die besonders geeignet sind, um *svābhāvika*-Krankheiten abzuwehren. Sie wehren den Tod durch die Kraft der Heilmittel hinsichtlich von *rasa* und *vīrya* ab.

Wichtig für Ḍalhaṇas Verständnis von SU, Sū 28,5 ist das Kompositum *rasavīryauṣadhaprabhāveṇa*, das den Wirkmechanismus des *rasāyana*s beschreibt, aber mit Ausnahme des Begriffs *auṣadha* aus Termini besteht, die in verschiedenen āyurvedischen Begriffsfeldern auftreten. Die Bedeutung des Begriffs *prabhāva* läßt sich aus Ḍalhaṇas weiterem Kommentar erklären, wo *tapaḥprabhāveṇa* 'durch *prabhāva* von Askese' erscheint. Das Wort hat daher keine medizinische Nebenbedeutung und kann mit '[einem Prozeß innewohnende] Kraft' übersetzt werden. Für *rasa* und *vīrya* bietet sich zunächst eine pharmakologische Interpretation an (vgl. MEULENBELD 1978: 5ff.). Allerdings spricht ihre Stellung im Kompositum gegen die einfachste Übersetzung als '*rasa* und *vīrya* von Heilmitteln' (hier würde man *auṣadharasavīrya*° erwarten), woraus sich die oben abgedruckte, etwas gezwungene Übersetzung ergibt.

### 1.4. Die *Standarddefinition* des *rasāyanas*

In den ersten Worten seines Kommentars zu SU, Ci 27,1 nimmt Ḍalhaṇa Bezug auf die *Standarddefinition* des *rasāyanas* in CA, Ci 1,1,8 (vgl. S. 50). Auf die pharmakologische Deutung, die das Wort *rasa* an dieser Stelle erfährt, hat ROŞU 1982: 364f. hingewiesen. Ob dem 'Autor' der SU die von Ḍalhaṇa angesetzte Bedeutung von *rasāyana* vorschwebte, läßt sich aus dem Haupttext nicht ableiten. Möglicherweise ist die Erwähnung der *Standarddefinition* von dem Wunsch inspiriert, die *rasāyana*-Abschnitte von SU und CA inhaltlich zu verknüpfen.

Obwohl die *Standarddefinition* in der SU nicht erwähnt wird, finden sich Textstellen, nach denen eine Abhängigkeit zwischen zunehmendem Alter und Fehlern im Verdauungsprozeß existiert. Eine dieser Passagen ist SU, Sū 14,19, wo die mit dem Alter abnehmende Nährwirkung des *annarasas* beschrieben wird: *sa evānnaraso vr̥ddhānāṃ paripakvaśarīratvād aprīṇano bhavati* 'Dieser *rasa* der Nahrung wird bei alten Menschen nicht nährend, weil der Körper "reif gekocht" ist.'

Zwei Gründe sprechen gegen eine vorschnelle Verbindung der hier vorgetragenen Theorie mit der *Standarddefinition*. So wird weder im Text noch im Kommentar die *rasāyana*-Therapie erwähnt. Daneben ist die exakte Bedeutung des Begriffs *rasa* an dieser Stelle schwer bestimmbar. Ḍalhaṇa interpretiert *rasa* als *poṣakarasa* (vgl. DAS 2003: 194ff., 215ff.), was nicht ohne weiteres mit dem *rasadhātu* der *Standarddefinition* gleichzusetzen ist. Die Passage liefert daher höchstens ein Indiz, aber keinen Nachweis dafür, daß der Kerngedanke der *Standarddefinition* auch in der SU bekannt war.

## 2. *Carakasaṃhitā*

In der CA ist die *rasāyana*-Therapie hauptsächlich mit der Lehre von den Körperelementen (*dhātu*) und damit der Theorie vom Nahrungs-Verdauungs-Zyklus verbunden. Diese Sicht auf die *rasāyana*-Therapie ist als *Standarddefi-*

*nition* rezipiert worden (unten, §2.1). Zumindest dem Kommentator Cakrapāṇidatta ist aber auch die aus der SU bekannte Verbindung von *rasāyana* und *svābhāvika*-Krankheiten geläufig (S. 52). Eine Passage im zweiten Ci-Kapitel schildert schließlich detailliert die Genese von Krankheiten, die eine *rasāyana*-Therapie nötig machen, und liefert möglicherweise eine Synthese von *Standarddefinition* und *svābhāvika*-Konzept (S. 58).

## 2.1. Die *Standarddefinition*

Die *Standarddefinition* des *rasāyana*s findet sich in CA, Ci 1,1,4-8, also ganz am Beginn des Ci. Die Passage wurde u.a. von ROȘU 1982: 364ff. besprochen und wird daher nur kurz behandelt. Ausgangspunkt ist die Aufteilung der Heilmittel (*bheṣaja*) in zwei Klassen (CA, Ci 1,1,4-5):

1. Mittel, die körperlich gesunde Menschen weiter kräftigen (*svasthasyorjaskaram*[13]).
2. Mittel, die bei 'echten' Krankheiten eingesetzt werden (*rogāṇām ... praśame*).

Zum Typ der kräftigenden Mittel gehört nach CA, Ci 1,1,5 das *rasāyana*, dessen klassische Definition sich in CA, Ci 1,1,7-8 findet:

> *dīrgham āyuḥ smṛtiṃ medhām ārogyaṃ taruṇaṃ vayaḥ* |
> *prabhāvarṇasvaraudāryaṃ dehendriyabalaṃ param* ||
> *vāksiddhiṃ praṇatiṃ kāntiṃ labhate nā rasāyanāt* |
> *lābhopāyo hi śastānāṃ rasādīnāṃ rasāyanam* ||
> Ein langes Leben, Erinnerungskraft, Intelligenz, Gesundheit, Jugendlichkeit, Glanz, [eine gesunde] Farbe, eine durchdringende Stimme, volle Kraft von Körper und Sinnen, *siddhi*-[Kräfte im Bereich] der Sprache (*vāksiddhi*), Gehorsam [anderer Menschen] und Schönheit erlangt ein Mann durch das *rasāyana*. Denn das *rasāyana* ist ein Mittel, um guten *rasa* usw. zu erlangen.

Bei der Beurteilung des *rasāyana*s sollte man allerdings in Betracht ziehen, daß nach CA, Ci 1,1,6 die Heilmittelklassen 1 und 2 in der Praxis nicht immer eindeutig getrennt werden können. So lassen sich Arzneien der Klasse 1 auch

[13] Zum Begriff *svastha* siehe HARA 1995. Der Begriff scheint an dieser Stelle der CA aber eindeutig die körperliche Gesundheit zu beschreiben.

bei Krankheiten (*vyādhi*) einsetzen, wie der Text bei der Diskussion des Adverbs *prāyas* in CA, Ci, 1,1,6 bemerkt: *prāyaḥśabdo viśeṣārtho hy ubhayaṃ hy ubhayārthakṛt* 'Der Begriff "im allgemeinen" dient nur zur Differenzierung [der Klassen]. Denn beide [Klassen] können zu beiden Zwecken eingesetzt werden.'

Zur Differenzierung der beiden Klassen schlägt Cakrapāṇidatta ein empirisches Kriterium vor. Arzneien sollten derjenigen Klasse zugeordnet werden, deren Wirkung sie in der Mehrzahl ihrer Anwendungen (*bāhulya*) zeigen:

> *brūmaḥ bāhulyena svasthorjaskaratvaṃ vyādhiharatvaṃ ca vyavasthāpyate. na ceha sarvārtarogaharasya svasthorjaskaratvam iti pratijñāyate*
> Wir sagen [zu diesem Problem]: Die Fähigkeiten, Gesunde zu kräftigen und Krankheiten zu beseitigen, werden durch die Mehrzahl der Fälle festgelegt. Denn es gilt, daß nicht jede [Substanz], die Krankheiten bei Kranken beseitigt, auch die Fähigkeit besitzt, Gesunde zu kräftigen.

Möglicherweise liegt hier ein Reflex der in der SU vorgetragenen Auffassung vor, daß *rasāyana* nicht nur gegen *svābhāvika*-, sondern als 'Notfallmedizin' auch gegen unheilbare *śārīra*-Krankheiten eingesetzt werden kann (S. 47). Auch die Tatsache, daß Ḍalhaṇa keine abschließende Definition der *svābhāvika*-Klassen $S_2$ und D bieten kann (S. 37), läßt sich wahrscheinlich mit der anwendungsorientierten Natur dieser pharmakologischen Basisdefinition erklären.

Eine Verbindung zwischen *Standarddefinition* und *svābhāvika*-Konzept stellt Cakrapāṇidatta in seinem Kommentar zu CA, Ci 1,1,4 her. Dabei erklärt er das pharmakologische Paar *ūrjaskara* und *rogahara* mit dem Konzept der *svābhāvika*-Krankheiten:

> *svasthatvena vyavahriyamāṇasya puṃso jarādisvābhāvikavyādhiharatvena ... ūrjaḥ praśastaṃ bhāvam ādadhātīti svasthasyorjaskaram. ārtasya roganuditi viśeṣaṇena jvarādinārtasya jvarādiharam*
> [Die Phrase] 'den Gesunden kräftigend' bedeutet, daß bei einem Mann, der durch den Zustand der Gesundheit beschrieben ist, [das *rasāyana*] den positiven Zustand der 'Kraft' (*ūrjas*) hervorruft, indem es *svābhāvika*-Krankheiten wie Alter usw. beseitigt ... .'Beim Kranken Krankheiten entfernend' heißt zur Differenzierung, daß [diese Arznei] bei an Fieber usw. Erkrankten das Fieber usw. beseitigt.

Ob auch der 'Verfasser' der CA wie sein Kommentator Cakrapāṇidatta die

These vertritt, daß die in der *Standarddefinition* beschriebenen Krankheiten letztlich mit dem Krankheitstyp der *svābhāvika*s identisch sind, läßt sich aus CA, Ci 1,1,4-8 nicht ableiten. Nach einer Übersicht über das *svābhāvika*-Konzept in der CA (§2.2) wird diese Frage auf S. 58 noch einmal aufgegriffen.

### 2.2. *svābhāvika*-Krankheiten in der *Carakasaṃhitā*

Neben der *Standarddefinition* ist der CA auch das Konzept der *svābhāvika*-Krankheiten bekannt, die von Kommentatoren mit dem *rasāyana* assoziiert werden. Eine mögliche 'etymologische' Interpretation des Begriffs *svābhāvika* bietet dann CA, Sū 30,25-26 mit der Gleichung *svabhāva* = Tod (S. 56).

#### 2.2.1. Śārīrasthāna 1,115

CA, Śā 1,110-114 beschäftigt sich mit zeitbasierten (*kālaja*) Krankheiten, die z.B. im Laufe der Jahreszeiten oder durch den Wechsel von Tag und Nacht entstehen. Direkt im Anschluß findet sich in CA, Śā 1,115 eine Definition von *svābhāvika*-Krankheiten, die ebenfalls vom Verstreichen der Zeit verursacht werden:

> *kālasya pariṇāmena jarāmr̥tyunimittajāḥ* ।
> *rogāḥ svābhāvikā dr̥ṣṭāḥ svabhāvo niṣpratikriyaḥ*
> Durch das Verstreichen der Zeit lassen sich *svābhāvika*-Krankheiten beobachten, die aus den Ursachen von Alter und Tod entstehen. Die eigene Natur ist unheilbar (d.h. gegen die eigene Natur läßt sich nichts ausrichten).

Wie in der *svābhāvika*-Definition der SU (S. 42) bezeichnet auch hier der Begriff *kāla* andere Zeiteinheiten als die Jahreszeiten usw., von denen in CA, Ci 1,110-114 die Rede ist. Die *svābhāvika*-Krankheiten sind daher nicht mit den regulären zeitbasierten Krankheiten zu identifizieren, worauf Cakrapāṇidatta in seinem Kommentar hinweist: *svābhāvikān api kālapariṇāmavyajyamānatayeha kālaje 'varodhayitum āha kālasyetyādi* '[Im Text] heißt es "*kālasya*" usw., um hier (*iha*) die *svābhāvika*-[Krankheiten] gegen die *kālaja*-[Krankheiten] abzugrenzen, indem auf das Verstreichen der Zeit besonders hingewiesen wird (°*vyajyamānatayā*).'

Um die Bedeutung von Cakrapāṇidattas Aussagen richtig einzuordnen, sollte man sich kurz die in der CA dominierenden Modelle zur Pathogenese vergegenwärtigen. Die Darstellung kann an dieser Stelle nur eine Skizze bleiben; schon JOLLY 1901: 47 hat auf die fehlende Konsistenz dieser Theorien hingewiesen.

Gemäß CA, Sū 1,54 (~ CA, Śā 2,40) werden Krankheiten durch drei Arten von Ursachen (*hetu*; = *nidāna*, vgl. CA, Ni 1,3) hervorgerufen: Zeit (*kāla*), (Kontakt mit) Sinnesobjekten (*artha*) und mentale Faktoren (*buddhi*). Mithilfe von CA, Ni 1,3 kann man die Gleichungen *kāla* = *pariṇāma*, *artha* = *asātmyendriyārthasaṃyoga* und *buddhi* = *prajñāparādha* aufstellen, die z.B. im Kapitel CA, Sū, 11 (*Tisraiṣaṇīya*) detailliert erläutert werden. CA, Sū 11,42 betont in diesem Zusammenhang nochmals, daß mit den Begriffen *kāla* bzw. *pariṇāma* die zyklischen Phänomene der Jahre oder Jahreszeiten gemeint sind.

Die zwei wichtigsten Krankheitsklassen *āgantu* und *nija* leiten sich nach CA, Sū 20,4 aus Verletzungen oder dem Einfluß übermenschlicher Kräfte (*āgantu*) bzw. einem Ungleichgewicht der *doṣa*s ab.[14] CA, Sū 20,5 verbindet jetzt die Konzepte der drei *hetu*s und der zwei Krankheitsklassen zum ersten Krankheitsmodell (= $M_1$). Danach sind die drei *hetu*s die Ursachen der beiden Krankheitsklassen: *dvayos tu khalv āgantunijayoḥ preraṇam asātmyendriyārthasaṃyogaḥ prajñāparādhaḥ pariṇāmaś ceti* 'Die Ursache[15] der beiden, von *āgantu*- und *nija*-[Krankheiten], sind Kontakt mit ungeeigneten Sinnesobjekten, Fehlverhalten[16] und Verstreichen [der Zeit].' Doch trotz der Eindeutigkeit des Textes sind Zweifel an der Aussage angebracht, ob wirklich alle Arten von *āgantu*-Krankheiten durch einen der drei *hetu*s verursacht werden.

Die Theorie $M_1$ läßt sich so darstellen:

---

[14] Daneben existieren andere Klassifikationsschemata. Siehe z.B. CA, Sū 11,45, wo als dritte Klasse *mānasa*-Krankheiten erwähnt werden; siehe auch Cakrapāṇidatta zu CA, Ni 1,4, wonach die *āgantu*-Klasse ebenfalls zu den *tridoṣa*-Krankheiten gehört. Die Mischung der Krankheitsklassifikation läßt vermuten, daß zur Kompilationszeit des Textes die Theorien zur Pathologie noch nicht gefestigt waren.

[15] Cakrapāṇidatta: *preraṇa* = *kāraṇa*.

[16] Die Übersetzung geht von den Resultaten einer mentalen Fehlleistung aus, wie sie z.B. in CA, Śā 1,102 geschildert sind; vgl. u.a. auch ROṢU 1978: 109f., wo eher die Fehlleistung betont wird. Zu *prajñāparādha* siehe auch DAS 1992: 173f.

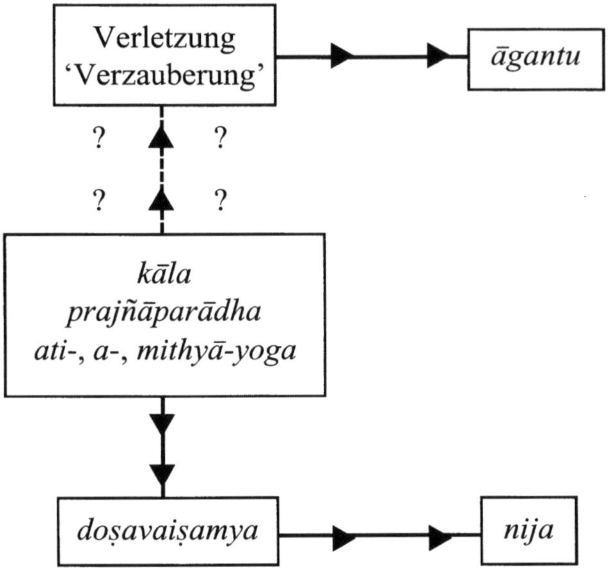


Eine andere Theorie zur Pathogenese (= $M_2$) wird in CA, Sū 28,4-7 angedeutet. Einen entscheidenden Anteil an der Enstehung von Krankheiten hat danach die Nahrung (CA, Sū 28,5[17]), die sich während des Verdauungsprozesses in *rasa* und *kiṭṭa* aufspaltet und in diesen Formen die Körperbestandteile (*avayava*) stärkt (CA, Sū 28,4). Genauso, wie der Körper seine Existenz der Nahrung verdankt, werden auch die Krankheiten von dem hervorgerufen, was der Mensch zu sich nimmt.

Dem 'Verfasser' der CA war der Widerspruch zwischen den beiden Theorien $M_1$ und $M_2$ durchaus bewußt, wie sich besonders klar aus CA, Sū 28,7 ablesen läßt. In CA, Sū 28,6 bringt Agniveśa gegenüber Ātreya die Klage vor, daß die Medizin keine exakte Wissenschaft sei: Selbst die genaue Befolgung der Vorschriften garantiere keinen Heilungserfolg, und andererseits erhebe sich manch Totgesagter wieder vom Krankenbett. Besonders die Ernährung (*āhāra*), die für viele Experten an der Wurzel der *tridoṣa*-Theorie steht, scheint für Agniveśa keine rational nachvollziehbare Wirkung auf die menschliche Gesundheit zu haben. In seiner Antwort weist Ātreya zunächst die universelle Gültigkeit eines rein ernährungsbasierten Krankheitsmodells zurück. Neben Faktoren wie der Konstitution des Patienten macht er dann vor allem das erste Modell der Pathogenese ($M_1$) für den Widerspruch zwischen theoretischem An-

---

[17] *aśitapītalīḍhakhāditaprabhavāś cāsmiñ charīre vyādhayo bhavanti.*

spruch und ärztlicher Praxis verantwortlich:

> *na ca kevalaṃ hitāhāropayogād eva sarvavyādhibhayam atikrāntaṃ bhavati. santi hy ṛte 'py ahitāhāropayogād anyā rogaprakṛtayaḥ. tad yathā kālaviparyayaḥ prajñāparādhaḥ śabdasparśarūparasagandhāś cāsātmyā iti. tāś ca rogaprakṛtayo rasān samyag upayuñjānam api puruṣam aśubhenopapādayanti. tasmād dhitāhāropayogino 'pi dṛśyante vyādhimantaḥ.*
>
> Die ganze Furcht vor Krankheiten ist nicht allein durch die Anwendung richtiger Nahrung überstanden. Denn neben der Anwendung falscher Ernährung existieren auch andere Krankheitsursachen wie der Verlauf der Zeit, Fehlverhalten und unpassende (*asātmya*) Geräusche, Berührungen, Formen, Geschmackssorten und Gerüche. Und diese Krankheitsursachen bringen Unglück über einen Menschen, auch wenn er die *rasa*s [der Nahrung] richtig anwendet. Deshalb lassen sich [Leute] beobachten, die trotz Anwendung richtiger Nahrung krank sind.

Kehren wir zu den *svābhāvika*-Krankheiten in CA, Śā 1,115 zurück. Cakrapāṇidatta betont, daß der Terminus *kāla* an dieser Stelle nicht im Sinne der *kālaja*-Krankheiten aus $M_1$ gebraucht wird. Damit billigt er den *svābhāvika*-Krankheiten eine Sonderstellung innerhalb der Pathologie zu. Im folgenden verknüpft er sie dann mit der *rasāyana*-Therapie:

> [1] *jarāmṛtyurūpān nimittāj jātā jarāmṛtyunimittajāḥ mṛtyuśabdeneha yugānurūpāyuḥparyavasānabhavakālamṛtyur grāhyaḥ. kiṃvā jarāmṛtyvor yan nimittaṃ tasmāj jātā jarāmṛtyunimittajāḥ. jarāmṛtyunimittaṃ ca prāṇināṃ sādhāraṇadehanivartakabhūtasvabhāvo 'dṛṣṭaṃ ca.* [2] *atha svābhāvikānāṃ kā cikitsety āha svabhāva ityādi.* [3] *niṣpratikriya iti sādhāraṇacikitsayā rasāyanavarjyayā na pratikriyate. rasāyanena tu pratikriyata eva tena.* [4] *asya prayogāc cyavanaḥ suvṛddho 'bhūt punaryuvā ityādirasāyanaprayogeṇa samaṃ na virodhaḥ. kiṃvā svābhāvikā jarādayo rasāyanajanitaprakarṣād uttarakālaṃ punar avaśyaṃ bhavanti.*
>
> [1] *jarāmṛtyunimittajāḥ* [bedeutet], daß [diese Krankheiten] aus einer Ursache entstanden sind, die die Form von Alter und Tod hat. Durch den Begriff 'Tod' sollte man den Tod zu einem Zeitpunkt definieren, der das Ende einer dem [jeweiligen] *yuga* angemessenen Lebensdauer ist. Oder (d.h.: eine andere Definition ist): Was die Ursache von Alter und Tod ist, daraus entstanden [sind diese Krankheiten, deshalb heißen sie] *jarāmṛtyunimittajāḥ*. Die Ursache von Alter und Tod der Lebewesen ist die allgemein vorhandene eigene Natur, die den Körper vernichtet, und das *adṛṣṭa*. [2] [Auf die Frage,] welche Heilmethode es für *svābhā-*

*vika*-[Krankheiten] gebe, sagt [der Text]: 'die eigene Natur'. [3] [Sie ist] 'unheilbar', d.h., durch gewöhnliche Heilmethoden mit Ausnahme von *rasāyana* kann sie nicht geheilt werden. Durch *rasāyana* aber kann sie[18] sicherlich geheilt werden. [4] Im Einklang mit der Anwendung des *rasāyana*s [in der Aussage] 'Durch seine Anwendung wurde Cyavana im hohen Alter wieder ein junger Mann' gibt es keinen Widerspruch [zwischen der Aussage, daß *svābhāvika*-Krankheiten prinzipiell nicht heilbar seien, und der, daß sie heilbar seien, denn beides ist durch autoritative Aussagen überliefert]. Oder aber [es gibt aus einem anderen Grund keinen Widerspruch]: Alter usw. kehren als *svābhāvika*-[Krankheiten] nach [Ablauf] der vom *rasāyana* erzeugten [zusätzlichen] Zeitspanne (*prakarṣa*[19]) unvermeidlich wieder[, wodurch die prinzipielle Nichtheilbarkeit der eigenen Natur bestätigt wird, auch wenn eine zeitweilige Heilung möglich ist].

Bemerkenswert ist die Interpretation der Phrase *svabhāvo niṣpratikriyaḥ*. Während die 'eigene Natur', d.h. *svābhāvika*-Krankheiten nach Aussage von CA unheilbar sind, können sie nach Cakrapāṇidatta mit dem *rasāyana* behandelt werden. Wie aus Satz [4] des Kommentars hervorgeht, zeigt nach Cakrapāṇidattas Meinung das *rasāyana* aber keine dauerhafte Wirkung. Ob diese Einschränkung nur getroffen wurde, um den Begriff *niṣpratikriya* zu erklären, läßt sich anhand von CA, Śā 1,115 nicht feststellen. Cakrapāṇidattas Aussage wird aber von der Tatsache relativiert, daß in den *rasāyana*-Rezepten der CA Präparate erwähnt werden, die eine extrem lange oder sogar endlose Lebensspanne verleihen.[20]

### 2.2.2. *svabhāva* = Tod

Einen Zusammenhang zwischen der Bestimmung der verbleibenden Lebensdauer mithilfe von *ariṣṭa*s, d.h. ungewöhnlicher körperlicher Veränderungen, die auf den nahenden Tod hindeuten, und dem Terminus *svabhāva* stellt CA,

---

[18] Die 'eigene Natur'.

[19] Als Terminus technicus in dieser Bedeutung u.a. an folgenden Stellen benutzt: CA, Sū 12,10 (*paramāyuḥprakarṣāya*), CA, Vi 1,22 (°*kālaprakarṣa*°). Das Wort wird im Zusammenhang mit Zeitspannen zur Beschreibung des *rasāyana*s eingesetzt, z.B. in CA, Ci 1,1,73 (*āyuḥprakarṣa*)

[20] Ein Beispiel für eine sehr lange Lebenszeit liefert CA, Ci 1,3,13 (*jīved varṣasahasrāṇi*). Eine endlose Lebenszeit wird in CA, Ci 1,1,54 und CA, Ci 1,2,20 versprochen. – Zur Bemessung der Lebenszeit nach einer *rasāyana*-Therapie und der Verbindung mit verschiedenen Formen des *karman*s siehe auch Cakrapāṇidattas Kommentar zu CA, Vi 3,33-35.

Sū 30,25-26 her. Die Passage ist Teil eines längeren Abschnitts, der sich mit dem Selbstbild des Āyurveda beschäftigt.:

> 25: *pramāṇam āyuṣas tv arthendriyamanobuddhiceṣṭādīnāṃ vikr̥tilakṣaṇair upalabhyate 'nimittaiḥ. ayam asmāt kṣaṇāt ... saṃvatsarād vā svabhāvam āpatsyata iti. tatra svabhāvaḥ pravr̥tter uparamo maraṇam ... ity eko 'rthaḥ. ity āyuṣaḥ pramāṇam. ato viparītam apramāṇam ariṣṭādhikāre. dehaprakr̥tilakṣaṇam adhikr̥tya copadiṣṭam āyuṣaḥ pramāṇam āyurvede.* 26: *prayojanaṃ cāsya svasthasya svāsthyarakṣaṇam āturasya vikārapraśamanaṃ ca.*
> 25: Die Bemessung der Lebensdauer[21] aber wird durch grundlose Zeichen [krankhafter] Veränderungen am Körper (*artha*[22]), an den Sinnen, dem *manas*, der *buddhi*, den Handlungen usw. durchgeführt. [Daraus resultiert das Ergebnis:] 'Dieser [Mensch] wird nach diesem Moment ..., nach diesem Jahr zu seiner eigenen Natur gelangen'. Die 'eigene Natur' ist synonym (*eko 'rthaḥ*) mit dem Aufhören der Aktivität, mit dem Tod .... So [wird] die Bemessung der Lebensdauer [durchgeführt]. Im Kontrast dazu [steht] die Nicht-Bemessung, wenn keine *riṣṭa*s vorliegen.[23] [In

[21] Das Wort *pramāṇa* tritt hier in einer Doppelbedeutung als Nomen actionis (= Vorgang des Messens, falls *riṣṭa*s – siehe Anm. 23 – vorliegen) und als Ergebnis des Meßprozesses auf. Die Übersetzung als Nomen actionis wurde gewählt, um den Begriff *a-pramāṇa* angemessen übertragen zu können.

[22] Cakrapāṇidatta gibt als Beispiel den Blumengeruch, den ein Todgeweihter verströmt; vgl. die Beschreibung des *puṣpita*s in Ca, In 2,3-9.

[23] Cakrapāṇidatta verwendet mehrmals den Terminus *riṣṭa*, und schreibt *ato viparītam apramāṇam iti riṣṭahīnaṃ na niścitapramāṇam āyur ariṣṭādhikāra ity arthaḥ.* Das läßt darauf schließen, daß er das Kompositum *ariṣṭādhikāre* als *a-riṣṭa-adhikāre* auffaßt und das Wort *riṣṭa* mit *ariṣṭa* gleichsetzt. Dieser Auffassung folgt die obige Übersetzung. Man könnte dem entgegenhalten, daß diese Analyse in zweierlei Hinsicht problematisch ist. Erstens ist das Wort *riṣṭa* in der *Carakasaṃhitā* nicht als Synonym von *ariṣṭa* belegt. Zweitens kann der Begriff *adhikāra* bei dieser Auflösung nicht in seiner üblichen Bedeutung als 'Kapitel' oder 'Abschnitt' übersetzt werden. Man könnte deshalb überlegen, *ariṣṭādhikāre* mit 'im *ariṣṭa*-Kapitel' zu übersetzen ('Im Kontrast dazu [steht] die Nicht-Bemessung, [wie sie] im *ariṣṭa*-Abschnitt [beschrieben wird]').

Obwohl beide Einwände vollständig zutreffen, halte ich die obige Übersetzung auf Grundlage der logischen Struktur des Abschnitts trotzdem für korrekt. Im ersten Teil von Ca, Sū 30,25 (*pramāṇam ... ity āyuṣaḥ pramāṇam*) wird die Diagnose des nahenden Todes mithilfe von *ariṣṭa*s beschrieben (zur Wortwahl vergleiche z.B. Ca, In 1,7). Nach Aussage der einleitenden Worte des zweiten Abschnitts (*ato viparītam ...*) wird jetzt eine Diagnosemöglichkeit

diesem Falle] ist die Bemessung der Lebensdauer unter Bezug auf den Körper, die Konstitution (*prakṛti*) und [äußere] Merkmale im Āyurveda das geeignete Mittel (*upadiṣṭam*). 26: Ihr Einsatzgebiet ist die Bewahrung der Gesundheit bei einem Gesunden und die 'Beruhigung' von Krankheiten bei einem Erkrankten.

CA, Sū 30,25-26 ist zunächst eine Anweisung für den Umgang mit *ariṣṭa*s, wie sie ähnlich z.B. in CA, In. 1 zu finden ist. Falls ein Arzt *ariṣṭa*s diagnostizieren kann, wird der Patient in relativ naher Zukunft sterben. Andernfalls kann seine verbleibende Lebensdauer mithilfe weiterer Indikatoren wie der 'Konstitution' (*prakṛti*) abgeschätzt werden. Nach Angaben der SU (siehe S. 47) können von *ariṣṭa*s begleitete Krankheitszustände, die unweigerlich zum Tod führen, medizinisch allein durch das *rasāyana* geheilt werden. Es liegt deshalb nahe, den Begriff *svabhāva* in seiner Bedeutung als 'Tod' für die Erklärung des *svābhāvika*-Konzepts heranzuziehen. Eine naheliegende Übersetzung als 'tödliche [Krankheit]' trifft den Inhalt des Begriffs *svābhāvika* allerdings nicht, da dieser ja auch Erschöpfung oder Hunger umfaßt. Eher kann er gedeutet werden als eine krankhafte oder einfach nur störende Erscheinung, die wie der Tod zur *Natur* des Menschen gehört und daher unausweichlich (und unheilbar) ist.

Getrübt wird diese Interpretation durch den Umstand, daß weder im Text der CA noch im Kommentar *svābhāvika*-Krankheiten oder sogar *rasāyana* erwähnt werden. Die Konzentration auf den *āyus*-Komplex, die Erwähnung der *riṣṭa*s und die Verbindungen zum therapeutischen Einsatz, die sich in CA, Sū 30,26 finden und die pharmakologischen Ideen der *Standarddefinition* widerspiegeln, lassen die Deutung aber zumindest als möglich erscheinen.

### 2.3. Cikitsāsthāna 1,2,3

Innerkörperliche Veränderungen, die eine Behandlung mit dem *rasāyana* erforderlich machen, werden in CA, Ci 1,2,3 beschrieben. Durch Anwendung des *rasāyana*s, so die Erzählung, gewannen Cyavana und andere Ṛṣis Jugend, Potenz und körperliche Kraft zurück. Ohne eine verbindende Überleitung fährt

---

dargestellt, die der ersten Möglichkeit entgegengesetzt ist, also nicht auf *ariṣṭa*s beruht. Solch eine Methode, bei der u.a. die *prakṛti* untersucht wird, wird aber wohl gerade nicht 'im *ariṣṭa*-Abschnitt' der CA dargestellt. Trotz der wichtigen sprachlichen Gegengründe halte ich daher meine obige Analyse für korrekt.

der Text mit der Aussage fort, daß körperliche Mängel und Verfallserscheinungen (*śarīradoṣa*[24]) auf falsche Ernährung und unkorrektes Verhalten zurückzuführen seien: An der Wurzel des körperlichen Verfalls stehe *grāmyāhāra*, also ein Ernährungsproblem, daneben aber auch die stereotyp wiederholten negativen Angewohnheiten des zivilisierten Lebens wie Völlerei, übermäßiger Schlaf und der Sexualtrieb. Kommen jetzt noch die üblichen mentalen Verwirrungen (*bhaya*, *krodha* usw.) hinzu, setzt eine Kettenreaktion krankhafter Prozesse ein, die im Verfall des *ojas* gipfelt und damit körperlichen Krankheiten das Feld bereitet. Die Beschreibung ist im folgenden Diagramm zusammengefaßt:

*grāmyāhāra*, zuviel Sex usw.
hohes Alter (?)
↓
Störung der *dhātus* {
*śithilībhavanti* ***māṃsāni***
*vimucyante* ***sandhayaḥ***
*vidahyate* ***raktam***
*viṣyandate ...* ***medaḥ***
*na sandhīyate* ***asthiṣu majjā***
***śukraṃ*** *na pravartate*
*kṣayam upaity* ***ojaḥ***
↓
Erschöpfung, mentaler Verfall,
Anfälligkeit für Krankheiten
↓
Patient kann volles *āyus* nicht erreichen

CA, Ci 1,2,3 schließt mit dem Ratschlag, die beschriebenen Fehler in Ernährung und Verhaltensweisen zu beseitigen (*apāsya*) und *dann* die *rasāyana*-Therapie anzuwenden, um – so kann man ergänzen – die Jugendkraft zurückzuerlangen.

Zwei Punkte verdienen besondere Beachtung. Der erste ist die im Mittelteil des Diagramms dargestellte Störung der *dhātu*s. Falls man die Reihenfolge der krankhaften Veränderungen, die sich vom Fleisch (*māṃsa*) bis hin zum *ojas*

[24] Die nicht-technische Übersetzung des Begriffs *doṣa* läßt sich mit dem letzten Satz von CA, Ci 1,2,3 rechtfertigen, wo die körperlichen Verfallserscheinungen so bezeichnet werden.

zeigen, als zeitlichen Ablauf interpretiert, liegt hier eine relativ klare Parallele zur Umwandlung von Nahrung in Samen (und dann weiter in *ojas*) vor, wie sie z.B. in CA, Sū 28,4 beschrieben wird.[25] Im Sinne der *Standarddefinition* kann man folgern, daß *rasāyana* die geschilderten Veränderungen rückgängig macht und damit den *rasa*, der in CA, Ci 1,2,3 nicht erwähnt wird, in CA, Sū 28,4 aber am Beginn des Verdauungsprozesses steht, wieder 'zum Laufen bringt'.

Allerdings besitzt des *rasāyana* nach CA, Ci 1,2,3 keine 'Wunderkräfte', denn *grāmyāhāra* und falsches Verhalten müssen *vor* Beginn der Therapie aufgegeben werden, was zum asketischen Grundton der Passage paßt. Ob die Störungen der *dhātu*s also durch die Verhaltensänderung oder durch *rasāyana* beseitigt werden, läßt sich deshalb nicht mit letzter Sicherheit feststellen.

Der zweite Punkt betrifft das Verhältnis von *Standarddefinition* und *svābhāvika*-Krankheiten. Aus der Angabe, daß die Ṛṣis in die Jugend zurückversetzt werden (*punaryuvatvam āpuḥ*), läßt sich ableiten, daß es sich um alte Männer handelt. Die Versuchung liegt nahe, CA, 1,2,3 als eine Synthese der *Standarddefinition* mit dem Konzept der *svābhāvika*-Krankheiten oder sogar als eine medizinische Beschreibung dieser Krankheitsklasse zu interpretieren. *Svābhāvika*-Krankheiten wären danach nichts anderes als intensive Störungen des Verdauungsprozesses auf Basis des *grāmyāhāra*s, die im Laufe des Lebens akkumuliert werden und dann im Alter hervorbrechen. Diese Interpretation würde das medizinische Bild der *svābhāvika*-Krankheiten um ihren innerkörperlichen Ablauf ergänzen, setzt aber voraus, daß CA, Ci 1,2,3 in allen Details als medizinisch exakte Beschreibung interpretiert werden kann.

Gegen diese Annahme sprechen zwei Gründe. So stellt der Text einerseits die beiden Motive vom hohen Alter der Ṛṣis und von der pathogenen Wirkung des *grāmyāhāra*s unvermittelt nebeneinander, ohne einen Hinweis auf einen inhaltlichen Zusammenhang zu geben. Andererseits ist CA, Ci 1,2,3 wie die inhaltlich ähnliche Passage CA, Ci 1,4,3-5 darum bemüht, *rasāyana* mit der Askese zu verknüpfen. Die Motive des hohen Alters und des *grāmyāhāra*s lassen sich daher zwangloser mit der *āśrama*-Theorie oder dem *grāma*/*araṇya*-Topos als mit einer medizinischen Theorie erklären.

---

[25] *puṣyanti tvāhārarasād rasarudhiramāṃsamedo'sthimajjaśukraujāṃsi.*

### 3. Zusammenfassung

Der therapeutischen Anwendung des *rasāyana*s liegen in SU, CA und ihren Kommentaren vier Konzepte zugrunde. Außer (1) zur Kräftigung und Wiederherstellung des Verdauungsprozesses (*Standarddefinition*) kommmt das *rasāyana* auch bei (2) *svābhāvika*-Krankheiten, bei (3) *śārīra*-Krankheiten und (4) als eine Art Notfallmedizin für unheilbare Fälle zum Einsatz. Obwohl im vierten Falle meistens unheilbare *śārīra*-Krankheiten vorliegen, besitzt *rasāyana* hier nicht den Charakter einer regulären āyurvedischen Medizin, die ja vorher offenbar versagt hat. Die Bereiche (3) und (4) können deshalb als differenzierbare Einsatzfelder angesehen werden.

Die *rasāyana*-Therapie wird in den untersuchten Texten unterschiedlich bewertet. Zur besseren Übersicht sind in der folgenden Tabelle die Einsatzgebiete des *rasāyana*s nach allen besprochenen Passagen zusammengestellt. Ein massiver Punkt (•) gibt an, daß das *rasāyana* sicher in der angegebenen Funktion benutzt wird. Mit einem Kreis (◦) markierte Funktionen sind dagegen nicht eindeutig zu erschließen oder stellen in der angegebenen Passage nur einen Teilaspekt dar. Ḍalh. = Ḍalhaṇa, Cakr. = Cakrapāṇidatta.

| Konzept Nr.: | (1) | (2) | (3) | (4) |
|---|---|---|---|---|
| SU, Sū 1,24-25 | | • | | |
| Ḍalh. zu ~ | | | • | |
| SU, Sū 24,4-7 | | • | | |
| Ḍalh. zu ~ | | • | | |
| Ḍalh. zu SU, Sū 1,27 | | | • | |
| Ḍalh. zu SU, Sū 15 | ◦ | | | |
| SU, Sū 33,3 | | | | • |
| SU, Sū 28,5 | | | | • |
| CA, Ci 1,1,4-8 | • | | | |
| Cakr. zu ~ | • | ◦ | ◦ | |
| Cakr. zu CA, Śā 1,115 | | • | | |
| CA, Ci 1,2,3 | • | ◦ | | |

Betrachtet man zunächst nur SU und CA, fällt der Unterschied in der theoretischen Bewertung der Therapie klar ins Auge. Während *rasāyana* in der CA vor allem im Rahmen der *Standarddefinition* eingesetzt wird, konzentriert sich die SU auf seine Wirkung gegen *svābhāvika*-Krankheiten und als Notfallmedizin. Dagegen zeigen die Kommentare die Tendenz, die Konzepte von SU und CA zu vermengen und um den Einsatz bei regulären körperlichen Krankheiten (*śārīra*) zu erweitern. Dies kann als Indiz für eine fortschreitende Standardisierung der altindischen Medizin gedeutet werden, wie sie MEULENBELD 1991 am Beispiel der *doṣa*s aufgezeigt hat.

Das Konzept der *svābhāvika*-Krankheiten hat daneben Einblick in Theorien zur Pathologie gewährt, die vom allgemein geläufigen Modell aus *nidāna*, Verdauung und *tridoṣa* abweichen. Zum einen lassen sich *svābhāvika*-Krankheiten klar von Krankheiten der Klasse *śārīra* → *kālaja* unterscheiden, da den beiden Klassen unterschiedliche Zeitmodelle zugrundeliegen. Kultur- oder religionswissenschaftliche Ansätze sollten diese Tatsache zumindest bei der Deutung des *rasāyana*s in der SU berücksichtigen.

Daneben greift die Klasse der *svābhāvika*-Krankheiten – wenigstens nach den hier besprochenen Textstellen – nicht in den Aufbau der Körperelemente aus dem *rasa* ein und verändert auch nicht das 'Gleichgewicht' der *doṣa*s. Vielmehr entfalten diese Krankheiten ihre Wirkung auf eine andere, nicht dargestellte oder darstellbare Weise. Zwar deuten Passagen wie SU, Sū 14,19 darauf hin, daß āyurvedischen Texten ein Zusammenhang zwischen zunehmendem Alter und Abnahme der nährenden Funktion des *rasa*s bekannt war (S. 49). Das Urteil, ob sich solche Aussagen zur Interpretation der *svābhāvika*-Krankheiten und der *rasāyana*-Therapie heranziehen lassen, bleibt einer detaillierten Studie der āyurvedischen Pathologie vorbehalten.

## Summary

The Āyurvedic therapy of *rasāyana* is usually defined as a means to refresh and strengthen the digestive cycle of the human body. This interpretation is based on the easily understandable 'etymology' of *rasāyana* as *rasasya ayanam*, and the passage *Carakasaṃhitā*, Cikitsāsthāna 1,1,8, which defines *rasāyana* as *lābhopāyo ... śastānāṃ rasādīnām*, i.e. 'a means to get good *rasa* etc.'. A closer examination of passages contained in the *Carakasaṃhitā* and the

*Suśrutasaṃhitā* dealing with the theory of *rasāyana* reveals at least three probably independent notions about the working of *rasāyana*.

1. In the *Suśrutasaṃhitā*, *rasāyana* is closely associated with the class of *svābhāvika* diseases. Diseases of this class are not caused by a malfunction of the digestive system, but rather by uncontrollable factors, such as advanced age or external influences such as deities or fate. Although the *Suśrutasaṃhitā* does not describe the exact mode of operation of *svābhāvika* diseases and their pathogenic factors, these diseases are definitely not caused by the *tridoṣa*. *rasāyana* is regarded as the only treatment to undo their effects.
2. Several passages of the *Suśrutasaṃhitā* consider *rasāyana* to be a kind of panacea for otherwise incurable diseases of the *śārīra* class. This class is usually treated with regular Āyurvedic therapies which influence the balance of *tridoṣa* and thereby the digestive cycle. Failure of these regular treatments requires the application of *rasāyana*. The use of *rasāyana* in this context underlines its somewhat special or even 'irrational' character.
3. By contrast, the *Carakasaṃhitā* emphasises the connection between the *rasāyana* therapy and the cycle of food, digestion and building of *dhātu*s. Hence, according to most passages in this text, *rasāyana* does not have an 'irrational' character, but is only one of several ways to treat a disease. Nevertheless, the relation between *rasāyana* and *svābhāvika* diseases was also known to the authors of the *Carakasaṃhitā*.

Unlike the classical texts of the *Carakasaṃhitā* and *Suśrutasaṃhitā*, later commentators (and modern scholars) tend to fuse the three layers into one theory which emphasises the effect of *rasāyana* on the digestive system, i.e. the doctrine of the *Carakasaṃhitā*. This tendency is a good example of the progressive standardisation of Āyurvedic teachings which suppresses diverging theories in favour of the dominant model of digestion and *tridoṣa*.

## Abkürzungen

AH = *Aṣṭāṅgahṛdayasaṃhitā*
CA = *Carakasaṃhitā*
Ci = Cikitsāsthāna/Cikitsitasthāna
In = Indriyasthāna
Ni = Nidānasthāna
Śā = Śārīrasthāna
SU = *Suśrutasaṃhitā*
Sū = Sūtrasthāna
Ut = Uttarasthāna/Uttaratantra
Vi = Vimānasthāna

## Bibliographie

DAS, Rahul Peter 1992: 'Indische Medizin und Spiritualität', *Journal of the European Āyur-*

*vedic Society* 2: 158-187.

— 2003: *The Origin of the Life of a Human Being. Conception and the Female According to Ancient Indian Medical and Sexological Literature*. Delhi: Motilal Banarsidass Publishers. Indian Medical Tradition 6.

HARA, Minoru 1995: 'A Note on the Sanskrit Word *Svastha*', *Journal of the European Āyurvedic Society* 4: 55-87.

JOLLY, Julius 1901: *Medicin*. Strassburg: Verlag von Karl J. Trübner. Grundriss der Indo-Arischen Philologie und Altertumskunde 3,10.

MAHDIHASSAN, S. 1979: *Indian Alchemy or Rasayana in the Light of Asceticism Geriatrics*. New Delhi: Vikas Publications.

MEULENBELD, G. J(an) 1974: *The Mādhavanidāna and its Chief Commentary. Chapters 1-10. Introduction, Translation and Notes*. Leiden: E.J. Brill. Orientalia Rheno-Traiectina 19.

— 1987: 'Reflections on the Basic Concepts of Indian Pharmacology', in: G. Jan Meulenbeld und Dominik Wujastyk (Hrsg.), *Studies on Indian Medical History. Papers presented at the International Workshop on the Study of Indian Medicine held at the Wellcome Institute for the History of Medicine 2-4 September 1985*. Groningen: Egbert Forsten. Groningen Oriental Studies 2, S. 1-17.

— 1991: 'The Constraints of Theory in the Evolution of Nosological Classifications: A Study on the Position of Blood in Indian Medicine (Āyurveda)', in: G. Jan Meulenbeld (Hrsg.), *Medical Literature from India, Sri Lanka and Tibet*. Leiden/New York/København/Köln: E.J. Brill. Panels of the VIITH World Sanskrit Conference 8, S. 91-106.

MÜLLER, Reinhold F.G. 1960: 'Die beiden indischen Götterärzte', *Archiv Orientální* 26: 399-413.

ROŞU, Arion 1975: 'Considérations sur une technique du *rasāyana* āyurvedique', *Indo-Iranian Journal* 17:1-29 und 395.

— 1978: *Les conceptions psychologiques dans les textes médicaux indiens*. Paris: Institut de Civilisation Indienne / Diffusion E. de Boccard. Publications de l'Institut de Civilisation Indienne, série in-8° 43.

WHITE, David Gordon 1996: *The Alchemical Body. Siddha Traditions in Medieval India*. Chicago/London: The University of Chicago Press.

ZIMMERMANN, Francis 1975: 'Ṛtu-sātmya. Le cycle des saisons et le principe d'appropriation', *Puruṣārtha. Recherches de sciences sociales sur l'Asie du sud* 2: 87-105.

— 1982: 'Yoga et alchimie', *Zeitschrift der Deutschen Morgenländischen Gesellschaft* 132: 363-379.

# Classification of Diseases in the Tamil Medical Work *Vaittiyacintāmaṇi*-800 of Yūkimuṉi

## *I: Introduction**

MUHAMMED MAJEED and DAMODARAN SURESH KUMAR

The Tamil language has a rich treasure of medical literature.[1] Though in its basics indistinguishable from Āyurveda, through the ages the Tamil tradition incorporated many elements of the alchemical practices of the Jains, Buddhists and Śaivites.[2] Attempts were also made by Tamil physicians to study the therapeutic value of many plants predominant in the South and not utilised by Āyurveda.[3] As a result its practitioners made many innovations in materia medica, pharmacy, nosology and therapeutics. The present-day Tamil medicine or Siddha system, as it is popularly called, is thus a veritable depository of medical knowledge.

A typical Tamil medical text describes the preparation of medicinal formulations and mentions only their indications. The entire text is mostly in one single body without divisions into sections or chapters. Though such works always mention numerous disease entities, no attempt is made in them to help the practitioner identify these entities. *Vaittiyacintāmaṇi*-800[4] of Yūkimuṉi (VC-800) is an exceptional work entirely devoted to nosology.

### Plan of the Text

VC-800 is authored by Yūkimuṉi, a disciple of the Tamil mystic Tēraiyar. This work was composed to satisfy a long-felt need, and as far as we are aware,

---

* Unless otherwise mentioned all technical terms used in this communication are in the Tamil language. But the names of deities are given in the Sanskrit form.

[1] NIRMALĀTĒVI 1983: 1-111.

[2] PILLAI 1931: 1-114.

[3] KUMAR 1995.

[4] It is customary in the Tamil medical tradition to mention the number of *pāṭal*s in a text, appended to the title of the text.

this is the only Tamil medical work devoted to nosology. It consists of 800 *pāṭal* or verses. Three published versions of the text are available.[5]

The author states in the opening verse that he has described clearly all the information contained in the *Vaittiyacintāmaṇi*. Thereafter, he traces the lineage of his school of thought. This is followed by explanations of the fundamental principles (*tattuvaviti*). Fever (*curam*) is the first disease to be classified, and the work ends with the nosology of anal fistula (*pavuttirarōka nitāṉam*). The contents of VC-800 are briefly listed in Appendix 1.

Each disease group is classified in a systematic manner. First of all, the names of the various sub-groups are mentioned. The listing of the causative factors follows this. Thereafter, the author describes in detail the characteristic symptoms and signs of the sub-groups. Finally, a prognosis is provided.

The author of VC-800 is of the opinion that transgression of propriety or morality is the root cause of all diseases. This is best exemplified by the listing of the aetiological factors of desiccation (*kṣayam/cayam*)[6]. Persons who outrage the modesty of women, speak false, steal or covet the wealth of others, wish harm to others, humiliate a destitute Brahmin scholar, cheat relatives, reply to slander with slander and spread rumours are said to contract the disease (*pāṭal* 672).[7]

## Āyurvedic Roots

The history of Tamil medicine is an extremely sensitive issue and, as KNÜPPEL 2001 has rightly observed, a dispassionate discourse on the topic is often impossible on account of the Tamil nationalist sentiments expressed by many contemporary authors. In keeping with this, links with Āyurveda are often denied, or else Āyurveda is derived from Tamil medicine.[8]

---

[5] NĀYAṈĀR 1932, TIYĀKARĀCAṈ 1976 and RĀMACCANTIRAṈ 1998.

[6] Though *cayam* is the form usually used, *kṣayam* too appears in the text. We shall use only *cayam* henceforth.

[7] This is reminiscent of Sanskrit *karmavipāka*- works, though here the transgressions need not be those of a previous birth.

[8] An example of the latter is MADHAVAN 1984: 35, referring to the sage Akattiyar (Agastya in Sanskrit): '…It is a well known fact that the compilers of the Ayurveda and their patrons

However, the author of VC-800 states at several places in the text that he composed this work in the Tamil language after studying in detail all the 'northern texts' of *āyuruvētam*. It is obvious that the words 'northern language' (*vaṭamoḻi*) and 'northern texts' (*vaṭamoḻiyin nūlkaḷ*) denote respectively the Sanskrit language and Sanskrit texts. The relevant evidence is presented in Appendix 2.

That the author depended on Sanskrit texts is evident from the medical terms used in VC-800. For example, the word used to denote skin disease is *kuṣṭam*. Some other striking examples are *antakacaṉṉi* (*antakajvara-* in Sanskrit), *uruttirakacaṉṉi* (*rugdāhajvara-* in Sanskrit), *cittapiramaicaṉṉi* (*cittavibhramajvara-* in Sanskrit), *cītāṅkacaṉṉi* (*śītāṅgajvara-* in Sanskrit) and *kaṇṭapuccaṉai* (*kaṇṭhakubjajvara-* in Sanskrit[9]) (*pāṭal* 159-167). Interestingly, several Sanskrit terms are used with little change. Examples are *tāpam*, *cantāpam*, *rātri*, *uṣṇam*, *carīram* and *piramēkam* (*pāṭal* 143, 148, 150, 170, 171, 422).

The order in which diseases are described also follows to some extent the tradition observed in Sanskrit texts. For example, fever (*curam*) is the first disease to be described. It is followed by *aticāram* (*pāṭal* 137-199). Similarly, morbid pallor (*pāṇṭurōkam*) is followed by jaundice (*kāmālai*) and oedema (*cōpairōkam*) (*pāṭal* 546).

## Problems of Nosology

Yūkimuṉi states several times in the text that he composed VC-800 after studying all northern texts meticulously. If that is the case, then one is at a loss to explain significant differences to the classical Āyurvedic texts in the noso-

---

had sent men to the South and East to gather materials to be assimilated in their then proposed Ayurvedic system. The greatness of Tamilian culture in all its branches and their very high philosophy which guided their life were well known to the Aryans just arrived in the north. They wanted to enrich their culture by the assimilation of the highly civilised culture of the Tamilians. So they sent the best of their men to gather materials from different sources. The man who was sent to the south i.e., Tamilnadu, was the sage Agasthiya (This fact lies hidden in the story of the marriage between Siva and Uma).'

[9] Cf. e.g. *Bhāvaprakāśa*, Jvarādhikāra 13 (MURTHY 2002: 69).

logy of several diseases like *cayam* (desiccation), *kācam* (respiratory disorders characterised by cough), *makōtaram* (enlargement of the abdomen), *kirāṇi* (diarrhoea), *kāmālai* etc.

As an example, we shall confine ourselves to Vāgbhaṭa's *Aṣṭāṅgahṛdaya*, as this is and seems for a long time to have been the most popular classical text in South India, so that Yūkimuṉi should have had access to it. This text states that *kāmalā-* (jaundice), when untreated, progresses into a condition called *kumbhakāmalā-*. Another variety of the disease mentioned by Vāgbhaṭa is *halīmaka-*, in which the body may acquire a greenish, brown or yellowish tinge.[10] However, VC-800 states that *kāmālai* can be divided into 13 types like *ūtukāmālai, varaṭkāmālai, vātakāmālai, pittakāmālai, cilēṭpakāmālai, vātacilēṭpakāmālai, pittacilēṭpakāmālai, tontakāmālai, mañcaḷkāmālai, aḻakukāmālai, ceṅkamalakāmālai, kumpakāmālai* and *kuṉmakāmālai* (*pāṭal* 528-545).

A similar deviation in nosology is also observed in the case of *makōtaram*. Vāgbhaṭa is of the opinion that *udara-* (and not *mahodara-*) is of eight types;[11] *mahodara-* is actually common in later texts. However, VC-800 describes 32 types of *makōtaram*, like *vātamakōtaram, pittamakōtaram, cilēṭpamakōtaram, kalmakōtaram, vilmakōtaram* etc. (*pāṭal* 554-594).

As these examples make clear, Yūkimuṉi's nosology is not identical with that of classical Āyurveda, even though he expressly mentions his indebtedness to Sanskrit Āyurvedic works. One explanation for this is that he might have depended upon other Sanskrit medical texts. Or he might have followed the nosological system adopted by the school of thought of his preceptor, or some other local school, and incorporated what he found in Sanskrit works into this. But basically this is speculation, since we have no concrete evidence regarding the actual cause.

## Śaivite Inclinations of the Author

Yūkimuṉi states that he reproduces the medical information as faithfully as

---

[10] UPADHYĀYA 1975: 266-268.

[11] UPADHYĀYA 1975: 263-266.

Śiva revealed it to Umā (*pāṭal* 552, 594). A survey of the verses of VC-800 unearths several other statements that suggest a Śaivite – and definitely Hindu – inclination of the author. These are listed below:

1) Those who speak impiously of Śiva will suffer from the eight kinds of *kuṉmam* (*pāṭal* 212).
2) Those who speak ill of elders, Brahmins and the Vedas will be afflicted by *vāta* diseases (*pāṭal* 243).
3) *Pittarōkam* attacks those who do not worship in temples and vandals who steal the property of Śiva (*pāṭal* 346).
4) *Kaparōkam* will flare up in persons who relieve themselves facing the Sun and show hostility to Śiva and Viṣṇu (*pāṭal* 395).
5) *Mēkarōkam* appears in persons who indulge in sexual intercourse with Brahmin women, speak ill of the Vedas and who do not worship the Sun (*pāṭal* 454).
6) Those who desecrate Śiva temples and blaspheme him will join the group of people suffering from *kuṭṭarōkam*[12] (*pāṭal* 496).
7) Persons who steal the property of Śiva will be afflicted with *pāṇṭurōkam* (*pāṭal* 521).
8) *Kirāṇirōkam* appears in those who oppose the worship of Śiva, Pārvatī, Subrahmaṇya and Viṣṇu (*pāṭal* 610).
9) Those who humiliate a destitute Brahmin scholar will contract *cayam* (*pāṭal* 672).
10) Persons who blaspheme Śiva will suffer from *vippurutirōkam* (*pāṭal* 755).
11) Those who ignore the path of Śiva and indulge in stealing and cheating will be afflicted with anal fistula (*pavuttirarōkam*), lose all their wealth and undergo great suffering (*pāṭal* 790).

Similar statements are found in other Tamil medical texts as well. The Tamil sage Pōkar states in *pāṭal* 998 of his celebrated work *Pōkar*-7000 that he has explained alchemy in lucid style so that society does not get influenced by the

[12] Though *kuṣṭam* is the commoner form, *kuṭṭam* too appears in the text.

Buddhists.[13]

Nevertheless, it seems that Tamil medical texts contain plenty of medical information dating from the Jain and Buddhist period of Tamil history.[14] But after the suppression of these beliefs in the Tamil country in the 7th century A.D.,[15] an attempt seems to have been made to remove even traces of Buddhist or Jainistic influences from all sections of Tamil literature and to bring the laity to the fold of Śiva worship; medical texts can hardly have been an exception.

## Discussion

The antiquity of Tamil medicine has been a subject of interest to philologists. Based on a comparative study of references to the 'three faults' discussed in the Tamil work *Tirumantiram*, some Pali medical texts and the treatises of Caraka and Suśruta, SCHARFE 1999 concludes that the theoretical foundation of the medicine of the Tamil *cittar*s, denoted by the terms *muttōcam* and *mukkuṟṟam*, is based on the later development of the doctrinal principles found, e.g., in the *Carakasaṃhitā* and *Suśrutasaṃhitā*.[16]

The *Tirukkuṟaḷ*, a philosophical treatise usually assigned to the third century A.D., but maybe actually from the sixth century, states in *kuṟaḷ* 941 that imbalance of 'the three starting with wind' causes diseases. It is significant that the word *nūlōr* (the learned books) implies the existence of a well-developed

[13] *nittarmaya mākavētāṉ paciya ṭakka, nērāka vātamuṟai cuḷuvāyc coṉṉṉēṉ / puttarmaya mākāmal nūluk kuḷḷē, pōtittēṉ vekupērkkup pōtit tēṉē* (cf. TĒVAR 1975: 290).

[14] The authors are thankful to Prof. Kenneth G. Zysk of the University of Copenhagen and Prof. Ulrike Niklas of the University of Cologne for a stimulating discussion on references to Buddhism in Tamil medical literature.

[15] Cf. SASTRI 1964: 19-108.

[16] DAS 2001: 155 note 18 criticises SCHARFE 1999 for painting a picture of philosophical doctrines in the classical Āyurvedic texts based on a-prioristic suppositions on their having borrowed ideas eclectically from various philosophical systems, suppositions made, moreover, without critically examining the texts as to their internal chronology and coherence. However, this criticism does not directly bear on the issue mentioned above.

medical system anterior to the *Tirukkuṟaḷ*.[17]

Though no ancient Tamil medical texts are available to us, certain Sangam (Caṅkam) works (around A.D. 400) like *Tirikaṭukam*, *Ciṟupañcamūlam* and *Ēlāti* are named after reputed medicinal formulae of Āyurveda. *Cilappatikāram* (approx. A.D. 450) mentions that *āyuḷvētar* (experts in Āyurveda) used to live in the city of Kāviripūmpaṭṭiṇam next to priests and astrologers.[18] Emperors of the Cōḻa dynasty (A.D. 850-1280) established and financed hospitals and medical schools. A stone inscription unearthed from Tiruvāvaṭuturai and dated to A.D. 1121 states that the students of such medical schools were taught *Aṣṭāṅgahṛdaya* and *Carakasaṃhitā*.[19]

VENKATRAMAN 1990 is of the opinion that alchemy and tantrism, which are hallmarks of the Tamil Siddha medical system, owe their origin to influences from northern India. Around A.D. 1200 the Buddhist monasteries of Udantapura and Vikramaśīla (in present-day Bihar) were destroyed by invaders and the monks fled southwards, carrying the esoteric knowledge. Nāthism or the cult of Nāthasiddhas, which was already in existence in the north, rose to prominence following the downfall of Buddhist institutions. These Nāthasiddhas are held to be directly responsible for the development of the Tamil Siddha system. The Tamil Siddha Koṅkaṇar states in *Koṅkaṇar nāṭi* that pulse diagnosis was a gift from the Nāthasiddhas.[20] Similarly, Caṭṭaimuṉi states in *Caṭṭaimuṉi nikaṇṭu*-1200 that alchemy and 'the secret of arsenics' were propounded by the Nāthasiddhas.[21] The author of VC-800 also seems to belong to the same lineage, as he pays obeisance to yogins of the Nātha order (*pāṭal* 552).

After examining the contents of nearly 633 Tamil Siddha medical texts, Venkatraman concludes that these texts which constitute the bulwark of the

---

17 VENKATRAMAN 1990: 117, MADHAVAN 1984: 11

18 VENKATRAMAN 1990: 116, SCHARFE 1999: 610.

19 VENKATRAMAN 1990: 116.

20 VENKATRAMAN 1990: 119.

21 VENKATRAMAN 1990: 39.

present-day Siddha system are not older than the sixteenth century A.D.[22] Nevertheless, the study of texts like VC-800 indicates that these works contain medical information of greater vintage. As Scharfe asked, could these treatises be the written reflections of an oral tradition that goes back to the hoary past?[23] It is interesting to note at this point that Tamil medical literature includes many works attributed to unusual authors like Acuviṉi, Tūrvācar, Camatakkiṉi, Kācyapamuṉi, Patañcali, Pulattiyar, Tilōttamai, Ūrvaci, Vālmīkar, Vaciṣṭar and Viyācar.[24] It is quite possible that the study of Tamil medical texts could provide interesting insights into the evolution of Āyurveda, especially its nosology.

All authoritative Sanskrit texts of mainstream Āyurveda follow a relatively rigid pattern of classification of diseases. The *Suśrutasaṃhitā*, *Carakasaṃhitā*, *Aṣṭāṅgasaṅgraha* and *Aṣṭāṅgahṛdaya* follow more or less the same nosology. This orthodox pattern is evident in most of Āyurvedic literature even up to present times. However, in VC-800 one observes a heterodox approach to the classification of many diseases like *kācam*, *kāmālai*, *kirāṇi*, *makōtaram* etc. This indicates that Tamil medicine was not constrained by the rigours of Āyurvedic dogmatism. Socio-historical factors prevalent in older times[25] might have contributed to this development.[26]

## Appendix 1

*Contents of VC-800 arranged according to* pāṭal *(verse) numbers*

| | |
|---|---|
| 1-3 | Introduction |
| 4-7 | Names of the various diseases |
| 8-13 | Description of *pañcapūtam* (five primordial principles) |
| 14-128 | Pulse examination |
| 129-130 | Characteristics of the body under the influence of *vātam*, *pittam* and |

[22] Venkatraman 1990: 42-75.

[23] Scharfe 1999: 611.

[24] Nirmalātēvi 1983: 1-111, Madhavan 1984: 57-158.

[25] On these cf. e.g. Sastri 1964: 19-108, Venkatraman 1990: 148-156.

[26] We are grateful to Prof. Rahul Peter Das for reading the manuscript critically and offering valuable suggestions that helped us in its revision.

| | |
|---|---|
| | *kapam* |
| 131-136 | Examination of speech, eye, stool, urine and tongue |
| 137-158 | Characteristics of *curam* (fever) |
| 159-173 | Characteristics of *caṉṉirōkam* (complicated type of fever characterised by coma and delirium) |
| 174-177 | Curable and incurable types of *caṉṉi* |
| 178-186 | Origin of a class of fever called *tōṣacuram* |
| 187-191 | Characteristics of *aticāram* (dysentery) |
| 192-199 | Prognosis of *aticāram* |
| 200-207 | Characteristics of individuals whose pulse cannot be examined correctly |
| 208-2107 | Characteristics of individuals who should not be subjected to *laṅkaṉam* (fasting) |
| 211-222 | Characteristics of *kuṉmam* (lumps in viscera) |
| 223-226 | Causes of *cūlai* (pricking pain) |
| 227-242 | Characteristics of various types of *cūlai* |
| 243-244 | Causes of *vātarōkam* |
| 245-253 | Seasons in which *vātam* increases or decreases in the body |
| 254-432 | Characteristics of 84 types of *vātarōkam* |
| 343-392 | Characteristics of 42 types of *pittarōkam* |
| 393-421 | Characteristics of 21 types of *cēṭparōkam* (diseases caused by *kapam*) |
| 422-450 | Characteristics of 21 types of *piramīyam* (urinary diseases) |
| 451-483 | Characteristics of 20 types of *mēkarōkam* (venereal afflictions) |
| 484-489 | Prognosis of *mēkarōkam* |
| 490-493 | Dietary and behavioural restrictions for 20 types of *mēkam* |
| 494-514 | Characteristics of *kuṣṭam* (skin diseases) |
| 515-518 | Causes and prognosis of *kuṣṭam* |
| 519-527 | Characteristics of *pāṇṭurōkam* (morbid pallor) |
| 528-543 | Characteristics of *kāmālai* (jaundice) |
| 544-545 | Prognosis of *kāmālai* |
| 546-553 | Characteristics of various types of *cōpai* (oedema) |
| 554-591 | Characteristics of various types of *makōtaram* (enlargement of abdomen) |
| 592-594 | Prognosis of *makōtaram* |
| 595-597 | Causes of *viṣapākarōkam* (allergic rashes) |
| 598-606 | Characteristics of various types of *viṣapākarōkam* |
| 607-635 | Characteristics of 25 types of *kirāṇi* (diarrhoea) |

| | |
|---|---|
| 636-638 | Prognosis of *kirāṇi* |
| 639-665 | Characteristics of 21 types of *mūlam* (haemorrhoids) |
| 666-669 | Prognosis of *mūlam* |
| 670-684 | Characteristics of various types of *cayam* (desiccation) |
| 685-688 | Prognosis of *cayam* |
| 689-704 | Characteristics of various types of *kācam* (respiratory disease) |
| 705-707 | Prognosis of *kācam* |
| 708-716 | Characteristics of *uḷaimāntai* (indigestion) |
| 717-724 | Characteristics of *perumpāṭurōkam* (dysfunctional bleeding) |
| 725-734 | Characteristics of *kallaṭaippu* (urinary stones) |
| 735-743 | Characteristics of *mūttirakiricciram* (dysuria) |
| 744-752 | Characteristics of *irumal* (dry cough) |
| 753-763 | Characteristics of *vippuruti* (abscess) |
| 764-775 | Characteristics of various types of *karappāṉ* (eruptions on the skin of children) |
| 776-782 | Characteristics of various types of *catti* (emesis) |
| 763-787 | Characteristics of various types of *vikkal* (hiccup) |
| 788-800 | Characteristics of various types of *pavuttiram* (anal fistula) development. |

## Appendix 2

*Evidence, in translation, from VC-800 suggesting Āyurvedic origins*

*Pāṭal* 1: I narrate in this *Vaittiyacintāmaṇi* the principles of *āyuruvētam* as revealed by the god Tanvantari.

*Pāṭal* 3: Tēraiyar passed it on to me, Yūki, the sage, and I record it hereby for the benefit of mankind. After studying the northern language and after receiving the blessings of the elders of that region, I hereby recite that knowledge after studying it meticulously.

*Pāṭal* 392: Pulattiyar passed it on to Tēraiyar and he passed it to me Yūkimuṉi. The knowledge which came from the northern language has been narrated by me without concealing any point. With the blessings of the great master the details of the 42 *pittam* are hereby concluded.

*Pāṭal* 422: Akattiyar passed on the knowledge to Pulattiyar. He passed on this great *āyuruvētam* to the sage Tēraiyar. Tēraiyar passed on this knowledge to me. I hereby narrate the characteristics of *piramēkam*.

*Pāṭal* 450: Pulattiyar passed on the knowledge to Tēraiyar, who revealed it to me, Yūki. I, Yūkimuṉi, delved deep into the mystical *āyuruvētam*, compiled the knowledge and recorded it clearly and faithfully as the words of Śiva.

*Pāṭal* 451: Devī stood respectfully in front of Śiva, and said that he was the one to bless *āyuruvētam*. She requested him to reveal the knowledge of *mēkarōkam* for the benefit of all living beings.

*Pāṭal* 493: After studying the words of Śiva, and after consulting the various works in the northern language, I hereby conclude in Tamil language the knowledge of *mēkarōkam* described in *āyuruvētam*.

*Pāṭal* 552: I have described the classification of *pāṇṭu*, *kāmālai* and *cōpai*. Thus, after consulting the texts in the northern language and after listening to the words of yogins of the Nātha order, I, Yūkimuṉi, have explained *āyuruvētam*, just as Śiva revealed it to Maṉoṉmaṇi for the benefit of mankind.

*Pāṭal* 553: I have explained the gist of *āyuruvētam* in mellifluous Tamil language. I, Yūkimuṉi, thus composed this work so that even young children could understand the subject easily.

*Pāṭal* 594: For the benefit of all people I, Yūkimuṉi, hereby record for posterity the knowledge received from texts of the northern language, as faithfully as Śiva narrated it to Umā.

*Pāṭal* 640: Tēraiyar organised this body of knowledge and passed it on to me, Yūki. For the benefit of mankind I hereby dedicate *āyuruvētam*, after paying homage to all sages.

*Pāṭal* 669: Akattiyar passed on the knowledge to Pulattiyar. Pulattiyar revealed it to the great sage Tēraiyar, who handed it over to me. After studying the works in the northern language I composed these verses in Tamil for the benefit of the world.

*Pāṭal* 688: For the benefit of the world Tēraiyar passed on the entire body of *āyuruvētam* to me, Yūkimuṉi. He created this garland of pearls in Tamil and revealed it for the knowledge of all, so that all living beings benefit.

*Pāṭal*743: The knowledge of healing is the foremost among the six bodies of knowledge (*cāttiram*). It is the knowledge of *āyuruvētam*. It is enshrined in 700,000 texts. I, Yūkimuṉi composed this work after meticulous study of texts of the northern language and after receiving the blessings of the master.

## Bibliography

DAS, Rahul Peter 2001: '[Review of] Meulenbeld, G. Jan: *A History of Indian Medical Literature I-II* (Groningen: Egbert Forsten 1999-2000)', *Traditional South Asian Medicine*

(Wiesbaden) 6: 145-158.

KNÜPPEL, Jens 2001: '[Review of] Zvelebil, Kamil V.: *The Siddha Quest for Immortality* (Oxford: Mandrake 1996)', *Traditional South Asian Medicine* (Wiesbaden) 6: 192-194.

KUMAR, D. Suresh. 1995: 'Some Preliminary Observations on the Chronology of Tamil Medical Works', in: P. Pushpangadan, Ulf Nyman and V. George (eds.), *Glimpses of Indian Ethnopharmacology*. Thiruvananthapuram: Tropical Botanic Garden and Research Institute, pp. 77-84.

MADHAVAN, V.R. (ed.) 1984: *Siddha Medical Manuscripts in Tamil*. Madras: International Institute of Tamil Studies. Publication, International Institute of Tamil Studies 89.

MURTHY, K.R. Srikantha (ed.) 2002: *Bhāvaprakāśa of Bhāvamiśra (Text, English Translation, Notes, Appendeces* ⟨sic⟩ *and Index). Vol. 2 (Madhya and Uttara Khaṇḍa)*. Reprint. Varanasi: Krishnadas Academy.

NĀYAṈĀR, Mārkkaliṅka (ed.) 1932: *Yūkimā muṉivarāṟ ceyyappaṭṭa Vaittiyacintāmaṇi*. Ceṉṉai: Śrī Ātimūlam Accukkūṭam.

NIRMALĀTĒVI, Irā. (ed.) 1983: *Tiruvaṉantapuram kēraḷap palkalaik kaḻaka tamiḻc cuvaṭikaḷ aṭṭavaṇai*. Ceṉṉai: Ulakat Tamiḻārāycci Niṟuvaṉam.

PILLAI, T.V. Sambasivam 1931: *Tamil-English Dictionary of Medicine, Chemistry, Botany and Allied Sciences. Based on Indian Medical Science. Volume 1*. Madras: Research Institute of Siddhar's Science.

RĀMACCANTIRAṈ, Es.Pi. (ed.) 1998: *Yūkimā muṉivar Vaittiya cintāmaṇi 800. Mūlamum uraiyum*. Ceṉṉai: Tāmarai Nūlaikam.

SASTRI, K.A. Nilakanta 1964: *The Culture and History of the Tamils*. Calcutta: K.L. Mukhopadhyay.

SCHARFE, Hartmut 1999: 'The Doctrine of the Three Humors in Traditional Indian Medicine and the Alleged Antiquity of Tamil Siddha Medicine', *Journal of the American Oriental Society* 119: 609-629.

TĒVAR, Pā. Kaṅkātarat (ed.)1975: *Pōkar Ēḻāyiram. Mutalāmāyiram*. 2. patippu. Ceṉṉai: Aruḷmiku Paḻani Taṇṭāyutapāṇi Cuvāmi Tirukkōyil Citta Maruttuvanūl Veḷiyīṭṭuk Kuḻu. Veḷiyīṭṭuttoṭar 14.

TIYĀKARĀCAṈ, Irā. 1976: *Yūki muṉivar Vaittiya cintāmaṇi (perunūl 800). Mutal pākam*. Iraṇṭām patippu. Ceṉṉai: Aruḷmiku Paḻani Taṇṭāyutapāṇi Cuvāmi Tirukkōyil Citta Maruttuva Nūl Veḷiyīṭṭuk Kuḻu. Veḷiyīṭṭut Toṭar 21.

UPADHYĀYA ⟨sic⟩, Yadunandana (ed.) 1975: *Aṣṭāṅga Hṛdaya of Vāgbhaṭa. Edited with the 'Vidyotinī['] Hindī Commentary by Kavirāja Atrideva Gupta Vidyālaṅkāra*. Varanasi: The Chaukhambha Sanskrit Sansthan. The Kashi Sanskrit Series 150.

VENKATRAMAN, R. 1990: *A History of the Tamil Siddha Cult*. Madurai: Ennes Publications.

# A Khotanese Medical Text on Poultices: Manuscripts P 2893 and IOL Khot S 9*

MAURO MAGGI

*In memory of Barbara Goss***

Besides large portions of Late Khotanese prose translations of Ravigupta's *Siddhasāra* and the so-called *Jīvakapustaka*, there are also remains, mostly fragmentary, of other Āyurvedic texts in Khotanese.[1] Among the works that were left unfinished by the late Ronald E. Emmerick there is a provisional critical edition and translation of almost half of one of such texts, an extensive but incomplete Late Khotanese collection of prescriptions that is entirely devoted to poultices. It is one of two Khotanese texts from Dunhuang that were written on the reverse of a discarded Chinese roll which contained Chinese Buddhist texts on the obverse, the Paris ms. Pelliot chinois 2893 (= P 2893; henceforth Pelliot ms.). The Khotanese side was published but not translated by Harold W. Bailey (BAILEY 1956, 3: 82-93). The medical text occupies ll. 32-267 and is preceded by a Buddhist text. Emmerick's provisional edition covers ll. 32-163, corresponding to §§ 1-58 in his numbering, while his translation stops at l. 161, corresponding to his § 57.[2] The last changes made by Emmerick to the relevant

---

* A preliminary version of this article was presented at the 'Giornate orientalistiche cagliesi III: Workshop on Current Research in Iranian Studies', Cagli, April 14-15, 2007. I am grateful to Hélène Vetch for information on ms. P 2893, and to Ursula Sims-Williams for information on ms. IOL Khot S 9 and for a photograph of its bottom line without the silk covering it from the repair, which I could use in the photomontage in fig. 2. – Abbreviations: ms(s). = manuscript(s), l(l). = line(s).

** This article is dedicated to the memory of my dear friend Barbara Goss (Mount Gambier, Australia 1942 – Rome, Italy 2007) as a token of gratitude and esteem. A gentle and kind-hearted person, she revised the English of most of my articles, including the present one, in a very skilled and careful manner. Discussing with her how to translate particulars of my works often enabled me to improve my own understanding of the subject matter itself.

[1] See EMMERICK 1992: 42-45; MEULENBELD 1999-2002, 2A: 126, 146-148, 2B: 144f., 166-170; MAGGI forthcoming: 413-416.

[2] According to the new numbering (see p. 81f. below), Emmerick's edition covers §§ 1-22

files date from June 17, 2001. This means that he worked on this text in parallel with the *Siddhasāra*, the medical text to which he attached the utmost importance and on which he continued working until his last days.

In 2006 I began completing the interpretation of the medical text of the Pelliot ms., and I would like to present some of the progress I have made in this study.

While comparing other Khotanese medical texts that are fragmentarily preserved, it occurred to me that the end of the Pelliot ms., which is mutilated, might join on to the beginning of ms. IOL Khot S 9 (= Ch. 00265) of the Stein Collection in London (henceforth Stein ms.), which also contains part of a Khotanese medical text on poultices on the reverse of a Chinese roll from Dunhuang and, like the Pelliot ms., makes a peculiar use of punctuation signs in that the single prescriptions are mostly divided by means of a double colon. The London ms. was first published by Bailey, and then re-edited with a working translation by Prods Oktor Skjærvø in his recent catalogue of the Khotanese manuscripts in the British Library.[3] Although I had photographs of the Pelliot ms. but not of the Stein ms., I was encouraged to pursue my hypothesis by the fact that, according to Skjærvø, the latter is written in a 'very regular cursive ductus' (SKJÆRVØ 2002: 487), which also applies to the former.

Since Chinese Buddhist texts on the obverse of manuscripts are usually otherwise known and may enable one to decide whether incomplete manuscripts belong together, I asked the advice of Hélène Vetch, who is working on the volume of the catalogue of the Chinese manuscripts in the Pelliot Collection that will include a description of the Pelliot ms. under consideration. Her reply was exciting. She informed me that the Stein ms. does not join on to the end of the Paris one but, surprisingly enough, 'inserts itself between the 5th and the 6th sheets of Pelliot chinois 2893. Line 91 of the Paris Khotanese text is the

---

and 42-78, and his translation covers §§ 1-22 and 42-77.

[3] BAILEY 1956, 3: 17-19 and SKJÆRVØ 2002: 487-489. The manuscript, which has 54 columns of Chinese on the obverse, measures 95 × 26 cm (ENOKI 1962: 245), and consists of 'two pieces joined together, each 46.3 × 26 cm. … the Khotanese was definitely written on the sheets when they were already stuck together, as one line spans two sheets' (Ursula Sims-Williams, letter of November 14, 2006).

dividing one: the very first line of Ch 00265 [i.e. IOL Khot S 9] completes its upper part, the last line completes its lower part.'[4]

In fact, the right half of l. 91 of the Pelliot ms. is odd in appearance (see fig. 1). Nevertheless, Harold W. Bailey in his edition was able to read it so as to obtain an acceptable sense, and Bailey's reading was provisionally accepted by Emmerick, though he underlined the unusual condition of the manuscript in his critical apparatus:[5]

§ 22 (P 2893.91-92) *mākṣī̧na vasva uysmä paherā̧ñä . ā* ***vā***[1]***vę́śtī̧ñe*** [2]***ā *nauka***[2] ***kūṭāñä*** . ***mā̧***kṣī̧'na paherā̧ñä cu jara strīśtä . vara bañā̧ñä ṣai' vasū̧je ::*

1. The paper containing the lower halves of the akṣaras of *vę́śtī̧ñe* has been physically split and the lower halves are no longer correctly positioned below their upper halves. 2. '*ā n(au)ka* not clear' (Bailey). The lower half of *ā* and the upper vowel mark for *au* are no longer visible.

Bailey's reading resulted in the following translation by Emmerick: 'Pure clay must be moistened with honey or alternatively (the clay) must be put in or finely ground (and then) mixed with honey. If the liver stiffens, (the poultice) must be tied on. It will remove (the swellings).' One may notice that this is a fairly tautological wording that is unexpected in an Āyurvedic work.

However, if we follow Hélène Vetch's hint and term ll. 91a and 91b the upper and lower parts of the fictitious line 91 of the Pelliot ms., and insert the Stein ms. between them as is shown in the virtual restoration of fig. 2, we obtain a perfectly legible and meaningful text. As can be seen, the fragmentary ll. 1 and 42 of the Stein ms. join on to the fragmentary ll. 91a and 91b respectively of the Pelliot ms. without any gap. The resulting new reading and translation of the joints of the two manuscripts is as follows:[6]

§ 22 (Pelliot ms. 91a + Stein ms. 1-2) ***mākṣī̧na vasva uysmä paherā̧ñä . ā vā*** *krreṃgī̧ñe āha'na ārrdä māṃgä paherā̧ñä . heṃje haśä tcabe'jā̧kä pęṇḍai ::*

**Pure clay must be moistened with honey, or alternatively** ground green gram

[4] Hélène Vetch, letter of May 27, 2006.

[5] Below, my **bold** print marks the odd-looking akṣaras.

[6] Emmerick's edition and translation are in **bold** characters. In the absence of a known original, the Sanskrit equivalents given in parentheses in the translation are hypothetical.

(*mudga*) must be moistened with a fowl's (*dakṣa*) egg (*aṇḍa*). [This] poultice (*piṇḍaka*) [is] a disperser of red swelling.

§ 42 (Stein ms. 42 + Pelliot ms. 91b-92) (1) *hauṣka gūra* . (2) *rṵ̄nai* . (3) *mahā-baujä* . (4) *haṃga* . *hạmagä vīśtạ̄ñä* . ***nauka kūṭāña . mākṣ̄ī'na paherạ̄ñä cu jara strīśtä . vara bañạ̄ñä ṣai' vasṵ̄je*** ::

(1) Dry grapes (*drākṣā*), (2) Indian madder (*mañjiṣṭhā*), (3) liquorice (*madhu-ka*), (4) bladder sorrel (*amlavetasa*) must be put in equally, be **finely ground [and then] mixed with honey. If the liver stiffens, [the poultice] must be tied on. It will** purify it (i.e. the liver).

The Pelliot and Stein mss. share a further formal peculiarity in addition to the use of double colons to divide the single prescriptions. In the Pelliot ms., the double colons at the end of §§ 44-46, 49 and 56 (ll. 96, 98, 100, 108 and 122) and the single dot at the end of § 47 (l. 102) are highlighted by means of a mark in pink ink, and a similar mark highlights the double colon in l. 19 of the Stein ms. at the end of § 28.

That parts of the same manuscript reached different collections is not uncommon in the case of Khotanese and other manuscripts from Chinese Central Asia, but one wonders how the fictitious l. 91 of the Pelliot ms. came into existence. As is known, Chinese rolls may consist of one single sheet to many sheets of paper glued together to form rolls up to several metres in length. As Hélène Vetch showed me during a visit to the Bibliothèque Nationale de France in May 2007, some of the joints between the sheets forming the Pelliot ms. are very fine and neat in that the paper overlaps for just a millimetre or a little more, whilst other joints are much rougher, the overlap of the sheets being definitely broader. On the other hand, both the fine and the rough joints were in her opinion made by means of an ancient, dark glue, which signifies that the original manuscript fell apart and was reassembled in ancient times. It was on that occasion that the Stein ms. also got detached from the rest of the roll, but was overlooked and omitted when the other detached parts were glued together again to obtain the Pelliot ms. with its wrongly joined l. 91. The fact that the reassemblage took place in ancient times rules out the hypothesis that the Pelliot ms. was 'restored' by the Taoist priest Wang Yuanlu, the self-appointed guardian of the Dunhuang caves who sold part of the Dunhuang manuscripts to Stein in spring 1907, and subsequently sold other manuscripts, including our Pelliot ms., to Paul Pelliot in 1908.[7] It must be added that the akṣaras of the Khotanese text retain their original shape in connection with the fine joints – which also applies to the only joint in the Stein ms. (l. 20) – but are slightly lost in the rough joints due to the broader overlap of the sheets, and that the Chinese text never spans two sheets in connection with the fine joints and only in a few instances marginal parts of the Chinese characters are lost in the rough joints. This reveals that the Khotanese text was written after the first assemblage of the roll containing the Chinese text, but before its falling apart and reassembly.

Recognition of the correct sequence of the folios makes it possible to restore the correct sequence of the paragraphs, that is otherwise illogical in the Pelliot ms. In fact, should the Stein ms. be left out of account, Emmerick's §§ 22-28, that contain prescriptions for the liver, would come within the section on swellings which, in § 16, is introduced by its own heading just like all other sections: Pelliot ms. 82-83 *ttī vā haśi va pęṇḍą̄* 'These [are] poultices (*piṇḍaka*) for swelling' (Emmerick). The only understandable exception is the very first section in §§ 2-8, which is not introduced by a special heading because it is preceded by the general heading of the text in § 1 (see below). In actual fact, the section containing prescriptions for the liver has its own heading in § 36: Stein ms. 32-33 *tti vā jarä bidāṣṭä pįṇḍą̄* 'These [are] the poultices [for placing] on the liver'.

The following table shows the contents of the text and its new paragraph numbering:

| *Emmerick* | *New* | *Contents*[8] |
|---|---|---|
| § 1 | § 1 | General heading: 'Now the poultices and prescriptions for various diseases are explained separately' |
| §§ 2-8 | §§ 2-8 | Poultices for eye diseases (without heading) |
| §§ 9-15 | §§ 9-15 | 'The following are poultices for the stomach' (§ 9) |
| §§ 16-22… | §§ 16-35 | 'These [are] poultices for swelling' (§ 16) |

[7] See the brief account of Wang Yuanlu's transactions with Stein and Pelliot in HOPKIRK 1980: 158-169, 182-185.

[8] Translations of the headings in §§ 1-16 and 50-78 are Emmerick's.

| | | |
|---|---|---|
| §§ ...22-28[9] | §§ 36-49 | 'These [are] the poultices [for placing] on the liver' (§ 36) |
| §§ 29-35 | §§ 50-56 | 'These [are] the poultices [for placing] on the spleen' (§ 50) |
| §§ 36-42 | §§ 57-63 | 'These (are) the poultices [for placing] on the navel' (§ 57) |
| §§ 43-56 | §§ 64-77 | 'These [are] poultices for hernia and for diseases [involving] downward [motion]' (§ 64) |
| §§ 57-...[10] | §§ 78-84 | 'These [are] the poultices for piles' (§ 78) |
| | §§ 85-101 | 'These [are] prescriptions and poultices for itches' (§ 85) |
| | §§ 102-116 | 'These [are] poultices for rheumatism' (§ 102) |
| | §§ 117-128 | 'Now poultices and prescriptions of each and every kind are explained' (§ 117). |

Though the last preserved paragraph is incomplete, it is likely that the text, which has not been identified so far, is almost entirely extant, since one may presume that the partially preserved miscellaneous section on 'poultices and prescriptions of each and every kind' that follows the specialised sections on poultices for particular organs or diseases was the closing one.

### Bibliography


BAILEY, H.W. 1956: *Indo-Scythian Studies being Khotanese Texts*. Volume III. Cambridge: University Press.

EMMERICK, Ronald E. 1992: *A Guide to the Literature of Khotan*. Second edition. Tokyo: The International Institute for Buddhist Studies. Studia Philologica Buddhica, Occasional Paper Series 3.

ENOKI, Kazuo 1962: 'Appendix. Chinese Manuscripts', in: Louis de la Vallée Poussin, *Catalogue of the Tibetan Manuscripts from Tun-huang in the India Office Library*. London: Oxford University Press, pp. 239-269.

HOPKIRK, Peter 1980: *Foreign Devils on the Silk Road. The Search for the Lost Cities and Treasures of Chinese Central Asia*. London: John Murray.

MAGGI, Mauro forthcoming: 'Khotanese Literature', in: Ronald E. Emmerick and Maria Macuch (eds.), *Persian Literature. Companion Volume 1. The Literature of Pre-Islamic Iran*. London. In the press, pp. 330-417.

MEULENBELD, G. Jan 1999-2002: *A History of Indian Medical Literature*. 3 volumes in 5 parts. Groningen: Egbert Forsten. Groningen Oriental Studies 15.


[9] The ellipses indicate the insertion point of the Stein ms. The second half of Emmerick's § 22 corresponds to the second half of the new § 42.

[10] Emmerick's edition stops at § 57.

SKJÆRVØ, Prods Otkor 2002: *Khotanese Manuscripts from Chinese Turkestan in The British Library. A Complete Catalogue with Texts and Translations*. With contributions by Ursula Sims-Williams. London: The British Library. Corpus Inscriptionum Iranicarum 2, Inscriptions of the Seleucid and Parthian Periods and of Eastern Iran and Central Asia 5, Saka Texts 6.

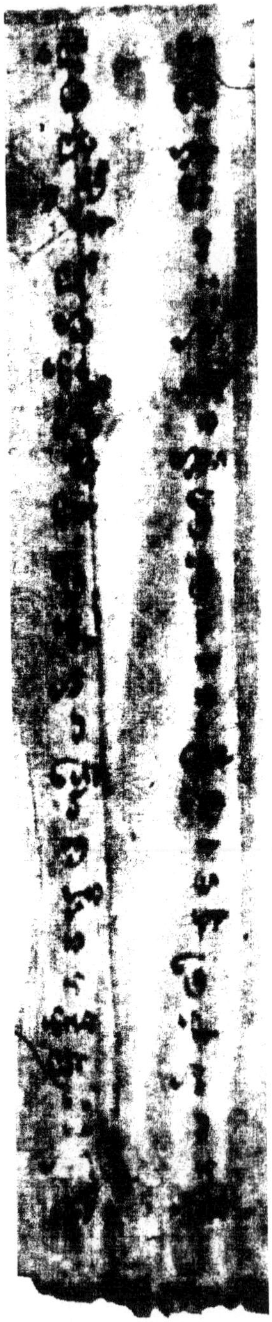

**Fig. 1:** P 2893.91-92
Courtesy of the Bibliothèque Nationale de France

**Fig. 2:** P 2893.91a + IOL Khot S 9.1-2, and IOL Khot S 9.41-42 + P 2893.91b-92
Courtesy of the Bibliothèque Nationale de France and The British Library

# The Three Channels in Tibetan Medicine

## *With a Translation of Tsultrim Gyaltsen's 'A Clear Explanation of the Principal Structure and Location of the Circulatory Channels as Illustrated in the Medical Paintings'*[*]

FRANCES GARRETT and VINCANNE ADAMS
with assistance from
JAMPA KELSANG, YUMBA and RENCHEN DHONDUP

This article comments on a centuries-old controversy in Tibetan literature: how the complex descriptions of the human circulatory system found in Buddhist tantric contemplative texts can be reconciled with descriptions of the circulatory system in Tibetan medical texts. In the essay translated below (= TG), the eminent twentieth-century Tibetan scholar of religion and medicine Tsultrim Gyaltsen (Tshul khrim rGyal mtshan)[1] addresses this problem with recourse to texts dating back to some of the earliest periods of Tibetan literary history. Tsultrim Gyaltsen's voice thus adds a contemporary flavour to an ancient debate.[2] In the following introductory words, we will contextualise the translation with a brief overview of Tibetan medical and religious views on the human circulatory system.

### The Circulatory System in Tibetan Medical Texts

The circulatory system portrayed in early Tibetan medical literature is

---

[*] This project was supported in part by grant T32 AT00052 from the National Center for Complementary and Alternative Therapies (NCCAM), U.S. National Institutes of Health. – The translation for this article was begun by Vincanne Adams with the help of Jampa Kelsang, Yumba and Renchen Dhondup. Their initial draft was brought to completion by Frances Garrett, who also added most of the introductory comments.

[1] This article uses the Extended Wylie transliteration scheme for transliterating Tibetan words . See <*http://www.thdl.org/collections/langling/tibetan-transliteration.html*> for a discussion of Extended Wylie – based on Wylie, the most commonly used transliteration scheme in use today – and other transliterations of Tibetan.

[2] GYATSO 2004 discusses mediaeval occurrences of debates on this topic.

roughly based on the classical Indian Āyurvedic tradition.[3] Āyurvedic medicine describes a network of hundreds of large and small ducts, or channels, variously named *nāḍī-, sirā-/śirā-, srotas-* or *dhamanī-* in Sanskrit, that transport nutrients, wastes, respiration and other substances throughout the body. These channels connect internal organs and are responsible for digestive and other physiological processes, they permit movement of joints and limbs, and they carry information that allows sense organs to function. The precise enumeration of various types of channels and their functions, however, is a contested topic, and debates among Indian medical scholars concerning the circulatory system are common.[4]

The structure of the circulatory system in medical texts is significantly different than that of the circulatory system described in Indian tantric texts. Unlike in medical texts, tantric physiology begins with a vertical spinal column in which, or along which – this too is debated – are three primary channels. At each of four points along this vertical column, at the throat, heart, navel, and genitals, is a channel nexus or 'wheel' (*'khor lo;* Skt. *cakra-*), and all subsidiary channels of the body are connected to this vertical column. Although over the centuries some Tibetan writers have tried to unite medical and tantric accounts of anatomy and physiology, descriptions of the body in South Asian literature are so numerous and so complex that few differences are fully reconciled.

In Tibetan medical literature of the *Four Tantras*[5] tradition, descriptions of

---

[3] The maturity of the Tibetan system of pulse analysis, a means of diagnosis not present in Āyurveda until the twelfth century, suggests other influences as well, such as from Chinese traditions or indigenous Tibetan systems. See DUMMER 1994: 79, or SVOBODA/LADE 1999: 142-145.

[4] Cf. DAS 2003: 553, 560, 584-590. See DASGUPTA 1975: 344-357 for an overview of the circulatory system in classical Āyurveda, followed by a discussion of the same in tantric texts.

[5] The most important text in the history of Tibetan medicine, the *Gyushi* (*rGyud bzhi*), considered the principal medical text still today, is known in English as the *Four Tantras* (*bDud rtsi snying po yan lag brgyad pa gsang ba man ngag gi rgyud*) (edition used: [Lhasa]: Bod ljongs mi dmangs dpe skrun khang 2000). While the origins of this seminal text are debated, it is likely to have been arranged in the definitive form we know today in the eleventh century by the famous Tibetan physician Yuthog Yonten Gonpo (g.Yu thog Yon tan mGon po, 1112-

the human circulatory system focus on the circulatory channels (*rtsa*, equivalent to the channels variously named *nāḍī-, sirā-/śirā-, srotas-* or *dhamanī-* in Sanskrit). These are sometimes translated into English as 'veins', 'arteries', or 'nerves', although the term *rtsa* in Tibetan is not directly equivalent to any of these. The channels are the basis of the circulatory system of winds, blood, and other energies and fluids that connect all aspects of the body. The contemporary Tibetan medical scholar Thubten Phuntsok explains that in Tibetan medicine channels are classified in several ways (TP: 80). In one taxonomy of channels, there are said to be black channels (*nag rtsa*), also called blood channels, and white channels (*dkar rtsa*), also called water channels. Blood channels are further divided into 'pulsating' channels (*'phar rtsa*) and 'staying' channels (*sdod rtsa*), which are sometimes today translated as 'arteries' and 'veins' respectively. In Tibetan medical texts channels are also classified functionally, in which case there are four types: channels of formation (*chags*), channels of existence (*srid*), connecting (*'brel*) channels, and vitality (*tshe*) channels.

The fourth chapter of the *Explanatory Tantra,* the second book of the *Four Tantras*, presents this fourfold functional division of channels, beginning with three channels of embryonic formation. Called the water or white channel, the blood or black channel, and the wind channel, these three are said to grow outwards from the navel of the embryo. The water or white channel travels along the left side of the body, and the *Four Tantras* tradition states that it forms the

---

1203), probably following several centuries of development. This text spawned the composition of a large number of commentarial works over the centuries. The *Four Tantras* consist of one hundred and fifty six chapters arranged in four books: the *Root Tantra* (*rTsa rgyud*); the *Explanatory Tantra* (*bShad rgyud)*, with a description of the human body and general information about the causes of disease and the principles of therapeutics; the *Secret Oral Tantra* (*Man ngag rgyud*), containing specific instructions and methods of diagnosis; and the *Concluding Tantra* (*Phyi ma rgyud*), containing specific information about various types of treatments. Page numbers from the Lhasa 2000 edition (= FT) are cited in this article. Portions of the *Root Tantra* and the *Explanatory Tantra* are available in English translation in CLARK 1995. Other portions of the *Four Tantras* on topics such as nosology, etiology and pharmacology, have been selectively translated as well, as for example in the works of R.E. Emmerick.

brain; its functions and activities are thus primarily focused in the upper part of the torso and head. The blood or black channel is said to travel along the right side of the body and is related to liver function, as well as with the emotion of anger and the bile humour; its activities are thus concentrated in the central part of the torso. The third channel of formation is associated with the emotions of desire and attachment and the region of the sexual organs, as well as with the activities of the winds.[6] Although the issue is contested, some religious and medical scholars, including Lodro Gyalpo (Zur mkhar bLo gros rGyal po, 1509-1579), Desi Sangye Gyatso (sDe srid Sangs rgyas rGya mtsho, 1653-1703 or 1705), and the 20th-century scholar Tsultrim Gyaltsen, identify these three channels in the *Four Tantras* as the three channels of tantric physiology, as we will discuss below.

The second of the fourfold functional division of channels, the existence channels, are themselves of four types and are responsible for sensory engagement with the external world, emotional feelings and nourishment of the bodily constituents. Thubten Phunstok explains that in the *Four Tantras* tradition, once the channels of formation have been completely produced in the embryo, the existence channels develop in four locations in the body and branch out into hundreds of surrounding auxiliary channels. Situated in the brain, the first existence channel is responsible for the function of the sense organs. The second existence channel, in the heart region, is the basis of memory, conceptuality and awareness of the ego. The third channel is located at the navel and in this tradition is considered responsible for the embryonic body's growth. The fourth channel, in the area of the genitals, is referred to as the source of one's family lineage.[7] Although the *Four Tantras* do not use the term 'wheel' (*'khor lo*) in this context, Tsultrim Gyaltsen explains that the four existence channels and their surrounding auxiliary channels described in the *Explanatory Tantra* are the four wheels referred to in Buddhist tantric systems (TG: 84).

The two connecting channels are referred to as white and black, or water

---

6 The *Explanatory Tantra* discussion of the circulatory channels begins at FT: 22; for the translation see CLARK 1995: 56-58.

7 TP: 83-85 summarises the *Four Tantras* presentation.

and blood, channels. In the adult, hundreds of subsidiary channels branch off from these two main connecting channels, interlinking the limbs and organs throughout the entire body. As in the Āyurvedic tradition, Tibetan medical texts debate the precise pathways of these hundreds of channels. The black connecting channels are said to be filled exclusively with blood and, passing through the liver, are involved in the sustenance and development of the seven bodily constituents[8]; a subset of these are the channels used in blood-letting. The main white channel, also travelling from the brain to the coccyx bone, is white in colour. It and its branch channels, sometimes glossed as 'ligaments', 'tendons' or 'nerves', are responsible for many of the functions also attributed to the existence channels, such as regulating emotions, enabling physical movement, and allowing speech and mental functions. The sixteenth-century medical scholar Lodro Gyalpo associates the white existence channel with the tantric solitary channel (*rkyang ma*) running vertically along the left side of the body, and the black existence channel with the tantric flavour channel (*ro ma*) running along the right side of the body.[9]

The *Explanatory Tantra* states that there are three types of vitality channel: one type that works throughout the entire body, a second type that accompanies respiration, and a third that also pervades the entire body as a sort of 'life force'.[10] Thubten Phunstok explains that in the tradition of LG, the vitality channels are not 'real' (*dngos*) channels; rather, they refer to forces within the body that maintain life (TP: 101). Human life in this tradition is by definition dependent upon the continuation of three physiological functions: the 'radi-

---

[8] A physiological system derived from Indian Āyurveda, the seven bodily constituents (*lus zungs*, Skt. *dhātu-*) in Tibetan medicine are the nutritive essence (*dwangs ma*), blood (*khrag*), flesh (*sha*), fat (*tshil*), bone (*rus pa*), marrow (*rkang*) and the reproductive fluids (*khu ba*).

[9] Cited in TP: 108f. on the basis of Lodro Gyalpo's *Transmission of the Elders* (LG): 165. LG is the most famous medical work of the Zurlug (Zur lugs) school, or Southern Tradition, of Tibetan medicine, and is still widely used by medical students today. This sophisticated commentary on the *Four Tantras* addresses medical knowledge and philosophical debates from a variety of schools of Tibetan medical and religious thought, using Tibetan sources dating back to the eleventh century and translated Indian sources as well.

[10] FT: 23; CLARK 1995: 58.

ance' (*gzi mdangs*) of the body caused by the metabolised essence of the reproductive substance; the movement of the breath; and the digestive fire of the body (TP: 102). When these functions are discontinued, death results. The vitality channels therefore refer to the activity of these three functions in sustaining life.

Pervading the entire body, the first of the three vitality channels is the body's digestive fire (*me drod*), which separates and refines the essential nutrients and wastes during the digestive process, thereby maintaining the function of all the bodily constituents that ultimately produce the body's radiant sentience.

The second vitality channel is the 'innate wisdom' (*ye shes*) wind that accompanies respiration. The innate wisdom wind is distinguished from the karmic (*las*) wind; the *Transmission of the Elders* explains that the karmic winds are those breaths that move in and out of the nostrils regularly, whereas the innate wisdom wind is the special type of wind that is only controlled through advanced yogic manipulations (TP: 103). If the totality of the innate wisdom wind is incorrectly circulated through the respiratory system, a person may become severely ill or die; for this reason these yogic practices are considered dangerous and are restricted to advanced contemplatives.

The third type of vitality channel is the body's 'life force' (*bla*), which is physiologically defined as the distilled essence of the body's reproductive substance, the refined substance that results from the total metabolic system that creates each of the bodily constituents. This life force is said to migrate throughout the body along a predictable track over the duration of a month, although the precise course of this track differs according to the various tantras, medical texts and astrological texts in which this subject is discussed in detail.

Another important channel described in the *Four Tantras* tradition is the life channel (*srog rtsa*). This channel is not named in the *Explanatory Tantra*'s fourfold functional division of channels, enumerated in that book's fourth chapter, described above, but it is mentioned in the context of embryology, in the *Explanatory Tantra*'s second chapter. That chapter states that the life channel develops from the navel during the sixth week of gestation. The identification of this life channel in relation to the other circulatory channels operative in adult physiology was, and still is, hotly contested among medical and religious scholars. Some medical scholars claimed that this life channel corresponds to the black blood channel;[11] still others claimed it was the white channel or the spine itself.[12] Describing Lodro Gyalpo's position on this issue, Tsultrim Gyaltsen posits that the life channel that initiates embryonic growth is to be identified as the central channel (*dbus ma*) of the tantric traditions; these scholars state that the two terms are thus synonymous for the same circulatory function.

### The Circulatory Channels in Tibetan Buddhist Traditions

The definition and enumeration of the circulatory channels is clearly a matter of controversy in medical and religious texts from the origins of these literary and scholastic disciplines in Tibet to the present date. Descriptive explication of the human psychosomatic body is certainly one of the most complex and heavily theorised topics in Buddhist medical *and* religious scholasticism. In the twelfth century, the Sakya master Drapa Gyaltsen (Grags pa rGyal mtshan, 1147-1216) wrote that it is vitally important for religious practitioners to know about the body because the body is the basis for meditation practice. He cites the *Sampuṭi* tantra to say that, '[Even if you know all] the rituals of the 84,000 divisions of the *dharma*, without knowing the nature of the body none of those [teachings] would have any effect.'[13] Attempting contemplative practices without a clear understanding of the body, Drapa Gyaltsen continues, is like trying to milk an animal by tugging at its horns.

In Tibetan tantric contemplative systems, the basis of human physiology is the subtle architecture of channels, winds and quintessential essences (*rtsa, rlung* and *thig le*) and the four, five or six channel nexuses or wheels (*'khor lo*).[14] While tantric systems vary to some degree, in general the locations and

---

[11] TG: 85 attributes this position to the medical scholar Tashi Bum (bKra shis 'Bum), a student of Situ Panchen (Si tu Pan chen), who wrote a commentary on the *Four Tantras*.

[12] LG: 132 does not identify these scholars by name.

[13] Grags pa rGyal mtshan: *rGyud kyi mngon par rtogs pa rin po che'i ljon shing* (in: CW, vol. 3, 60a-b).

[14] In a system of physiology derived from Indian tantric texts, the term *rtsa* is equivalent

functions of the three channels are agreed upon. The central channel (*dbu ma*, Skt. *suṣumṇā-*) runs through the centre of the wheels from the genitals to the crown of the head. Control over the entry of the winds into the central channel and their maintenance within that channel, which is ordinarily empty, is the objective of many of the most advanced tantric contemplative practices.

Running vertically through the centre of the body to the left and right of the central channel are the solitary channel (*rkyang ma*, Skt. *piṅgalā-*) and the flavour channel (*ro ma*, Skt. *iḍā-*) respectively. The white-coloured solitary channel, along the left, is said to face downward, and the red-coloured flavour channel, on the right, is said to face upward. The upper tips of these two channels connect at the nostrils, and it is through these channels that ordinary respiration travels. The bottom ends of these two channels approach the lower tip of the central channel, but ordinarily they do not enter the central channel; it is the aim of many advanced tantric practices to cause the ends of the right and left channels to touch the central channel so that the respiration may enter the central channel during the course of contemplative practice. The lower tips of the right and left channels are also associated with expelling waste matter from the body: in men and women of good health, urine emerges from the solitary channel and, for women, menstrual blood from the flavour channel. The central channel is similarly associated with the release of reproductive fluids (TP: 107).

Many volumes of text in Indian and Tibetan literature are occupied by discussion of the three channels, their functions, their relationship to other aspects of the body psychologically and physiologically, and the techniques for controlling their functions during meditative practice. Nonetheless, in the dialogue between medical and religious traditions over the centuries, the existence of these three channels is questioned. Lodro Gyalpo cites an unidentified

---

to terms for 'channels' variously named *nāḍī-*, *sirā-/śirā-*, *srotas-* or *dhamanī-* in Sanskrit, *rlung* in general is equivalent to the terms for 'winds', *prāṇa-* or *vāyu-* in Sanskrit, and *thig le*, often translated into English as 'drops' but here translated as 'quintessential essences', is equivalent to the Sanskrit *bindu-*, *tilaka-* or *śukra-*. Different traditions of Tibetan Buddhist tantra have different ways of describing these physiological substances and functions, a complex topic that extends beyond the scope of this article.

Vajrayāna scholar to assert that the tantric presentation of three channels is a trope developed to enhance contemplative practice, and that in fact the three channels do not exist in the body (LG: 132). Summarising Lodro Gyalpo's argument, Tsultrim Gyaltsen asks how a transformative effect could possibly occur as a result of completing such tantric practices if the three channels did not even exist in the body (TG: 88). Other unidentified scholars claimed that if these three channels really existed, they ought to be clearly visible in a cadaver. Again Tsultrim Gyaltsen points out that many elements of the body, such as aspects of the bodily constituents or forces of illness, are invisible, and yet their effects prove their existence (TG: 89).

## The Reality of these Controversies Today

These very debates echoed still in the seminar rooms of the International Academic Conference on Tibetan Medicine held in Lhasa in 2000. Scholars questioned their ability to "prove" the material existence of channels that have no apparent physical correlate in anatomical dissection, and physicians wondered whether Tibetan medicine should simply abandon discussion of such channels, since they have no obvious bearing on physical outcomes of medical interventions. Within the halls of Lhasa's Tibetan medical college and premier clinical institution, *Mentsikhang* (*sMan rtsis khang*), there is a growing tension between those scholars who remain committed to explications of Tibetan medicine that require acceptance of the three channels, and those who do not.

Many of these controversies have heightened importance today as *Mentsikhang* and Medical College scholars attempt to modernise their medical traditions by borrowing from and entering into dialogue with Western medicine. Curious about the medical writings addressing the contested topic of the circulatory system at present, the authors of this article made inquiries with Tibetan scholars in Lhasa. When the renowned medical historian and former director of Lhasa's *Mentsikhang*, Jampa Trinlay, was asked about the status of controversies over the three channels in Tibetan medicine, he commented that the debate has been resolved, conclusively, by the famous medical scholar Tsultrim Gyaltsen. He directed us to Dr. Gyaltsen's skillfully expressed and beautifully written scholarly article, translated below, appearing in a Tibetan volume of essays on medical research published in the late 1990s. Tsultrim Gyaltsen, one of the twentieth century's greatest Buddhist scholars of the Sakya school, also a distinguished scholar of medicine and highly regarded physician on staff at the *Mentsikhang*, passed away in Lhasa in 2001.

Tsultrim Gyaltsen divides his article, 'A Clear Explanation of the Principal Structure and Location of the Circulatory Channels as Illustrated in the Medical Paintings', (= TG) into three main sections. First, he briefly refers his readers to the paintings themselves. Second, the bulk of the article is devoted to a discussion of how the medical and tantric traditions explain the presence of the three channels in the human body. Finally, he addresses some additional scholastic debates about the role of the channels in the medical and tantric traditions. He relies heavily throughout the article on the views of Lodro Gyalpo, repeating many of the sixteenth-century scholar's arguments and citing many of the same scriptures.

Tsultrim Gyaltsen's position is that the medical tradition and the tantric tradition are ultimately in agreement on the existence of the three channels in the human body. Because medical texts address most centrally the healing of illness, however, the topic of the three channels is therefore only alluded to in the medical tradition, and it is within tantric texts, which teach meditation practices that are explicitly involved with the subtle body, that the three channels are explained at length. Tsultrim Gyaltsen insists, contrary to alternative opinions, that the presentation of the body found in tantric texts describes the ultimately true condition of the body, and that the Tibetan medical texts are in full agreement with that presentation.

## The Circulatory System in Tibetan Medical Paintings

TG begins as an explication of the traditional Tibetan anatomical medical paintings. This famous series of eighty medical paintings (*sman thang*) was commissioned by Desi Sangye Gyatso, the prolific regent of the Fifth Dalai Lama, founder of the *Chakpori* (*lCags po ri*) medical college in Lhasa, and author of the *Blue Beryl* (= SG), completed in 1688, a *Four Tantras* commentary that is very similar, and even at times identical, to LG. This series of medical paintings has been beautifully published with English annotations in DOR-

JE/MEYER 1992. There are a number of anatomical and physiological paintings in this collection. Paintings seven and eight include front and back views detailing gross skeletal anatomy; paintings nine, ten and eleven portray front and back views of the circulatory system. The twelfth painting depicts the locations and movements of the vitality channels (*tshe'i rtsa*).

As an example of what such depictions look like, on the following page an image from a thangka hanging in the Medical History Museum of the Factory of Tibetan Medicines, Nyangre Road, Lhasa, is reproduced; it depicts channels in the body. Unfortunately, the coloured original can only be reproduced here in black and white, with grey shades. A more detailed version of this image can be seen in AVEDON/MEYER/BOLSOKHOEVA/GERASIMOVA/BRADLEY 1998: 84.

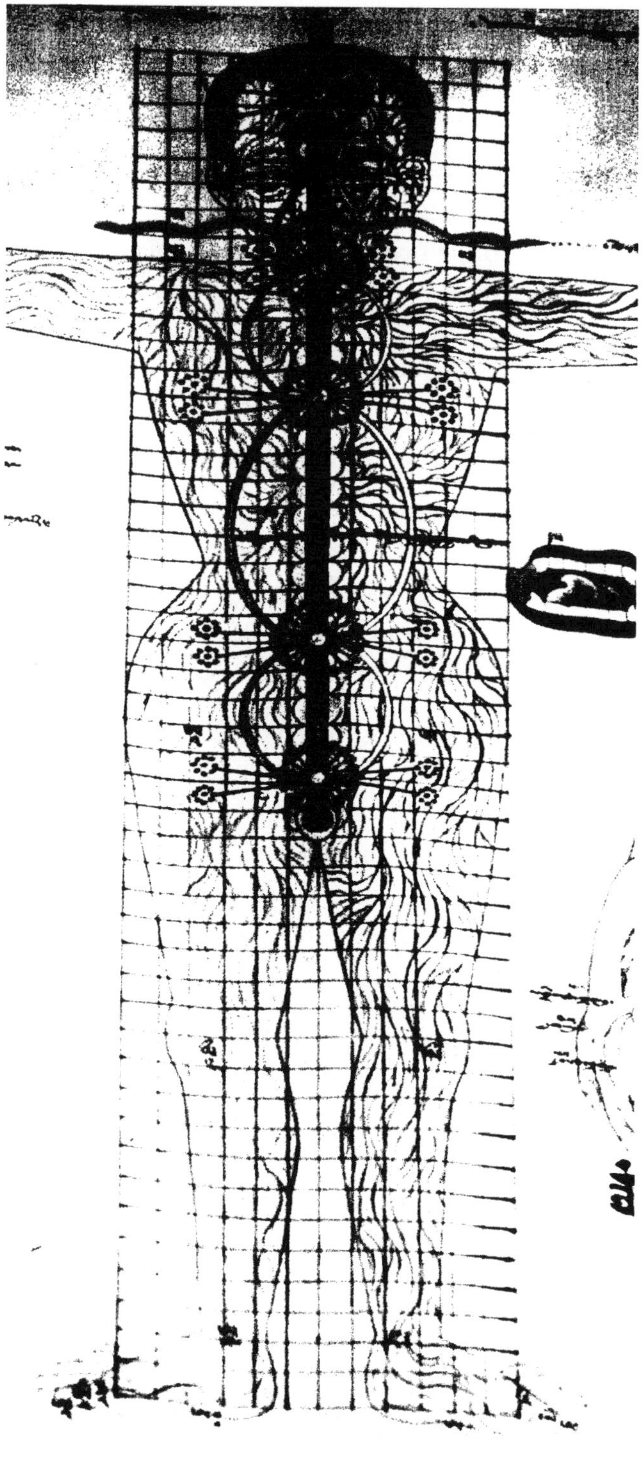

## *A Clear Explanation of the Principal Structure and Location of the Circulatory Channels as Illustrated in the Medical Paintings*

TSULTRIM GYALTSEN

Increase, decrease and disturbance of the humours, involving the natural elements, are external illnesses;
Disharmony of the bodily elements (*khams*), involving the channels, quintessential essences and winds, are internal illnesses;
Illusory cognitions, involving the three poisons, are secret illnesses.
I pay homage to the Medicine King, whose activities dispel all [these illnesses] without exception.[15]

Throughout the ages, many commentaries have been written on the *Four Tantras,* which is the principle text of the multitudinous scriptures of the Tibetan science of healing and the oral teachings of the Medicine Buddha, of Yuthog, and of an ocean-like assembly of sages. In particular, Miwang Pandita Sangye Gyatso gathered the best parts of the early commentaries and, skilfully drawing out the thoughts of Zurkhar [Lodro Gyalpo] on the earlier and later [commentaries], he wrote the commentary *Blue Beryl* [= SG]. In addition, he established the eighty medical paintings (*sman thang*) – an illustrated display of the phases of the basis [of illness, that is, the body], the symptoms [of illness], and the [methods of] healing, and a diagrammatic display of all the Accomplished Ones.[16] From among those, in order to identify the basis – where does illness enter [into the body]? – and the object – how is it treated? – according to the *Explanatory Tantra*'s teaching about the natural condition[17]

[15] In the first line of this introductory verse, *'phel zad 'khrugs* is a threefold expression in Tibetan medicine that refers to the increase (*'phel*), decrease (*zad*), and disturbance (*'khrugs*) of humours in the body, which causes illness. This topic is discussed in the eleventh chapter of the *Explanatory Tantra*.

[16] The medical paintings are ornamentally framed with images of Buddhas important to the medical tradition and with images of legendary and historical figures that played significant roles in the transmission of medical texts.

[17] We translate *gnas lugs* here as 'natural condition' – although it could also be 'basic condition', 'natural state', 'mode of abiding', etc. – rather than as 'anatomy', as is used by Barry Clark and other translators of medical texts, because the latter term has a historical meaning

of the body achieved [in a human birth], I will explain a bit about the natural condition of the circulatory channels. Here there are three [topics]: an introduction to the meaning of the illustrations, how these relate to scholastic theories, and a clarification of misconceptions therein.

### One: The Meaning of the Illustrations

We can understand this from the clear explanations labelling the illustrations of the eleventh and twelfth medical paintings.

### Two: Relating the Paintings to Scholastic Theory

Such illustrations are themselves the means by which scholars explained the meaning of the tantras in detail. Thus, because it is the case that having channels and wheels *is* the condition of the actual body, the presentation of the three channels and four wheels is explained in the medical tantras as well. If I were actually to explain all the terminology and theories – such as the names [of the channels], the uma (*dbu ma*)[18] and so forth, and the activities that generate innate wisdom (*ye shes*), and so on – for which the Vajrayāna traditions (*gsang sngags*) are well known, however, [then my presentation] would be confused with that of the highest tantras of Vajrayāna.

In general, then, all saṃsāric manifestations emerge from the channels, quintessential essences and winds within [the body], and the medical tantras and Vajrayāna tantra classes agree on the gross nature of the channels, winds, and quintessential essences of the body. The medical texts, which primarily explain the treatment of illnesses that emerge in the bodily elements via the increase, decrease and disturbance [of the humours], and the therapies that instigate physical health, are the ordinary sciences (*rig gnas*). [84][19] Therefore, because these [medical teachings] are *not* the teachings of the great secret path in

specific to Western medicine.

[18] The central channel.

[19] Page numbers for the Tibetan text are inserted in square brackets, representing the beginning of a new page in the Tibetan original.

which realisation is generated in the mind through having penetrated the key points of the body, [nothing is explained in the medical texts] other than that which is relevant to the healing of disease. The channels and so on – as that with which realisation is generated about the path, such as the way of bringing those [channels, winds and quintessential essences] to the path by utilising them skillfully, mantra, samādhi, the clairvoyance of knowing others' minds, and the appearance of exalted bodies and pure lands; and about the fruit[20] – are not necessary to explain here [in full, in the context of medicine], although they *are* referred to indirectly [in the medical texts]. The manner of formation and the functions that are explained in the Vajrayāna are *ultimately* the natural condition of the body. If [the nature of the body] were explained in the context of medicine in a way that *disagreed* with that [tantric presentation], this would be as irrational as classifying the features of an ox without [mentioning] its black dewlap. As Sakya Pandita[21] says:

> When explaining the natural condition
> Or classifying the features [of the body],
> If you were to present it such that it were not the *real* condition,
> How could you satisfy the scholars?

It would also be unreasonable [to offer a medical account of the body that disagrees with the tantras, because if the medical and tantric traditions were to disagree], there would be a contradictory relationship within the Tibetan scholastic traditions.[22]

---

[20] In the traditional Buddhist threefold categorisation of basis, path, and fruit (*gzhi*, *lam*, *'bras bu*), the subtle body is considered here to be the basis. The author is referring to a series of tantric practices that involve manipulation of the substances and energies of the subtle body.

[21] Sakya Pandita (Sa skya Pan di ta kun dga' rgyal mtshan, 1182-1251), one of the five great Sakya forefathers, was a prolific Tibetan scholar with a large corpus that includes several medical texts. We were unable to locate the source text for this citation.

[22] Tsultrim Gyaltsen explains here that because both the Buddhist tantras and the medical texts fall within the main Tibetan "sciences", therefore they cannot state contradictory positions. This is expressed as further evidence for why the medical and religious texts must be fundamentally in agreement.

The two mighty scholars, Jang and Zur,[23] explained this [issue] in a preliminary way, and their successors, such as Miwang Pandita[24] and Darmo Menrampa,[25] established it as their own system and wrote commentaries that analysed its subtleties. In particular, Mipham Rinpoche,[26] an actualisation of Mañjuśrī, in a commentary on the difficult points of the *Explanatory Tantra* negated the position of those who say that there are no channels and wheels in the body, and that it is illogical to include channels and wheels in the context of medicine. [Mipham] held to the theories of his own system, that of Zurkhar [Lodro Gyalpo] and his later successors. Having written this special explanation in which the manner of teaching the formation, abiding, and functions of the channel and wheels was established textually by the evidence of scriptures and reasoning, all the scholars who understood the rationale accepted it without argument.

Now, if you wonder where and how this [topic] is referred to in the [medical] texts, [it is as follows]. [The *Explanatory Tantra*] states: 'In the sixth [week of embryogenesis or gestation], the life (*srog*) channel is formed in dependence upon the navel.'[27] It is also stated [in the *Explanatory Tantra*]: 'There are three channels of formation that extend from the navel.'[28] Therefore, three channels *are* referred to [in the medical texts, and these are] the central channel (*dbu ma*) and so on. That which is called the 'life channel'

---

[23] Jangpa Namgyal Draksang (Byang pa rNam rgyal Grags bzang, 1395-1475) and Zurkar Nyamnyid Dorje (Zur mkhar mNyam nyid rDo rje, 1439-1475), the two founders of the so-called Northern and Southern schools of Tibetan medicine.

[24] Desi Sangye Gyatso. Praise of his name has been recently banned in Lhasa, so the author is referring to him obliquely as the 'Administrator-Scholar'

[25] Darmo Menrampa (Dar mo sMan rams pa blo bzang chos grags, 1638-1710), a medical scholar and the physician of the Fifth Dalai Lama.

[26] Jamgon Ju Mipham Gyatso ('Jam mgon 'Ju Mi pham rGya mtsho, 1846-1912), a famous religious thinker of the nonsectarian movement who has also written widely on medicine.

[27] FT: 18; CLARK 1995: 50.

[28] FT: 22; CLARK 1995: 56.

(*srog pa rtsa*) is the central channel, and it is the basis that connects the white and black life channels – the two channels, the [right side] flavour (*ro ma*) and the [left side] solitary (*rkyang ma*). According to [the following scriptural] citation [from the *Four Tantras*], the four wheels are indicated [in the medical texts as well]:[29]

> There are four types of great channels of existence (*srid pa*): the channel that causes the sense organs to apprehend their objects, located in the brain and surrounded by 500 tiny existence channels; the channel that causes clarity of the faculty of memory, located at the heart and surrounded by 500 tiny existence channels; the channel that causes the aggregates of the body to grow, located at the navel and surrounded by 500 tiny existence channels; and the channel that causes the family lineage to grow, located at the sexual organs and surrounded by 500 existence channels. These channels run straight up and down, holding together all the [various aspects] of the body.

Because the scholars previously mentioned have surveyed this topic in a mostly unified way in the scriptural and commentarial works, here, because it would be tedious to describe so many texts, I will [continue to] hold the *Explanatory Tantra* as the basis of discussion in these notes. [85] In order to better understand the citation from the aforementioned text, [the *Explanatory Tantra,* which states:] 'In the sixth [week of embryogenesis], the life channel is formed in dependence upon the navel', I will offer some additional information using eloquent commentarial accounts that also present [teachings on this topic]. In tantra classes such as the *Kālacakra*, [the transmigrating consciousness'] entry into the womb is taught according to the model of the ten incarnations of Viṣṇu, whereas here [in the medical texts], the functions of the winds and so forth are taught according to the Bodhisattva collections.[30] Alternatively, [embryogenesis is sometimes presented in the tantras] in three stages: the

---

[29] FT: 22; CLARK 1995: 57.

[30] In this case 'Bodhisattva collections' (*Byang chub sems dpa'i sde snod*) refers to Mahāyāna texts in general, being contrasted here to tantric texts. In particular, the Bodhisattvas Manjuśrī, Avalokiteśvara and Tārā are said to have authored medical texts; see RABGAY 1981.

fish, tortoise, and pig stages.[31] With regards to that, some scholars, such as Trabum[32], claim that the life channel is the black blood channel, and that the description of the central channel and so forth in the Vajrayāna tantra classes are *not* actually presented here [in the medical texts]. While the presentation of topics such as the central, flavour, and solitary channels have not been taught *in detail* according to the tantra classes, they *are* indicated indirectly [in the medical texts]. The [medical texts] are not like the treatises of the non-Buddhists, which contain *no* doctrine in which the very subtle key points of tantra are realised, but in fact, the [medical texts] are special oral teachings of the Vidyādhara of emptiness, the sages, and the Medicine Buddha, and [the topic of the circulatory system] is a topic that is taught just exactly like the [topic of the] body as established by those [great masters]. [The medical teachings] are not a *new* contemplative tradition in which there is no [spiritual] progress via the central, flavour, and solitary channels, nor any existence of those in the body, because, [to the contrary,] it is due to penetrating these important points – the channels, winds and quintessential essences that naturally exist in the Vajra body – that there is realisation, spontaneous and naturally emergent.

We may clarify this by taking up the later Zurkhar's[33] own system, [as follows]. Our subject is the [*Four Tantras*'] statement that the life channel emer-

[31] Some Indian and Tibetan tantric texts, such as the *Guhyasamāja* and *Kālacakra* tantras, and the many exegetical systems that grew around these tantras in Tibet, describe the development of the embryo in either three or ten stages. In the three-stage scheme, the embryo grows through a 'fish' stage, a 'tortoise' stage, and a 'pig' stage, each period comprising roughly a trimester of foetal development. In the ten-stage scheme, gestation is divided into ten month-long gestational periods named for the ten incarnations of Viṣṇu, the first two of which are the fish and the tortoise. Although these Indian tantric sources were available to Tibetan authors as they began to compose their own embryologies, interestingly there was little consistency across Tibetan literature when describing the stages of foetal development. Thus the three- or ten-stage schemes are but two of several methods for documenting gestation in Tibet. See GARRETT 2005.

[32] Trabum (bKra 'bum; dates unknown) was a medical scholar and author of a commentary to the *Four Tantras*, and a student of Situ Panchen.

[33] The 'later Zurkhar' refers to Zurkhar Lodro Gyalpo. At this point the author moves into the stylised form of Tibetan prose used in philosophical debate texts.

ges from the navel. The life channel is the central channel [for three reasons]: because it is the basis of the *a*-[syllable]-possessing life wind, because it is the life-tree[34] of the four or six wheels, and because it is the first of all the channels that are formed.

The first reason is proven by the *Avalokiteśvara Commentary*,[35] which states: 'Life (*srog*) is the kusuma (*ku su ma*) and it is called either "very empty" or "very pleasing".' It also asserts: 'Initially the basis of the formation of the body is the central channel together with the life wind.'

The second reason is proven by the *Saṃvarodaya* (*sDom 'byung*) and other tantras, which explain: 'It is located at the centre of all the channel-wheels, and it generates everything.' This claim is made because [the central channel] is said to be at the centre of the six wheels, 'running twelve finger-lengths in the middle and bending at the genitals and crown of the head.' It is also said that 'it travels through the middle of the lotus flower of the heart, it is empty like water and flowers, and it is a *ham*-syllable hanging face down.' The auto-commentary to the *Inner Meaning*[36] states: 'The basis of the life wind that generates the body is the central channel and so forth, and the basis of the consciousness (*kun gzhi'i rnam shes*) is the great life wind that exists in the cen-

---

[34] The life-tree (*srog shing*), or life pillar, is placed as an axis at the centre of a stūpa or a statue.

[35] *sPyan bzigs 'grel pa*. This text, commonly cited by the main early commentators of the *Four Tantras*, such as Lodro Gyalpo, may be a commentary on the *Kālacakra*, but we have not identified it. Its reference to *ku su ma*, generally understood to refer to saffron, is unclear.

[36] The Kagyu author Rangchung Dorje (Rang byung rDo rje, 1284-1339) wrote an auto-commentary to his *Profound Inner Meaning* (*Zab mo nang don)*, the *Zab mo nang gi don gsal bar byed pa'i 'grel pa*, publication data unknown. The *Profound Inner Meaning* (= PM), a text on yogic physiology and practice, is a commonly cited source in the important sixteenth-century *Four Tantras* commentary by Lodro Gyalpo. A source for fourteenth-century Tibetan views on the tantric body, this text contains twelve chapters, including topics such as the conception and formation of the body; explanations of the locations, functions, and movements of the channels, winds, and quintessential essences; the relationship of these to the consciousness; the link between the inner body and the external world; and the use of the subtle body features in contemplative practice.it is cited here from a xylographic print (1970?) from blocks preserved at Rum btegs (Rumtek) Karma chos sgar in Sikkim.

tral channel.' In this context the *Kālacakra* states: 'Above is Rāhu, below is the universe eater, and the root of all the winds is based on that.'[37]

The third reason is proven by the *Saṃpuṭi,* which states: 'It is located at the centre of the crown of the head, at the wheel, as an *e*-syllable. It is also located at the heart and throat, as a *bam*-syllable.'[38]

These names are assigned to the life channel [86] because it is the basis of the life wind and it is the channel that generates, sustains and dissolves the body. As it is said also by Saraha[39]: 'There is no doubt that when the winds and the respiration enter the great life channel, ordinary consciousness automatically stops.' Additional names include 'avadhūti' (*a wa dhu ti*), 'kusuma' (*ku su ma*), 'kundarma' (*kun 'dar ma*), 'subtle form' (*phra ba'i gzugs*), 'life channel' (*srog pa'i rtsa*), 'uma' (*dbu ma*), 'internal wood' (*nang gi shing gcig*), 'life thread' (*srog gi skud pa*), 'great path' (*lam po che*), 'downward-reaching great conch' (*mar snar dung can ma*), and 'upward- reaching Rāhu' (*yar snar sgra gcan*).

Now, to comment on the [*Four Tantras'*] statement that in the twenty-fifth [week of embryogenesis] the movement of winds occurs:[40] every one of those

---

37 In Hindu mythology Rāhu (sGra gcan) is known as a demon who tried to capture the sun and moon but was subdued, whereupon he became one of the planets; he is thus held responsible for eclipses. The 'universe eater' (*dus me*) is said to be one of three types of fire in Hindu mythology: fire for cooking; 'horse face fire' for evaporation; and the 'time fire' (*dus me*) that can burn the entire universe. The precise meaning of this citation is obscure, although it seems to refer at least generally to a moon-like element existing at the top of the central channel, in the area of the head, and a fire-like element existing at the bottom of the channel, in the area of the genitals. 'Moon' and 'fire' often refer to the male and female reproductive substance; cf. DAS 1992: 412, but also DAS 1992: 407 and DAS 2003: 521ff.

38 *Saṃpuṭi* is the *Sampuṭanāmamahātantra*, identified as Toh. 381 in UI 1934, and also as No. 26 in the Peking edition of the *Kangyur* (bKa' 'gyur).

39 Saraha is one of the great Indian *mahāsiddha*s and a master in the *mahāmudrā* lineage. This citation does not come from the *Do ha mdzod kyi glu*, Saraha's best known work in Tibetan, and we have not identified the source text.

40 This is a paraphrase of a verse from the *Explanatory Tantra* that explains when in gestation the respiration first begins to travel through the nostrils. FT: 19; CLARK 1995: 51.

winds merely branches out from the life wind. The channels generated throughout the entire body emerge from only the central or life channel. The *Saṃpuṭi* states: 'From the very limits of the feet to the crown of the head, from one to the other, a [connecting] thread occurs.' It is also said: 'The fact that the life wind emerges from the consciousness-element is something that must be known.'

[The *Explanatory Tantra*] explains that: 'There are three channels of formation that extend from the navel.'[41] As for the channels that produce the body, the navel wheel emits three separate tips. From among those, the channel in which water circulates, or the moon channel, proceeds along the left side of the body and gathers at the heart, throat, and crown of the head wheels. Expressed alternatively, this is the white channel, which, as it travels outwards, is the basis of the formation of the brain. The brain is the substantial cause (*nyer len*) and cooperative condition (*lhan cig byed rkyen*) of both ignorance and the phlegm humour. This is why it feels as if ignorance is located in the brain, and it also seems like dullness, heaviness, cloudiness and so forth emerge predominantly from the head. Phlegm is produced from ignorance, and therefore it is established that the causes, conditions, and results [of phlegm illnesses] reside in the upper part of the body.

The channel in which blood circulates, or the fire-element (*me khams*) channel, is transmitted along the right side of the body. It joins the channel that carries the nutritive essences (*dwangs ma*) at the great region of the liver in the middle of the body, and branching into two, it goes to the thirteenth vertebra; based on that, the black life channel and its branches develop. Blood is the substantial cause and cooperative condition of both hatred and the bile humour, and hatred occurs in dependence upon the black life channel and blood. Because bile is produced from hatred, the middle of the body is the location of its cause, condition and effect. Thus, when hatred is suddenly generated, it feels as if it has been stirred up and emitted from the middle of the body. That ac-

[41] FT: 22; CLARK 1995: 56. The following three paragraphs are closely borrowed from sections of the *Transmission of the Elders*'s commentary on the *Explanatory Tantra*'s verses on the channels of formation (LG: 145-184).

tual red channel that touches the middle is gathered at the centres of the wheels of the heart, the throat, and the crown of the head, and it is that which branches out throughout the body.

The channel in which wind circulates, or the wisdom-element (*ye shes kyi kham*) channel, goes directly straight up in the middle of the body. One end precisely touches the previous [right and left channels] at the bottom of the navel. From that, the secret place in which the bliss-element flows is formed. The wind [humour] is located in the lower part of the body and the quintessential essences are the substantial cause and cooperative condition of both desire-attachment (*'dod chags*) and the wind [humour]. For that reason, desire-attachment is based on the quintessential essences, [87] because the wind [humour] is produced from that desire-attachment. The causes, conditions, and effects [of wind diseases] are all located in the lower part of the body, and so, when desire-attachment is suddenly generated, it feels as if it has been stirred up and emitted from the lower part of the body.

So, the brain is the substantial cause of ignorance and phlegm, blood is the substantial cause of bile and hatred, and the quintessential essences are the substantial cause of desire-attachment and the wind [humour]. Therefore, the causes are the three afflictions, the conditions are the brain, blood and the quintessential essences, and the effects are the three humours; they are respectively located in the upper, middle and lower parts of the body. This explanation of the central channel and so forth is correct according to the system of Mati (Ma ti).[42]

Aside from this, another way of teaching the flavour and solitary channels is as presented in the commentary, which states: 'it moves through association with the breath.'[43] The karmic winds are the breaths that constantly move in the nostrils via the pathways of the flavour and solitary channels.[44] The innate

---

[42] This refers to the system of Zurkhar Lodro Gyalpo.

[43] The following explanation is directly modelled after LG's commentary on the *Explanatory Tantra* discussion of the life channels (LG: 145-184).

[44] Ordinary, or karmic (*las*), breath, or wind, is being contrasted to exalted, or innate wisdom (*ye shes*), breath.

wisdom winds travel through the central channel pathway. [These latter winds] divide into two, one of which produces the power of the life wind, and the other of which circulates by mixing with the karmic wind. When yogins hold that very wisdom wind, possessing the nature of life (*srog*), within [the central channel] by means of the 'vase' contemplative practice (*bum can sbyor*), immortality results.[45] Ordinary people, however, exhale the wisdom wind. One's lifespan is shortened when [the breath] flows outside continuously. It is said that if one were to circulate 21,600 [breaths] per day, one would die after that. This is explained in the *Profound Inner Meaning* as follows:

> The explanation of the external circulation [of the breath is as follows]:
> From among all the openings of the sense organs and body hairs,
> The two great channels travel through the nostrils,
> Which are the special openings through which breath circulates.
> On the right is the sun, the winds of the poisons, and
> On the left is the moon, nectar.
> These are the nature of 'means and wisdom' (*shes rab*).[46]
> The 10,462 and one half winds each day [through each nostril]
> Are known as the winds of the sun and moon.
> The 675 winds that move through the central channel between those two are [known as the]
> Winds of Rāhu, the sky, wisdom (*ye shes*), and
> The heart of non-duality.[47]

---

[45] The 'vase', 'jar' or 'pot' contemplative practice is a tantric practice in which the winds are gathered into the centre of the body such that one's abdomen is like a 'pot' or container for those winds. The related 'vase initiation' (Skt. *kalaśābhiṣeka-*), aimed at cleansing the channels, is a tantric ritual involving consecration and empowerment of a series of vases containing various substances. See SNELLGROVE 1987, 1: 223-227.

[46] The phrase 'means and wisdom' refers to the Mahāyāna Buddhist integrated approach to practice that joins 'skill in means' or 'skill in liberative technique' (Skt. *upāya-*), which is the efficacious expression of compassionate activity toward sentient beings, with 'wisdom' (Skt. *prajñā-*), which is the realisation of the true nature of all phenomena as empty of inherent existence.

[47] This citation is found in the fourth chapter of PM: 11b.1-11b.3.

The *Vajra Essence* commentary[48] also states: 'When the life wind enters the central channel for the period of a day and a night, disease will disappear. If the life wind is held [within the central channel] for fifteen days, a pure land (*mkha' spyod*) [contemplative state] is conferred. If the life wind is held at the heart for a month, the yogin will attain immortality.' The tantras also claim: 'Having held it equally at the top, bottom and middle, all the body will be filled by the winds. In seven days, death will be taken away.' And, it is said in the *Kālacakra*: 'The sun and the moon are blocked, and they proceed equally and unequally; fire will enter into the central channel; by both the life wind and the downward elimination wind, the sun travels [into the central channel], as a result of which one deceives death (*'chi blu*) in an untimely way.'[49]

In this context, the *Transmission of the Elders* and *Blue Beryl* are in agreement: the way the central channel forms up to and including the navel is presented in this way in the second chapter of the previously mentioned [text, the *Four Tantras*]. In addition, the citation, 'three channels of formation radiate out from the navel', indicates the solitary and flavour channels and the central channel up to below the navel. [88] The channel that produces phlegm and so forth is the [left side] solitary channel, in which the water-element moves; the channel that causes the production of bile and so forth is the [right side] flavour channel, in which the fire-element moves; and the channel that produces wind and so forth is that part of the central channel that goes up to the bottom of the navel and is the channel that contains the wind-element. The central channel touches the two lower ends of the right and left channels; the theories of the *Kālacakra* refer to this as three points of the channels at both the top and bottom of the navel. The primeval Buddha [text, the *Profound Inner Meaning*], explains:

The three tips [facing] downwards,
And likewise also the three tips [facing] up,
Exist as the middle of the Rāhu tip,
The right tip of the sun,

[48] We have been unable to identify to which text named *rDo rje snying* this citation refers.

[49] This citation is found in chapter four of the *Kālacakra* root text.

And the left tip of the moon.
From the right, left and middle lower ends,
[Which are respectively those of] the winds of water, fire, and space,[50]
Move faeces, urine, and reproductive fluids.
Channels that are like fastened shackles
Are the three pathways of existence and elimination.[51]

Finally, according to the great commentarial teachings that were revealed [by Mipham], all channels are summarised as a collection of three types: wind channels, blood channels and water channels. Moreover, it is reasonable to say that it is exclusively the case that all wind channels radiate out from the central channel, all blood channels radiate out from the [right side] flavour channel, and all water channels radiate out from the [left side] solitary channel.

If it is explained other than this, that is, if one makes a claim that goes against the theories of the subtle meaning of the tantras that explains the natural condition of the body's channels, then a thesis that invalidates the scriptures would be established. Therefore it is best to abandon personal arrogance and follow the experts.

### Three: Clarification of Misconceptions

Some writers claim that because the presentation of the channels and wheels is taught in the higher tantra classes such as the highest yoga tantra class (*bla na med pa'i rgyud*), it cannot be associated with medical texts. To the contrary it is quite suitable to do so because, for example, it is similar to instances when the power of medicines conquer illness in the non-Buddhist Vedic scriptures, the Vinaya scriptures, sūtras such as the *Golden Light*,[52] the

[50] In the Rumtek edition of PM, this line of the verse says *chu dang me dang nam mkha' rgyu*, whereas here the text says *chu dang me dang nam mkha' rlung*.

[51] In the Rumtek edition of PM, this line of the verse says *srog dang thur sel lam gsum nyid*, whereas here the text says *srid dang thur sel lam gsum nyid*. This citation is found in the third chapter of PM: 6a.6-6b.2.

[52] The *Golden Light* (*gSer 'od*) referred to here is a sūtra found in the Tibetan *Kangyur (bKa' 'gyur)*, known in Sanskrit most commonly as the *Suvarṇaprabhās(ottam)asūtra*; see SS. This sūtra contains a chapter on medicine. The entire text is translated in EMMERICK 1996.

Primeval Buddha [text, the *Kālacakra*], and tantras such as the *Cakrasaṃvara*. The explanation of how the body's actual structure is formed is systematised in the sūtras, tantras *and* the sciences, and all these presentations are the same. Moreover, when the issue is set forth as an object of logical establishment, manifestly it is not disproved by perceptual cognition; secretly, it is not disproved by inferential cognition; and very secretly, it is not disproved by scriptural cognition. Therefore it can be said that it is correctly proven.

Some writers claim that the channels and wheels that are explained in the tantra classes do not exist other than in meditation.[53] If they did *not* exist fully in the body, which is the Vajra basis for a secret *mantra* [practitioner], however, then what would be the transformed effect finally, after the contemplative has [completed the practice of] piercing the key points [of the body, if there were no channels originally]? This manner of objection is [89] quite unreasonable, because, as Sakya Pandita says: 'Those who make claims such as that the channel knots do not exist, are those who do not understand the theories of the tantra classes; they[, that is, the channels,] are very important.'

Some writers claim that according to the medical tantras' explanation of how the channels and wheels develop, they must not exist in the ordinary person's body. If they did, they ought to appear in a corpse, but since they do not, they should not be presented in the [texts of the medical] sciences. Although it is true that we cannot see them with our ordinary eyes, however, it cannot be proven that they do not exist just for that [reason]. If that were the case, it could be said that many other things in our bodies do not exist, like tiny insects, and illnesses, and aspects of the bodily constituents and wastes. Indeed, things that we previously could not see are visible [today] in reliance upon chemicals and scientific machines and so forth. There are countless objects of knowledge that cannot be understood by apprehending them [using the ordinary senses or new technologies], such as the very subtle secrets of the channels, winds and quintessential essences. It is therefore like the famous Dhar-

---

[53] Zurkhar Lodro Gyalpo addresses this same objection in LG: 132, with much the same conclusion. Tsultrim Gyaltsen's line of discussion in this section is closely modelled after this argument in LG.

makīrti said: 'It is not the case that things do not exist because we do not see them.' The channel structure itself is merely a proliferation of all channels of the body from the flavour, solitary and central channels; from among the many channels [of the body, those three] are the roots, and they are the main channels that cause the generation, growth and abiding of the body, above and below. As one takes to heart the way this expansion occurs, it is drawn like a map, and so as soon as it is experienced just like this, there is no need to see it. In addition, about the central channel the tantras declare: 'Because the central channel is the channel of wisdom (*ye shes*), it pervades all channels.' The *Tantra of the Union*[54] states: 'A channel lies along the centre, with the capacity for clarity or obscurity [depending on the abilities of the observer], indivisible and extremely tiny.' The *Mahāyoga* (*rNal 'byor chen po*) tantra identifies it as 'the finest of the fine, supremely excellent'. For this reason it is said that ordinary people cannot see [the channels].

The proofs that have been established here are described in brief, and they should be expanded upon elsewhere.

For whomever is suffering bodily pain,
What else is there than medicine, the most excellent protective friend?
For this reason beings uphold, preserve and spread this science,
Making efforts for the benefit of others.

The science of medicine, the excellent essence of the ocean of the Buddha's word and the commentarial treatises,
The jewel that is the lord of the Nāgas, sages and Vidyādharas,
(The victorious wish-fulfilling lord, the glorious *Four Tantras*), was
Offered to this land by that supreme guide, Yuthog.

Pray by this excellent tradition,

[54] This text's title is here simply rendered as *Kha sbyor*. LG quotes this same citation, calling the text, *kun tu Kha sbyor*. There are also a tantra known as *Kha sbyor* with the full title *rNal 'byor ma bzhi'i kha sbyor gyi rgyud ces bya ba*, No. 24 in the Peking canon; a text, *'Phrul 'khor nyi zla kha sbyor gyi rtsa 'grel*, by Vairocana (Pe cin: Mi rigs dpe skrun khang 1993); the *Kha sbyor brtag pa bcu'i don bshad pa* by Kun dga' snying po (1092-1158), published in the *Sa skya'i gsung 'bum* (ed. rDo rje Rin chen and Nor bu Kun 'grub, Lan kru'u: Kan su'u mi rigs dpe skrun khang 1994), vol. 1: 454-476. We have not identified the source of this citation.

Displayed at the tip of the victory banner of faith, without confusion.
Those fortunate ones who satisfy the welfare, happiness, and desires of themselves and others
Practise the glorious [*Four Tantras*].

Although you are born as the inheritor of such an excellent jewel,
When you turn the mind toward mere stones,
Verbally refuting [the medical tradition], citing hundreds of faults,
Why make vows to these lineage holders?

The land of snows shines radiantly as the holder of merit.
The science of medicine is a river, and the great compendium of tantras is the ocean;
The analysis of difficult issues is invoked by the winds –
Observe the play of movement of the waves in their eloquent explanations.

Those who are mistaken do not consider the Buddhas and Bodhisattvas to be genuine,
And they thereby establish that which is not deluded to be deluded.
Do not entrust yourself to such people!
Maintain accordingly the medical scriptures and the thought of the Medicine King.

## Bibliography and Abbreviations

AVEDON, John F.; MEYER, Fernand; BOLSOKHOEVA, N.D.; GERASIMOVA, K.M.; BRADLEY, Tamdin Sither 1998: *The Buddha's Art of Healing. Tibetan Paintings Rediscovered.* New York: Rizzoli Publications.

CLARK, Barry 1995: *The Quintessence Tantras of Tibetan Medicine.* Ithaca, NY: Snow Lion Publications.

CW = *The Complete Works of the Great Masters of the Sa skya Sect of the Tibetan Buddhism.* Compiled by Bsod Nams Rgya Mtsho. Tokyo: The Toyo Bunko 1968-1969. Bibliotheca Tibetica 1.

DAS, Rahul Peter 1992: 'Problematic Aspects of the Sexual Rituals of the Bauls of Bengal', *Journal of the American Oriental Society* 112,3: 388-432.

—— 2003: *The Origin of the Life of a Human Being. Conception and the Female According to Ancient Indian Medical and Sexological Literature.* Delhi: Motilal Banarsidass. Indian Medical Tradition 6.

DASGUPTA, Surendranath 1975: *A History of Indian Philosophy.* Volume 2. Delhi: Motilal Banarsidass.

DORJE, Gyurme; MEYER, Fernand (ed.) 1992: *Tibetan Medical Paintings. Illustrations to the Blue Beryl Treatise of Sangye Gyamtso (1653-1705)*. 2 vols. New York: Harry N. Abrams 1992.

DUMMER, Tom 1988: *Tibetan Medicine and Other Holistic Health Care Systems*. New Delhi: Paljor Publications 1994.

EMMERICK, R.E. 1996: *The Sūtra of Golden Light. Being a Translation of the Suvarṇabhāsottamasūtra*. 3rd (revised) edition. Oxford: The Pali Text Society 1996.

FT: Lhasa 2000 edition of the *Four Tantras*; see note 5.

GARRETT, Frances 2005: 'Ordering Human Growth in Tibetan Medical and Religious Embryologies', in: Elizabeth Lane Furdell (ed.), *Textual Healing. Essays on Medieval and Early Modern Medicine*. Leiden: Brill, pp. 32-52.

GYATSO, Janet 2004: 'The Authority of Empiricism and the Empiricism of Authority: Medicine and Buddhism in Tibet on the Eve of Modernity', *Comparative Studies of South Asia, Africa and the Middle East* 24,2: 83-96.

LG = Lodro Gyalpo (Zur mkhar bLos gros rGyal po): *rGyud bzhi'i 'grel pa mes po'i shal lung*. Lhasa: Khrung go'i pod kyi shes rig dpe skrun khang 1991.

PM = *Profound Inner Meaning*; see note 36.

RABGAY, Lobsang 1981: 'The Origin and Growth of Medicine in Tibet', *Tibetan Medicine* 3: 10f.

SG = Desi Sangye Gyatso (sDe srid Sangs rgyas rGya mtsho): *gSo ba rig pa'i bstan bcos sman bla'i dgongs rgyan rgyud bzhi'i gsal byed baidur sngon po'i malli ka zhes bya ba bzhugs so*. Dharamsala: Tibetan Medical & Astro Institute 1994.

SNELLGROVE, David 1987: *Indo-Tibetan Buddhism. Indian Buddhists and their Tibetan Successors*. Boston: Shambala.

SS = *'Phags pa Gser 'od dam pa mdo sde'i dbaṅ po'i rgyal po źes bya ba theg pa chen po'i mdo. The Suvarṇaprabhāsottamasūtrendrarāja-nāma-mahāyānasūtra in its Tibetan Translation by Paṇḍita Jinamitra, Śīlendrabodhi, and the Locchava Bande Ye-śes-sde*. Reproduced from a print from Zur-maṅ Rdo Dgon-pa Thub-bstan-'phel-rgyas-chos-gliṅ prepared by Ras-sprul Karma-mkhyen-rab-phun-tshogs. Bir, H.P.: D. Tsondru Senghe 1984.

SVOBODA, Robert; LADE, Arnie 1999: *Chinese Medicine and Ayurveda*. Delhi: Motilal Banarsidass 1999.

TG = Tsultrim Gyaltsen (Tshul khrim rGyal mtshan): 'sMan thang las 'brel pa rtsa yi gnas lugs kyi dpe ris skor gsal bar bshad pa', in: *Krung go'i mtho rim bod sman shib 'jug bgro gleng 'dzin grwa'i rtsom yig gces bsdus*. [Lhasa]: Bod rang skyong ljongs sman rtsis khang n.d. (probably in the late 1990's), pp. 83-91.

TP = Thubten Phuntsok (Thub bstan Phun tshogs): *Gso bya lus kyi rnam bshad*. Pe cin: Mi rigs dpe skrun khang 1999.

UI, Hakuju (ed.) 1934: *A Complete Catalogue of The Tibetan Buddhist Canons (Bkaḥ.-ḥgyur and Bstan-ḥgyur)*. Sendai: Tôhoku Imperial University.

# Sound and the Musician's Body*

MAKOTO KITADA

As mentioned in KITADA 2003, the musicological work *Saṅgītaratnākara* (= SR) of Śārṅgadeva treats human anatomy in its section 1,2 (*Piṇḍotpattiprakaraṇa*). It explains the anatomical process of vocal production in the human body in verses 3-10ab of section 1,3 (*Nādasthānaśrutisvarajātikuladaivatarṣicchandorasaprakaraṇa*). According to these verses, sound/voice (*nāda-*) arises through the following process: the abdominal fire drives the vital wind upwards; the vital wind strikes the twenty-two tubes (*nāḍī-*) which, radiating from the heart, stretch obliquely or horizontally within the rib cage;[1] through this, the twenty-two microtones, of which the octave consists, are produced. In this presentation the human body seems to be compared to a string instrument, or *vīṇā-* (harp[2]). The striking of the tubes by the vital wind corresponds to the plucking of the catgut strings of a harp by the fingers of a musician.[3]

Thus, the twenty-two microtones constituting the octave are explained as being a result of the human organism. The dramaturgical work *Bhāvaprakāśana*, which also contains passages on musical theory, even considers vocal manifestation to be a result of metabolism, in associating these microtones with the twenty-two vessels (*sirā-*) carrying the seven body elements (*dhātu-*) arising in the transformative process of metabolism.

By mentioning abdominal fire, vital wind and tubes radiating from the

---

* I express my thanks to Ms. Kazuyo Sakaki (Hokkaido) and Mr. John Perkins (Halle) for their significant suggestions on this article.

[1] SR 1,3,8cd-9:
*hṛdy ūrdhvanāḍīsaṃlagnā nāḍyo dvāviṃśatir matāḥ* (8cd)
*tiraścyas tāsu tāvatyaḥ śrutayo mārutāhateḥ*
*uccoccataratāyuktāḥ prabhavanty uttarottaram* (9)

[2] The term *vīṇā-* can denote various kinds of instruments. In the SR presentation referred to here, a bow-shaped harp is dealt with.

[3] For further information, see LATH 1978: 197-203.

heart, the SR seems to refer to the Haṭhayoga system. But the *Bhāvaprakāśana* is based on the Āyurvedic theory of metabolism and seven body elements (*dhātu-*), although works on Āyurveda neither mention these twenty-two vessels, nor contain the theory associating them with the twenty-two microtones. Indeed, this is a theory which could have been fabricated by the *Bhāvaprakāśana* itself in an Āyurvedic garb. But however this might be, in order to explain the association of sound and the human body, it is worthy of note that the two works on music rely on Haṭhayoga on the one hand and Āyurveda on the other.

## Division of the Octave

Let us now investigate the character and function of the microtone theory in ancient Indian music. The works on musical theory in Sanskrit usually divide the octave into twenty-two microtones (*śruti-*). Even today, Indian musicologists of the classical tradition refer to this division of twenty-two, despite the fact that we do not have any proof at all as to whether the modern interpretation of this theory is really the same as was originally intended. For a drastic change took place in Indian musical theory during the end of the first millennium A.D., and on a practical level the theory of the twenty-twofold division became obsolete.[4]

According to GOMPERTS 2002, the original character of this theory and its intended original function seem to have been as follows: This tuning system was a 22-tone equal temperament. I quote GOMPERTS 2002: 574: 'In early Indian music theory, the concept of a basic tuning system consists of 22 *śruti*-intervals. There were two primary scales (Sk. grāma) with seven tones (Sk. saptasvara) which consisted of interval sequences of 2-, 3-, and 4-*śruti*-intervals.' The concept of consonance and dissonance is defined by the difference in the microtonal intervals (*śruti-*). Consonant intervals (*saṃvādin-*) are defined as consisting of nine *śruti*-s (i.e. a fourth) and thirteen *śruti*-s (i.e. a fifth). Dissonant intervals (*vivādin-*), or intervals which are perceived as dissonant, are

[4] Or, musicians began to interpret it in a different manner

defined as consisting of two and twenty *śruti*-s: '… the Indian concepts of consonance and dissonance relations were observed by the ear and expressed in *śruti* intervals. They were not calculated in harmonical string length ratios like ancient Greek music' (GOMPERTS 2002: 576) .

As WIDDESS 1995 remarks, the Indian musical modes (*rāga*-) very often have a structure in which one and the same melodic line is shifted by the distance of a fourth or fifth interval.[5] Melodies are constructed on the basis of consonant relations. Consonance intervals were, therefore, one of the essential elements in a melodic structure or composition. Thus, the equal temperament with twenty-two *śruti*-intervals seems to have been conceived originally with the purpose of producing consonant relations with a harp-style instrument. It was a theory aiming at the facilitation of tuning, and was inseparably related to the theory of melody.

Therefore, the association of the twenty-two tubes in the chest with the microtones, as argued in the SR, implies something more than a mere sound arising in the human body. The sound/vocal manifestation is an organic phenomenon, which includes musical activities such as construction of melodies. In Indian thought, melody is also considered to be an organic phenomenon.

## Manifestation of Melody

By comprehending the theoretical background mentioned above, we are a-

[5] Cf. WIDDESS 1995: 210f, 231f. On p. 370 we find: 'The importance of melodic consonance foreshadows the tetrachordal symmetry and concomitant evolutionary processes described by Jairazbhoy for the rāgas of modern Indian music.' And on p. 170: 'The sequences of fourths and fifths perhaps suggest a harp-style [string instrument], since wide intervals can be played easily on that instrument; but the pairs of repeated notes perhaps point rather to instruments of the stick-zither family – either the fretless *ekatantrī* or fretted *kinnarī vīṇā* – which were plucked with two fingers in alternation. Instruments of this class had replaced the harps and short-necked lutes in the art-music tradition during the second half of the first millennium A.D., the period during which the rāga system developed; so we can perhaps assume that the ŚSR instrumental melodies would have been played on instruments of the stick-zither type. The fourth/fifth leaps might have been easier to execute on the fretted kinnarī, perhaps by lateral deflection of the string, than on the unfretted ekatantrī.'

ble to grasp the meaning of verse 82 in SR 3 (*Prakīrṇakādhyāya*),[6] which deals with the term *śārīra-* 'pertaining to the human body', denoting the inborn voice quality of a talented singer:

> *rāgābhivyaktiśaktatvam anabhyāse 'pi yad dhvaneḥ*
> *tac chārīram iti proktaṃ śarīreṇa sahodbhavāt*
> The ability of resonance (*dhvani*) to manifest musical modes (*rāga*) even without practising is called [the ability] pertaining to the human body, because of [its, i.e. resonance's] arising together with the human body.

A talented musician has the resonance, namely sound/voice, with which he is able to manifest musical modes,[7] namely construct or develop melodic structures, even if he does not practise.

The commentator *Kallinātha* explains this verse, adopting a vocabulary tinted with Tantrism, as follows: The relation of sound (*śabda-*) and the human body is that of a property and the proprietor of the property (*dharmadharmibhāva-*). He interprets the ability (*śakti-*) of manifestation of *rāga*-s to be the ability to develop a certain *rāga-*, without violating the theoretical musical prescriptions.[8] He expresses this ability as power (*śakti-*). This power of vocal

---

[6] This verse and its commentary are on pp. 137f. of the SR edition (Adyar edition).

[7] More correctly, he has the voice which is able to manifest modes. It might imply the idea that it is not the musician, but sound/voice itself, which arises in his body, that manifests modes. The term *abhivyakti-* is also a little problematic: does it mean that voice manifests *rāga*-s? Or that *rāga*-s manifest *themselves* in voice?

[8] *rāgasya grahāṃśādisvarasanniveśaviniveśavataḥ śrīrāgādeḥ abhivyaktiḥ avaisvaryeṇāsāṅkaryeṇa ca prakāśanam. tatra śaktatvaṃ śaktimattvam* 'The manifestation (*abhivyakti-*), of a *rāga-*, [such as] *Śrīrāga* etc., through insertion (*sanniveśa-*) and combination (*viniveśa-*) of the tones of *graha-, aṃśa-* etc., is expression (*prakāśana-*) without being out of tune and without mingling [the characteristics of other *rāga*-s into the *Śrīrāga* etc.]. The state of possessing ability/power [means] the state of being able in that regard.' The term *graha-* denotes the initial note, on which melodies should begin (WIDDESS 1995: 401). The *aṃśa-* is the predominant note in a melodic structure; WIDDESS 1995: 398 describes it as follows: 'The Predominant: in a jāti, one of several strong notes, each of which can serve as aṃśa; in a rāga, the single most important note. It occurs frequently and prominently, usually serving also as *graha*

and musical manifestation has the form of a seed (*bīja-*) for the manifestation/ development of a *rāga-*. Without it, the *rāga-* would not flow out, or even if the *rāga-* were flowing out, it would become ridiculous.[9] In the same manner, resonance (*dhvani-*) or sound/voice arises together with the human body; so does the resonance's ability of manifestation of *rāga-*s.[10] This ability cannot be acquired secondarily through practising.[11]

In this view, melodic structure (*rāga-*) seems to be considered to be inherent in voice itself. Melodic structure is not a human artificial invention, but rather a kind of natural phenomenon.

## The *Ā'īn-i Akbarī*

The idea of this *anāhata- nāda-* (not-struck sound) seems to have attracted the interest of Muslim musicologists too. The *Ā'īn-i Akbarī*, the famous historiography with encyclopaedic character in Persian by Abū 'l-Fażl ʿAllāmī, dedicated to the Muġal emperor Akbar, reports on the musical tradition of the Hindus[12]. Chapter 7 of volume 3 of this work also deals with music (AA2, 3: 260ff.). Abū 'l-Fażl calls Hindu music *sngyt* in the Perso-Arabic script, which is clearly *saṅgīt*, i.e. *saṅgīta-* with a New Indo-Aryan pronunciation, and states that this subject is dealt with *dar haft adhyāy* 'in seven chapters (*adhyāya-*)'.

---

and *vādī*.' So the commentary means a correct rendering of a *rāga-*, which fulfils the theoretical requirement of *rāga-* definition, furnishing a *rāga-* with its prescribed characteristics such as initial, predominant etc.

[9] Kallinātha on SR 3,82: *tatra śaktatvaṃ śaktimattvam. śaktir nāmātra rāgābhivyaktibīja-rūpaḥ saṃskāraviśeṣaḥ, yāṃ vinā rāga eva na prasaret, prasr̥taṃ vā hasanīyaṃ bhavet.*

[10] Ibid.: *yathā dhvaniḥ śarīreṇa sahodbhūto bhavati, tathā tasya rāgābhivyaktiśaktatvam api śarīreṇa sahodbhūtaṃ bhavati.*

[11] Ibid.: *na hy abhyāsenāgantukam.*

[12] This is, as is well known, a foreign geographic term applied to what pertains to the Indian subcontinent including the religion(s) predominating there, but by no means exclusive to the religious sphere. A Hindu can thus be an inhabitant of this region, as well as a person adhering to a certain autochthonous religion, the two categories often being immingled.

He seems to have consulted the SR, for this text is mentioned as the *Saptādhyāyī* in later works on music theory.[13] Though '(of) seven chapters' might possibly be a general denomination for the science of music, like the term *Aṣṭāṅga* was for medical science, it seems more probable that the term refers to the particular work by Śārṅgadeva. This is supported by the contents presented by Abū 'l-Fażl,[14] as they are very similar to the contents of the SR, and the titles of the chapters in Sanskrit reconstructed by AA2 are in accordance with those in the SR.[15]

Here only that part of Abū 'l-Fażl's text is quoted which contains topics relevant for our discussion.[16] It is given in translation, based on that of AA2, but modified for greater accuracy and precision. The translation takes into account word meanings current in South Asia, but not necessarily in Iran;[17] in cases of doubt the Urdu meanings have also been considered. Reconstructed Sanskrit terms are underlined:

> Saṅgīta is the art of various [types of] singing/melody (*naġma*), instrument(s) (*sāz*) and the movement of dance etc. These subjects are treated in seven chapters (adhyāya). The first is Svarādhyāya, the explanation of sound/voice (*āvāz*). They enumerate two kinds of it.
>
> Anāhata, the sound without a cause (*āvā-yi bē-sabab*). They consider it to be one and eternal (*qadīm*). Whenever one closes the orifices of one's ears with

[13] SHRINGY 1999: xii: 'S.R. has been known as *saptādhyāyī* on the model of Pāṇini's *Aṣṭādhyāyī* … .' In note 2, Shringy refers to the *Saṅgītasudhā* as an example mentioning the SR as the *Saptādhyāyī*.

[14] The word forms Abū 'l-Fażl gives presuppose a New Indo-Aryan pronunciation.

[15] The titles mentioned by Abū 'l-Fażl are the following, based on the transcription of AA2: *Svarādhyāya, Rāgavivekādhyāya, Prakirṇādhyāya, Prabandhādhyāya, Tālādhyāya, Vādyādhyāya* (AA2, 3: 260ff.). These are written in the original script as *svr adhyāy, rāg bbykāy adhyāy, prkyrnkādhyāy, prbndh adhyāy, tāl adhyāy* and *vādyā adhyāy* respectively. The correct transcription of the title of the third chapter seems therefore to be *Prakīrṇakādhyāya*.

[16] The original Persian text consulted is AA1: 134f.

[17] Also, the transliteration used for Persian here is for the older form still predominant in South Asia, not the more recent Iranian variety.

one's fingers, one perceives a sound/resonance (*ṣadā*[18]). [So] it has such a name. They believe [it to be] *Brahmā*.[19] When one is accustomed to this perception [of *anāhata* sound] and hears it without mediate aid, liberation (*mukti*[20]) appears.

*Āhata*, the sound which, [being provided] with a cause manifests itself. They consider that to be a phenomenon of air (*'arż-i havā*) like speech. And it is produced by striking (*ḫōrdan*[21]) and plucking/tearing (*kandan*[22]).

They say (*bar sar āyand*[23]) that in each of [the three locations of] the abdomen[24], the throat and the head (or: and the crown of the head) (*tārak*), twenty-two veins/vessels/sinews (*rag*[25]) have been applied by the hand of the divine (*qudrat*). The preliminary stadium (*sarāġāz*) of the accomplished/graceful movement (*čāliš*) of the wind (*bād*) arises from the navel. And a sound arises [according] to the degree of strength and weakness of the striking of it (i.e. of the *rag* like a string). They state that the fifth, sixth, eighteenth and nineteenth veins/vessels/sinews are not accomplished.[26] And they class the [remaining] eighteen into seven portions (i.e. intervals) (*laḫt*), in the following order … .

This reveals a theory of sound/voice manifestation which is almost the same as that in the SR. Still, several deviations are found. For instance, the following portion has no counterpart in the SR:

---

[18] This seems to translate Sanskrit *dhvani*.

[19] AA2: 'They believe this to proceed from *Brahmā*.'

[20] In the original script: *mkt*.

[21] Explained by AA2 as percussion. But it could equally refer to the striking of a string.

[22] AA2 translates this as 'protrusion'. However, it seems rather to refer to the plucking of a string.

[23] Literally: 'they come to the point', i.e. 'they conclude'?

[24] According to the SR, however, it should be the chest, or thorax.

[25] Cf. Kabīr's *sab rag taṃt rabāb tan* 'all veins/vessels/sinews are the strings, the [human] body is the stringed instrument' (SIṂH/SIṂH 1993: 40: *Birah ko aṃg*, verse 20).

[26] Literally: 'is not accomplished' (*na rasad*). AA2 has 'mute', but this does not make sense.

> Whenever one closes the orifices of one's ears with one's fingers, one perceives a sound/resonance. [So] it has such a name. They believe [it to be] *Brahmā*. When one is accustomed to this perception [of *anāhata* sound] and hears it without mediate aid, liberation appears.

Actually, this is a Haṭhayoga theory of practising by utilising the *anāhata- nāda-*. The parallel is found in *Haṭhayogapradīpikā* 4,81f. (cf. SINH 1980: 58f.):

> *karṇau pidhāya hastābhyāṃ yaṃ śr̥ṇoti dhvaniṃ muniḥ*
> *tatra cittaṃ sthirīkuryād yāvat sthirapadaṃ vrajet* (81)[27]
> *abhyasyamāno nādo 'yaṃ bāhyam āvr̥ṇute dhvaniṃ*
> *pakṣād vikṣepam akhilaṃ jitvā yogī sukhī bhavet* (82)
> One should make one's consciousness steady in the sound (*dhvani-*) which a sage hears, closing one's ears with one's hands, until [one's consciousness] attains a steady state. This sound (*nāda-*), being exercised, conceals/keeps off external sounds (*dhvani-*). In fifteen days, the Yogin should become happy, conquering all distractions.[28]

Abū 'l-Fażl probably was not able to resort to the original Sanskrit text of the SR, but only to let some pundit orally translate or summarise the Sanskrit into Persian or a New Indo-Aryan language he could understand. I surmise that this person additionally explained the notion of *anāhata- nāda-*, and that Abū 'l-Fażl included these comments in the *Ā'īn-i Akbarī* too.

---

[27] After this, a further verse is given:
*abhyasyamāno nādo 'yaṃ bāhyam āvr̥ṇute dhvaniṃ muniḥ*
*tatra cittaṃ sthirīkuryād yāvat sthirapadaṃ vrajet* (81)
It seems obvious, also from irregular metre, and the same numbering as in the case of the preceding verse, that this is a mistake. SINH 1980: 59 too acknowledges this by translating only the first verse 81.

[28] The same posture is mentioned in the embryological description of SR 1,2,34ff., which describe the state of the foetus in the seventh month after conception. 34cd says: *pālyantarita-hastābhyāṃ śrotrarandhre pidhāya saḥ* 'covering the openings of the ears with both hands, placed within the lap/lobes of the ears, he (the foetus) [meditates upon the means of liberation (*mokṣopāya-*)]'. It might imply that the foetus hears *anāhata- nāda-* in meditating. More information is contained in the notes on this passage in my dissertation on the chapter on embryology in the SR, which I hope to publish soon.

We also find other statements deviating from SR in Abū 'l-Fażl's text. This does mention the twenty-two vessels, but these are characterised as divinely created, which differs from the description in SR.

The last statement explaining the ratio of the seven musical tones/intervals in the octave, namely 'that the fifth, sixth, eighteenth and nineteenth veins/vessels/sinews are not accomplished', is also peculiar, not being mentioned in the SR.

Although I am not able to explain this latter statement by Abū 'l-Fażl, I would like to draw attention to the following: In the above-mentioned Indian theory of 22 *śruti*-s, the respective intervals of the seven tones (*svara-*) of the octave are measured as 4, 3, 2, 4, 4, 3, und 2 *śruti*-s.[29] All of the fifth and sixth, eighteenth and nineteenth 'veins/vessels/sinews', which Abū 'l-Fażl considers to be incomplete, belong to the two musical tones (*svara-*) consisting of 3 *śruti*-s, namely the second and sixth tones (*svara-*) of the octave. The pair of fifth and sixth 'veins/vessels/sinews' corresponds to the first and second of the three *śruti*-s constituting the third tone (*svara-*), while the pair of eighteenth and nineteenth 'veins/vessels/sinews' corresponds to the first and second of the three *śruti*-s constituting the sixth tone (*svara-*). Therefore we can conclude that this statement is most probably based on the Indian classical music theory of respectively attributing 4, 3, 2, 4, 4, 3, and 2 *śruti*-s to the seven musical tones (*svara-*).

Thus Abū 'l-Fażl's summary of the SR poses an intriguing problem: Its contents are in accordance with the original text of the SR, but it contains deviations. What are the reasons for and the background of these deviations? Unfortunately, I am unable to fully elaborate on this matter within the limits of this small article, but hope to investigate it in detail in the near future.

## Dārā Šikōh on the *anāhata- nāda-*

The Muġal prince Muḥammad Dārā Šikōh (1615-1659)[30] is well known for

---

[29] In the standard scale called *ṣaḍjagrāma-*. Cf. GOMPERTS 2002: 575.

[30] Šikōh is also transliterated as Šukōh, Šikūh and Šukūh.

his attempts to integrate Islam and Hinduism. His attempts crystallised in his theological work, *Mağma‘u 'l-Baḥrain* which deals with the comparative study of Islamic and Hindu cosmology.

In his argument on sound (*āvāz*),[31] Dārā Šikōh refers to *Qur'ān* 2,117: *fa-'innamā yaqūlu lahu kun fa-yakūnu* 'then indeed he says to it: "Be"; then it is.'[32] Then he attempts to connect this statement to the Indian argument on sound. He reports that Indian fakirs (*fuqarā-yi hind*) call it, namely sound, *Sarasvatī*.[33]

He continues that this sound (*āvāz*) is called *nāda*[34] by Indian monotheists (*muvaḥḥidān-i hind*), and that it is of three kinds: *anāhata, āhata* and *śabda*.[35]

Dārā Šikōh considers the Hindus' *anāhata* sound to be equivalent to the Sufis' *āvāz-i muṭlaq* 'sound of the Unlimited/Absolute' or 'absolute/unlimited sound', or *sulṭānu 'l-azkār* 'Sultan of the recitation exercises'.

Not being specialised in Islamic theology, I shall refrain from engaging in further argument on this matter.

### Music Therapy: Islamic and Autochthonous Thought

As observed above, Muslim intellectuals were interested in the Indian theory of music and sound, and tried to describe it with Islamic vocabulary, or to associate its notions with Islamic ones. Besides, we know that cultural exchange transcending religious boundaries flourished in northern India during the period of Islamic rule in various scientific fields such as medicine,[36] astro-

---

[31] For the Persian text see MAHFUZ-UL-HAQ 1982: 91f.

[32] Cf. MAHFUZ-UL-HAQ 1982: 47 note 2, 91 note 1.

[33] In the original Perso-Arabic script this is *srsty*. MAHFUZ-UL-HAQ 1982: 47 renders this as *sarastī*. However, this gives no proper sense. On the other hand, *sarsutī* would fit perfectly, as this is a common New Indo-Aryan equivalent of the Sanskrit *sarasvatī-*.

[34] In the original script *nād*, plainly *nāda-* in New Indo-Aryan pronunciation.

[35] Given as *anāht*, *āht* and *sbd*. Note the sibilant of the latter.

[36] Cf., e.g., BAGCHI 1997: 71-107, SHARMA 1992: 465-484.

logy[37] etc.

In the field of music, we sometimes also come across terms and notions which suggest such an exchange of ideas. For instance, the comparison of the human body with a stringed instrument is also found in Islamic music theory. Islamic musicologists, referring to the Pythagorean theory of mathematics and the Hellenistic theory of medicine,[38] associate the four humours contained in the human body with the four strings of the Arabian lute (*ʿūd*). SHEHADI 1995: 16 writes as follows :

> It would be of interest to mention a few of these writers in the Kindi-Pythagorean tradition in Islam. They are selected to show the spread in time from the Ninth Century, Kindi's own, down to the early Fifteenth Century, .... Al-Jāḥidh (d. 869) is actually a contemporary of Kindi, and in his book *al-Tarbīʿ wa l-tadwīr* (*Squaring and Circling*) he has a brief section on music, one of the oldest in Islam, that links "the strings, the elements and the temperaments". Ibn Khurradādhibah (d. 911) makes the links primarily between the *ʿūd* strings and the humors of the body, noting the influence for purposes of therapy.

According to AK 2006, in his research work on music therapy in the Turkish-Islamic culture and its possible influence on the European Renaissance, this Islamic music theory associating music and the human organism was even utilised in clinical practice. To each musical mode (*maqām*), a certain medical, psychosomatic effect[39] was prescribed, and diseases were treated according to prescription (pp. 132f). In hospitals in big cities such as Istanbul, Kairo etc., music was systematically utilised in psychiatric treatment (pp. 140f).[40]

---

[37] Cf. YANO 2005.

[38] On Hellenistic medical science and its use of music as treatment cf. KOCH 1995: 267-277.

[39] 'Effect' has been chosen to translate *etki* in *makamların ruha olan etkileri* 'the *maqāms*' effects on the soul'. It refers to something resulting from a 'medicinal' melody, i.e. a melody as a psychosomatic stimulant, which induces a certain feeling or reaction in the body.

[40] AK 2006: 140: 'Hospital General Valencia ve Londra'daki Bethlehem Hospital'den çok önce Selçuklu, Memlûklu ve Osmanlı Türklerinin Şam, Kahire ve Bursa'da tesis ettikleri has-

Today, sound therapy and music therapy are common phenomena (particularly in the field of alternative healing), also in India, where their origins are as a rule traced back to ancient Indian culture. I do not propose to enter into this discussion,[41] but shall, rather, comment on a particular aspect pertaining to possible cultural interaction.

Indian music theory allots a certain psychosomatic effect to every single mode or *rāga-*. However, we cannot trace the tradition of such a prescription back to an early period.[42] The early theory of *jāti-* which was in vogue up to the first half of the first millennium does not seem to be precise in correlating each mode with an effect.[43] Should this indeed be so, then it would mean that the tendency to exactly attribute certain psychosomatic effects to each mode started in the second half of the millennium, when similar developments were taking place farther to the West. This raises the question of whether there were exchanges between the Indian subcontinent and the Mediterranean/Middle East during the formative process of a new system of music theory in this period.

Koch 1995: 284-286 observes some parallelisms between the Indian aesthetic theory of *rasa-* and the European theory of emotions (Affektenlehre) which is a development from the Hellenistic four-humour theory. But no evidence is provided which would demonstrate that one theory influenced the

---

tanelerde akıl hastalarının insanî bir şekilde ilâçla, meşguliyetle ve müzikle İslâm psikiyatrisinin esaslarına göre tedavi edildikleri eski kaynaklarda bilhassa belirtilmektedir.' The gist of this is that in Islam, psychiatric institutions were built earlier than those in Europe; in these institutions, music was partly utilised as treatment for mental diseases. The author holds the Turco-centric view that only the Turks built these institutions.

[41] There are various publications – of uneven quality – on this subject, one of the more recent ones being Paul 2004. Basic to many such publications is the linkage of spirituality, sound and healing. For an overview on the importance of sound in religion or spirituality, particularly in the traditional Indian context, see, e.g. Beck 1993 and Beck 2006.

[42] Koch 1995: 289: 'Aufffällig ist ebenso die Beziehung der Affektenlehre zur Humoralpathologie und Temperamentenlehre, während dies in der indischen Musik, trotz ähnlicher Voraussetzungen, nicht vorhanden ist.'

[43] Cf. Widdess 1995: 39-45, particularly p. 39: 'It has to be said that the allocation of rasas to jātis is far from convincing, and can only be regarded as a theoretical construct.'

other, or that there was an exchange between them.

On the other hand, if music as mental treatment did indeed diffuse over the Islamic world, then we would inevitably have to expect that, later, the Yūnānī physicians in South Asia practised this method of music therapy too. It can also easily be imagined that famous works on music theory written by Muslim thinkers such as al-Kindī, al-Farābī etc. were collected in libraries and widely read during the period of Muslim domination in the Subcontinent.

However, this is all that can be said on the matter here without drifting off into speculation. It is obviously an extremely interesting field for furthter research.

### Bibliography and Abbreviations

AA1: The Áin-i-Akbarí by Abul-Fazl-i-ʾAllámí. Edited in the Original Persian by H. Blochmann. Vol. II. Reprint of the Edition Calcutta 1877. Frankfurt am Main: Institute for the History of Arabic-Islamic Science at the Johann Wolfgang Goethe University 1993. Publications of the Institute for the History of Arabic-Islamic Science, Islamic Geography 116.

AA2: *The Āʾīn-i Akbarī (A Gazetteer and Administrative Manual of Akbar's Empire and Part History of India)* by Abū ʾl-Faẓl ʿAllāmī. Vol. – I translated into English by H. Blochmann, edited by D.C. Phillott. Vol. – II & III. translated into English by H.S. Jarrett. Corrected and further annotated by Jadu Nath Sarkar. Reprinted edition. Calcutta: The Asiatic Society 1993.

AK, Ahmet Şahin 2006: Avrupa ve Türk-İslâm medeniyetinde müzikle tedavi. Tarihî gelişimi ve uygulamaları. Genişletilmiş II. Baskı. İstanbul: Ötüken.

BAGCHI, Asoke K. 1997: *Medicine in Medieval India. 11th to 18th Centuries*. Delhi: Konark Publishers.

BECK, Guy L. 1993: *Sonic Theology. Hinduism and Sacred Sound*. Columbia, South Carolina: University of South Carolina Press. Studies in Comparative Religion.

— (ed.) 2006: *Sacred Sound. Experiencing Music in World Religions*. Waterloo, Ont.: Wilfrid Laurier University Press.

*Bhāvaprakāśana*: *Bhāvaprakāśana of Śāradātanaya*. Edited by Yadugiri Yatiraja Swami & K.S. Ramaswami Sastri Siromani. Baroda: Oriental Institute 1930. Gaekwad's Oriental Series 45.

GOMPERTS, Amrit 2002: 'Indian Music, the Epics and Bards in Ancient Java', in: Ellen Hickmann, Anne D. Kilmer and Ricardo Eichmann (eds.), *Archäologie früher Klangerzeugung und Tonordnung. Vorträge des 2. Symposiums der Internationalen Studiengruppe Musikarchäologie im Kloster Michaelstein, 17.-23. September 2000. Musikarchäologie in der Ägäis und Anatolien. Vorträge des Internationalen Musikarchäologischen Kolloquiums des*

*Deutschen Archäologischen Instituts (Istanbul) in Zusammenarbeit mit der ICTM-Study Group on Music Archaeology und dem Institut Français d'Archéologie (Istanbul), Mimar Sinan Universität, Istanbul, 12.-16. April 1993.* Rahden/Westf.: M. Leidorf. Studien zur Musikarchäologie 3, pp. 573-596.

KAUFMANN, Walter 1981: *Altindien.* Unter Mitarbeit von Joep Bor, Wim van der Meer, und Emmie te Nijenhuis. Leipzig: VEB Deutscher Verlag für Musik. Musikgeschichte in Bildern 2(Musik des Altertums),8.

KITADA, Makoto 2003: 'Embryology, Asceticism and Music: *Yājñavalkyasmṛti* and *Saṅgītaratnākara*', *Traditional South Asian Medicine* 7: 111-113.

KOCH, Lars-Christian 1995: Zur Bedeutung der *Rasa*-Lehre für die zeitgenössische nordindische Kunstmusik. Mit einem Vergleich mit der Affektenlehre des 17. und 18. Jahrhunderts. Bonn: Holos-Verlag. Ravīndra Dhvani 2.

LATH, Mukund 1978: *A Study of Dattilam. A Treatise on the Sacred Music of Ancient India.* New Delhi: Impex India.

MAHFUZ-UL-HAQ, M. (ed.) 1982: *Majmaʿ-ul-Baḥrain or the Mingling of the two Oceans by Prince Muhammad Dārā Shikūh.* Edited in the original Persian with English translation, notes and variants. Reprinted. Calcutta: Asiatic Society. Bibliotheca Indica 246.

PAUL, Russill 2004: *The Yoga of Sound. Healing & Enlightenment through the Sacred Practice of Mantra.* Novato, CA: New World Library.

SAKAKI, Kazuyo 1999: 'Myōonkansōhō – Nāda no kansō to sūfī no zikuru', *Indo Tetsugaku Bukkyōgaku* 14: 217-230. [On the meditation on *nāda* and the *ḏikr* of sufis.]

—— 2000: 'Akubaru kaiten no tsutaeru vēdānta tetsugaku', *Indo Tetsugaku Bukkyōgaku* 15: 170-184. [On Vedānta philosophy in the *Akbarnāmah.*]

SHARMA, Priya Vrat (ed.) 1992: *History of Medicine in India. (From Antiquity to 1000 A.D.)* New Delhi: Indian National Science Academy.

SHEHADI, Fadlou 1995: *Philosophies of Music in Medieval Islam.* Leiden/New York/Köln: E. J. Brill. Brill's Studies in Intellectual History 67.

SHRINGY, R.K. 1999: *Saṅgīta Ratnākara of Śārṅgadeva. Sanskrit Text and English Translation with Comments and Notes. Chapter I.* English Translation by R. K. Shringy. Under the supervision of Prem Lata Sharma. Vol. I. New Delhi: Munshiram Manoharlal.

SIṂH, Jay'dev; SIṂH, Vāsudev (eds.) 1993: *Sākhī. Bhāvārth'bodhinī vyākhyā sahit.* Dvitīya saṃskaraṇ. Vārāṇasī: Viśvavidyālay Prakāśan. Kabīr Vāṅmay 3.

SINH, Pancham 1980: *The Hatha Yoga Pradipika. Translated into English.* Third edition. Delhi: Oriental Books Reprint Corporation.

SR: *Saṃgītaratnākara of Śārṅgadeva with the Kalānidhi of Kallinātha and the Saṃgītasudhākara of Siṃhabhūpāla. Vol. II – Adhyāyas 2-4.* Edited by Subrahmanya Sastri. Revised by V. Krishnamacharya. Third reprint. Madras: The Adyar Library and Research Centre 1976. The Adyar Library Series 43.

WIDDESS, Richard 1995: *The Rāgas of Early Indian Music. Modes, Melodies and Musical*

*Notations from the Gupta Period to c. 1250.* Oxford: Clarendon Press. Oxford Monographs on Music.

YANO, Michio (ed.) 2005: *Indo ni okeru isurāmu kagaku no genten kenkyū. Kadai bangō 14580008. Heisei 14 nendo ~ heisei 16 nendo kagaku kenkyūhi hojokin (kiban kenkyū c 2) kenkyū seika hōkokusho.* [Philological study of Islamic science in India. Report of grants-in-aid for scientific research, project no. 14580008. Sponsored by the Ministry of Education, Culture, Sports, Science and Technology, 2002-2004.]

# Sleep in Sanskrit Literature: *nidrā* and *svapna*[*]

MINORU HARA

The two terms *nidrā*[1] and *svapna* are often considered to be synonymous, both used in the sense of 'sleep'. Amarasiṃha's *Amarakośa* treats them as synonyms,[2] and commentators often gloss one by the other.[3]

But not only in the dictionaries and commentatorial literature, in actual literary contexts too the one is often replaced by the other. Thus the so-called *yoga-doṣa*s[4] are described in Vyāsa's discourse as follows (MBH 12,232,4):

*yoga-doṣān samucchidya pañca yān kavayo viduḥ*
*kāmaṃ krodhaṃ ca lobhaṃ ca bhayaṃ svapnaṃ ca pañcamam*
Having thoroughly cut off the five which the sages know as the hindrances to yoga, that is: desire, anger, greed, fear and sleep (*svapna*) as the fifth … .

Immediately after this, their remedy is given with the following words:

*krodhaṃ śamena jayati kāmaṃ saṅkalpa-varjanāt*
*sattva-saṃsevanād dhīro nidrām ucchettum arhati* (5)
…
*a-pramādād bhayaṃ jahyāl lobhaṃ prājñopasevanāt*
*evam etān yoga-doṣāñ jayen nityam a-tandritaḥ* (7)
A wise man conquers anger by tranquility, desire by giving up [all] intentions; and he should dispel drowsiness (*nidrā*) by waiting upon the good(?; *sattva-saṃsevana*). … He should abandon fear by means of mindfulness, greediness

---

* The gist of the contents of this paper was read at the 13th World Sanskrit Conference held in Edinburgh in July 2006. Special thanks are due to Professor Georges-Jean Pinault for his many kind remarks and useful suggestions. I can only regret that I could not use them all in this paper.

1 In this paper the stem form of Sanskrit words is not marked (e.g., *nidrā* and not *nidrā-).*

2 1,7,36: *syān nidrā-śayanaṃ svāpaḥ svapnaḥ saṃveśaḥ*. Cf. also 3,1,33: *svapnak śayālur nidrālur nidrāṇa-śayitau samau.*

3 Cf., e.g., Kullūka on MS 7,47 and 12,33, Śaṅkara on BHG 18,35 and Ānandagiri on BHG 14,8.

4 For *yoga-doṣa*, cf. HOPKINS 1901: 181.

by waiting upon the wise. In this way, one should constantly subdue these faults of yoga, unwearied.

As is evident, *svapna* in MBH 12,232,4 is replaced by *nidrā* in MBH 12, 232,7.[5]

Also, in Sūtrasthāna 21, CS uses the compound *divā-svapna* for daytime sleep (which may include a nap, but also more extensive sleep), which is usually expressed in MBH by *divā-nidrā*, as we shall see later.[6]

But despite the overlapping area of the semantic fields of *nidrā* and *svapna*, they have different connotations and thus are not exact synonyms. The situation can be best illustrated by passages where the two words appear one after the other in one and the same verse.

A Brahmin, Cyavana, says to king Kuśika (MBH 13,52,29):

*tataḥ sa bhagavān bhuktvā dam-patī prāha dharma-vit*
*svaptum icchāmy ahaṃ nidrā bādhate mām iti prabho*
Having finished his meal, the sage, conversant with duty, addressed the master and mistress of the house (the king and queen), saying, 'I desire to sleep (√*svap*), o powerful one, for drowsiness (*nidrā*) hinders me now.'

Here, √*svap* is an intentional action, as it is the object of one's will (*icchāmi*), whereas *nidrā* approaches the same person irresistibly. So we must allot the

---

[5] Cf. MBH 12,209,1:
*niṣ-kalmaṣaṃ brahma-caryam icchatācaritum sadā*
*nidrā sarvātmanā tyājyā svapna-doṣān avekṣatā*
He who constantly wishes to practise stainless chastity should by all means abandon *nidrā*, seeing the faults of *svapna*.
Cf. also MBH 12,187,35 (*svapna*) and 12,239,25 (*nidrā*), where the same *tāmasa-guṇa*s are enumerated:
*abhimānas tathā mohaḥ pramādaḥ svapna-tandritā*
*kathañ-cid abhivartante vividhās tāmasā guṇāḥ* (12,187,35)
*tathā mohaḥ pramādaś ca tandrī nidrā-prabodhitā*
*kathañ-cid abhivartante vijñeyās tāmasā guṇāḥ* (12,239,25)

[6] Both are also used as euphemisms for death; cf. *dīrgha-nidrā* (MP 7,13 and *Raghuvaṃśa* 12,81) and *svapsyanti nihatāḥ* (MBH 8,31,46), as well as *vinihatau kac-cin nā-svapatāṃ kṣitau* (MBH 10,8,4).

meaning 'to sleep' to *svaptum* and 'sleepiness' or 'drowsiness' to *nidrā*.[7]

Furthermore, *svapna* in the sense of 'dream' should be distinguished from *nidrā*, which never denotes a dream. When Sītā in exile saw Hanumat, the messenger of her husband, she wondered whether it was real or a dream (R 5, 30,5ab):

> *svapno 'pi nāyaṃ na hi me 'sti nidrā śokena duḥkhena ca pīḍitāyāḥ*
> But this cannot be a dream (*svapna*). For afflicted as I am with grief and sorrow, I never feel sleepy (*nidrā*).

Also, a passage quoted in Śaṅkara's commentary on BS 3,2,3 (p. 625,1) reads as follows (with Thibaut's translation):

> *kuruṣv aham adya śayāno nidrayābhiplutaḥ svapne pañcālān abhigataś cāsmin pratibuddhaś ca*
> Lying on my bed in the land of the Kurus I was overcome by sleep and went in my dream to the country of the Pañcālas, and being there I awoke.[8]

Thibaut has here translated *nidrā* as 'sleep', but it is clearly the state which precedes sleep and hence the dream.[9] This state is not sleep itself, but the process of leading to this. In the following, this state will be referred to as 'sleepiness' or 'drowsiness', to differentiate it from the state of sleep proper, which comes after the person has succumbed to the latter.

As is shown by these examples, despite the fact that *nidrā* and *svapna* are often treated as synonyms, their connotations differ.[10] To ascertain these, let us

---

[7] For *nidrā-vaśaṃ prāpta°* and *supta*, cf. MBH 10,1,31, and for the compound *svapna-nidrā-jñānālambana*, cf. YS 1,38.

[8] Cf. *Vikramorvaśīya* 2,10b (*katham upalabhe nidrāṃ svapne samāgama-kāriṇīm*) and MD 86cd (*mat-saṃyogaḥ katham upanamet svapna-jo 'pīti nidrām ākāṅkṣantīm ...*).

[9] In the context of Māyā's well-known dream, a passage of the *Nidānakathā* states: *siri-gabbhaṃ pavisitvā siri-sayane nipannā niddaṃ okkamamānā imaṃ supinaṃ addassa* (J 1,50,10-11). Also, we read in the *Mahāsupinajātaka*: *eka-divasaṃ kira Kosala-mahā-rājā rattiṃ niddūpagato pacchima-yāme soḷasa mahā-supine disvā bhīta-tasito pabujjhitvā* (J 1,334, 28ff.).

[10] In *Gauḍapādakārikā* 1,14, *svapna* is used in the sense of 'dream,' while *nidrā* means

examine the semantic content of both words in more detail.

### *Nidrā*

Unconscious

Depicting a thief at his work, KSS 77,57cd-58 says:

*pāna-matto 'dhva-klinnaś ca so 'pi jahre 'tha nidrayā*
*tataś ca supte sarvasmin bhukta-pīte jane śanaiḥ*
*sandhiṃ bhittvā viveśātra cauro vāsa-gr̥hāntare*

Intoxicated with [alcoholic] drink and tired from his journey, he was overpowered with sleepiness (*nidrā*). When all the people were asleep (*supta*) after eating and drinking, a thief made a hole in the wall and entered their apartment.

Tawney translated *nidrā* here as 'sleep', but 'sleepiness' in the sense detailed above on p. 132 is really meant.

Powerful

A somniloquous servant, Gorambha, tells the King in PT 1,150 (prose, p. 25,3-6):

*deva, dyūtāsaktayā rātri-jāgaraṇena sammārjanaṃ kurvāṇasya mama balān nidrā samāyātā. tayāviṣṭena kiñ-cij jalpitam. tan na vedmi. tat prasādaṃ karotu svāmī me para-vaśasyeti*

O king, having indulged in dice-play and thus being awake the whole night, I was forcibly (*balād*) induced to sleep while sweeping (your room). Being possessed by it, I may have spoken something, but I cannot remember it. Thus, the master should kindly forgive me who was under the control of others.

Irresistible

One can hardly resist a fit of this powerful drowsiness. It approaches the eyes slowly, unbeknownst and irresistibly (MITTWEDE 1993: 139). Thus it is said in CD 3,4 ≈ MK 3,8 (with Woolner's translation):

---

'sleep':

*svapna-nidrā-yutāv ādyau prājñas tv a-svapna-nidrayā*
*na nidrāṃ naiva ca svapnaṃ turye paśyanti niścitāḥ*

This passage has been discussed in more detail in note 59.

*iyaṃ hi nidrā nayanāvalambinī lalāṭa-deśād upasarpavatīva mām*
*a-dṛśyamānā capalā jareva yā manuṣya-vīryaṃ paribhūya vardhate*
Sleep descends upon mine eyes and from my brow creeps over me, unseen, elusive, like old age, that waxes greater as it saps a mortal's strength.

Describing king Vinītamati, KSS 72,181 reads (with Tawney's translation):

*tad eka-deśe tṛṣṇārto dūrādhva-klama-viklavaḥ*
*niṣaṇṇaḥ sa kṣaṇaṃ jahre sa-patnīko 'pi nidrayā*
Being thirsty and exhausted with the fatigue of the long journey[11] he reclined for a moment in a spot in this desert, and both he and his two wives were overtaken by sleep.

Here again, *nidrā* is to be translated by 'sleepiness' in the sense given on p. 132, instead of 'sleep'. For the compound *nidrārta* 'afflicted by drowsiness', cf. MBH 10,1,52.

Moha-maya

Approaching unbeknownst and irresistibly, *nidrā* deludes the mind (BÖHTLINGK 1966, 3721):

*nidrām imāṃ prabala-moha-mayīm apāsya*
*re re janāḥ kuruta śāśvata-vastu-kṛtyam*
*ete patanty aviratam praharāpadeśād*
*āyus-taror nibiḍa-mūla-bhidaḥ kuṭhārāḥ*
Casting off this sleep(iness), which forcibly causes delusion [of the mind], oh you people, perform the eternal and essential obligations. In the guise of the divisions of time (*prahara*), these axes fall incessantly, destroying the dense root of the tree of life.

Mind stolen

As such, it carries the mind (*manas*) away. Thus we read in the Sāvitryupākhyāna (MBH 3,281,69) (with the translation of BROUGH 1951: 55):

*tvayopagūḍhasya ca me nidrayāpahṛtaṃ manaḥ*
*tato 'paśyaṃ tamo ghoraṃ puruṣaṃ ca mahaujasam*

[11] Cf. *adhva-klinna* in KSS 77,57.

And while I was embraced by you, my mind was stolen away by sleep. Then I saw a fearful darkness, and a man of great strength.[12]

Sense-organs inoperable

When one is deprived of one's mind and deluded, all the sense-organs cease functioning. Thus we read in Bharadvāja's discourse (MBH 12,180,17):

*na paśyati na ca brūte na śr̥ṇoti na jighrati*
*na sa sparśa-rasau vetti nidrā-vaśa-gataḥ punaḥ*
Once coming under the control of sleepiness, it (*jīva*) stops seeing, speaking, hearing, and smelling. It loses [all] the perception of touch and taste.

Unable to react properly

Under such circumstances, one cannot react properly. When Aśvatthāman attacked Dhr̥ṣṭadyumna who was exhausted (*śrānta*) and sleeping confidently (*su-viśvasta*), the latter could hardly react properly because of *nidrā* (MBH 10, 8,17):

*sa balāt tena niṣpiṣṭaḥ sādhvasena ca bhārata*
*nidrayā caiva pāñcālyo nāśakac ceṣṭituṃ tadā*
Though kicked by him violently, Dhr̥ṣṭadyumna was unable to behave (properly) because of fear (*sādhvasa*) and drowsiness.

*Nidrābhibhūta* and others

Beside such expressions as *nidrayābhiplutaḥ* (Śaṅkara on BS 3,2,3) and *nidrā-vaśa-gata* (MBH 12,180,17),[13] as we have seen above, we have other compounded forms of similar purport.
— *Nidrābhibhūta* (MBH 13,11,12):

*lolām acokṣām avalehinīṃ ca vyapeta-dhairyāṃ kalaha-priyāṃ ca*
*nidrābhibhūtāṃ satataṃ śayānāṃ evaṃ-vidhāṃ strīṃ parivarjayāmi*

---

[12] One needs a special effort (*nigraha*) to resist it: *kṣarita-nīhāre nija-nilaya-nilīna-niḥśeṣa-jane nitānta-śīte niśīthe ... netra-niṃsinīṃ nidrāṃ nigr̥han ...*(*Daśakumāracarita* 236, 12-15).

[13] Cf. PT 2,94 (prose, p. 21,11): *tasya nidrā-vaśaṃ gatasya,* and 2,104 (prose, p. 22,10): *nidrā-vaśam upāgatasya.*

I avoid such a woman who is fickle and unclean, one who always licks the corners of her mouth, who is destitute of steadfastness, one who is fond of quarrelling, one who is given to drowsiness and always lying in bed.

— *Nidrārta* (MBH 10,1,52):

*nidrārtam ardha-rātre ca tathā naṣṭa-praṇāyakam*
*bhinna-yodhaṃ balaṃ yac ca dvidhā-yuktaṃ ca yad bhavet*
[One can attack] the army afflicted with drowsiness at mid-night, deprived of the commander, whose soldiers are scattered and divided in two ways.[14]

— *Nidrāndha*

In a fit of drowsiness, one can hardly see objects clearly, hence the compound *nidrāndha*. People experience this state of mind not only before, but also after *nidrā*.

Half-awake and half-asleep: After a day-long fight, soldiers, horses and elephants were too fatigued to continue to fight any more (MBH 7,159,12):

*nidrāndhās te mahārāja pariśrāntāś ca saṃyuge*
*nābhyapadyanta samare kāñ-cit ceṣṭāṃ mahārathāḥ*
Being fatigued (*pariśrānta*) by fighting and blind because of drowsiness, the great warriors did not understand what they were doing.

Stupefied by drowsiness (*nidrayā mohita*: 21), they could scarcely open their eyes (*nidrā-saṃsakta-locana*: 19). Seeing them in such a condition, Arjuna proposed to both armies to sleep for a moment, so that they might fight once again well refreshed.

Half-asleep and half-awake: In the well-known night-attack by Aśvatthāman, the Pāṇḍava soldiers were awakened suddenly from deep sleep (MBH 10,8,75):

*tatas tac-chastra-vitrastā utpatanto bhayāturāḥ*
*nidrāndhā naṣṭa-saṃjñāś ca tatra tatra nililyire*
Though they sprang up, they were threatened by his weapon and afflicted by fear, they perished here and there (without fighting properly), blinded by sleep-

[14] Cf. MBH 10,8,17: *sādhvasena ca bhārata nidrayā ... nāśakac ceṣṭitum.*

iness and deprived of consciousness (*naṣṭa-saṃjña*).[15]

*Nidrā* as a vice

Since *nidrā* carries one's mind away (*nidrayāpahṛta-manas*: MBH 3,281,69) and stupefies one's sense-organs, it appears in a list of vices, which are characterised by carelessness.[16] In a sense, it is akin to laziness and negligence.[17] — Thus, BHG 14,8 enumerates it together with *pramāda* and *ālasya* (with Edgerton's translation):

*tamas tv a-jñāna-jaṃ viddhi mohanaṃ sarva-dehinām*
*pramādālasya-nidrābhis tan nibandhnāti bhārata*
But know that darkness is born of ignorance, the deluder of all embodied (souls);
By heedlessness, sloth, and sleep, it binds, son of Bharata.[18]

— It is also enumerated as one of six faults (BÖHTLINGK 1966, 6615 = MBH 5,33,66 = *Hitopadeśa* 1,25):

*ṣaḍ doṣā puruṣeṇeha hātavyā bhūtim icchatā*
*nidrā tandrīr bhayaṃ krodha ālasyaṃ dīrgha-sūtratā*
Those who wish for success in this world should abandon the following six faults: drowsiness, idleness (*tandrī*), fear (*bhaya*), anger (*krodha*), laziness (*ā-*

[15] For the compound *nidrāndha*, cf. also MBH 1,137,19; 3,62,8; 7,159,14; 16; 20; 37.

[16] It brings about troubles not only to oneself, but also to other people. Thus, in the Sāvitryupākhyāna, Satyavat condemns *nidrā* (MBH 3,281,89) (with the translation of BROUGH 1951: 57):
*nidrāyāś cābhyasūyāmi yasyā hetoḥ pitā mama*
*mātā ca saṃśayaṃ prāptā mat-kṛte 'n-apakāriṇī*
I am annoyed at my sleep because of which my father and mother, through no fault of their own, have come into danger, and all because of me.

[17] Cf. *thīna-middha* (Pali) and *styāna-middha* (Buddhist Hybrid Sanskrit) in Buddhist texts. SS also enumerates it together with *tandrā, jṛmbha, klama, ālasya, utkleśa, glāni, gaurava, mūrchā, bhrama* in Śarīrasthāna 4,47ff. Cf. also ROȘU 1978: 186 (Vāgbhaṭa), and MEULENBELD 1999-2000, 1A: 248 and 2A: 62 (Mādhava).

[18] Cf. MITTWEDE 1993: 137. Cf. also BHG 18,39 (juxtaposition of *nidrā* with *ālasya-pramāda*). For the construction of *nidrā* with *alasa*, cf. *Ṛtusaṃhāra* 6,11 (*aṅgāni nidrālasa-vibhramāṇi*).

*lasya*) and slowness (*dīrgha-sūtratā*).[19]

— It appears in a list of five *yoga-doṣa*s, as we have seen above on p. 130. Of these five, the first three (*kāma, krodha* and *lobha*) are the well-known Hindu trinity of vices, whereas *bhaya* and *nidrā*[20] are not vices in the strict sense of the term, but simply instincts which human beings share with animals. When the parrot Vaiśampāyana uttered human speech, king Śūdraka wondered (KD 27,2f., with Riddings's translation):

> *prāyeṇa hi pakṣiṇaḥ paśavaś ca bhayāhāra-maithuna-nidrā-saṃjñā-mātra-vedino bhavanti*
> Generally, birds and beasts are only skilled in the science of fearing, eating, pairing, and sleeping.

— As an instinct, *nidrā* is apparently destitute of human dignity. Consequently, one should be careful not to submit oneself to it at ceremonial occasions (BÖHTLINGK 1966, 7566):

> *na hi karmāṇi catvāri sandhyā-kāle prayojayet*
> *āhāraṃ maithunaṃ nidrāṃ tathā svādhyāyam eva ca*
> Indeed, at the time of the [two] twilights (*sandhyā*), one should not commit oneself to the following four actions: eating (*āhāra*), mating (*maithuna*), sleepiness (*nidrā*), together with Vedic studies.[21]

— In the medical texts, however, *nidrā* is not always condemned. For example, CS divides it into two categories, proper (*yukta*) and improper (*a-yukta*). According to what is said, it functions positively as well as negatively (Sūtrasthāna 21,36):

> *nidrāyataṃ sukhaṃ duḥkhaṃ puṣṭiḥ kārśyaṃ balā-balam*
> *vr̥ṣatā klīvatā jñānam a-jñānaṃ jīvitaṃ na ca*
> Pleasure and pain, growth and decay, strength and weakness, manliness and

[19] For the juxtaposition of *nidrā* with *tandrī*, cf. also MBH 5,22,5; 5,88,93; 12,221,47.

[20] These two also appear in MBH 5,33,66; 12,289,47; 12,290,54f. Yet in BHG 18,35 *svapna* is enumerated together with *bhaya* (*yayā svapnaṃ bhayaṃ śokaṃ viṣādaṃ madam eva ca*).

[21] Cf. also BÖHTLINGK 1966, 1788 and 3710.

impotence, knowledge and ignorance, life and absence [of life]: all depend upon *nidrā* (sleep).

One should not resort to *nidrā* at an improper time (*a-kāle*) or more than necessary (*ati-prasaṅgāt*). If one takes *nidrā* at an improper time and more than necessary, it will deprive one of happiness (*sukha*) and vital power (*āyus*) as *kāla-rātrī* (21,36f.). But if one takes it properly (*yukta*), it furnishes one's body (*deha*) with both *sukha* and *āyus*, and provides one with proper judgement (*satyā buddhiḥ*) (21,37) (cf. MITTWEDE 1993: 139f.).

The word *ati-svapna* appears in BHG 6,16, and *yukta-svapna* in 6,17. Note that in BHG *svapna* is used instead of *nidrā* of CS.

Daytime sleep (*divā-nidrā*)

As Manu says, 'sleep' (*svapna*) is primarily intended for night (MS 1,65 = MBH 12,224,14) (with Bühler's translation):

*aho-rātre vibhajate sūryo mānuṣa-daivike*
*rātriḥ svapnāya bhūtānāṃ ceṣṭāyai karmaṇām ahaḥ*
The sun divides days and nights, both human and divine, the night (being intended) for the repose of created being and the day for exertion.

CS also says in Sūtrasthāna 21,59 that 'sleep' is natural at night:

*rātri-sva-bhāva-prabhavā matā yā tāṃ bhūta-dhātrīṃ pravadanti taj-jñāḥ*
*tamo-bhavām āhur aghasya mūlaṃ śeṣāḥ punar vyādhiṣu nirdiśanti*
Being considered as derived from the very nature of night (*rātri-sva-bhāva;* cf. 21,58), the connoisseurs advocate it (sleep at night) as the nurse of [all living] beings. But they say that [*nidrā* (21,58)] which is derived from *tamas* is the root of mishap (*agha*). Other people (non-connoisseurs), however, assign it to [various sorts of ] diseases.

As is evident, *nidrā* at night is natural and nourishing, but *divā-nidrā* is unnatural and even harmful. As such, it is condemned as one of the six sins (*pātaka*) for ascetics (BÖHTLINGK 1966, 2535):

*tāmbūlaṃ sūkṣma-vastrāṇi strī-kathendriya-poṣaṇam*
*divā-nidrā sadā-krodho yatīnāṃ pātakāni ṣaṭ*

The leaf of piper-betel (*tāmbūla*), delicate clothes, talk with women, nourishment of sense-organs, daytime sleep (*divā-nidrā*) and constant anger – these six are sins (*pātaka*) for ascetics.[22]

Further, MS 7,47 includes *divā-svapna* in the list of the ten vices of a king, together with hunting (*mṛgayā*), dice (*akṣa*), and others,[23] and 9,13 enumerates *svapna* (Kullūka comments: *akāla-svāpa*) among the six faults of women, as we have seen in note 22.

'Day-sleep' is not only faulty (*doṣa, pātaka*), but also unhealthy. It is particularly so in the early morning, for *nidrā* in *prabhāta* is enumerated in a list of six *prāṇa-hara*s (BÖHTLINGK 1966, 6498):

*śuṣkaṃ māṃsaṃ striyo vṛddhā bālārkas taruṇaṃ dadhi*
*prabhāte maithunaṃ nidrā sadyaḥ prāṇa-harāṇi ṣaṭ*
Dry (old) meat, old women, the morning sun, soured milk, sexual intercourse and sleep in the morning: these six instantly take away the vital energy.[24]

---

[22] Another set of six vices which causes ruin for women has *svapna* in place of *nidrā* (MS 9,13) (with Bühler's translation):

*pānaṃ dur-jana-saṃsargaḥ patyā ca viraho 'ṭanam*
*svapno 'nya-geha-vāsaś ca nārī-saṃdūṣaṇāni ṣaṭ*
Drinking (spirituous liquor), associating with wicked people, separation from one's husband, rambling abroad, sleeping (at an unseasonable hour), and dwelling in other men's houses, are the six causes of the ruin of women.

Cf. also *Strīdharmapaddhati* 25,11 (Leslie 1989: 49 and 275). Yet *su-nidra* is one of six *guṇa*s of a dog (BÖHTLINGK 1966, 4427):

*bahv-āśī svalpa-saṃtuṣṭaḥ su-nidraḥ śīghra-cetanaḥ*
*prabhu-bhaktaś ca śūraś ca jñātavya ṣaṭ śuno guṇāḥ*

[23] *mṛgayākṣo divā-svapnaḥ parivādaḥ striyo madaḥ*
*taurya-trikaṃ vṛthāṭyā ca kāma-jo daśako gaṇaḥ*

Kullūka comments: *sakala-kārya-vighātinī*.

[24] Early rising (*prātar-utthāna*) is recommended instead. One should learn it from a cock (BÖHTLINGK 1966, 5510):

*yuddhaṃ ca prātar-utthānaṃ bhojanaṃ saha bandhubhiḥ*
*striyam āpad-gatāṃ rakṣec catvāry etāni kukkuṭāt*

For a set of the six *prāṇa-kara*s, cf. BÖHTLINGK 1966, 6775.

CS uses the compound *divā-svapna* instead of *divā-nidrā*, as mentioned above on p. 131, but does not always condemn daytime sleep. Rather, it recommends it for those who need rest in order to recover the balance of the elements (*dhātu*).[25] According to what it says, a nap in summer when the night is short (*rātrīṇāṃ cāti-saṃkṣepāt*) is recommended as wholesome (*hita*), but otherwise – that is, in other seasons (*grīṣma-varjyeṣu kāleṣu*) – daytime sleep is condemned as unwholesome (*a-hita*). The *a-hita* sort of daytime sleep causes various disturbances, mental (*smr̥ti-buddhi-pramoha*) as well as physical.[26] Thus the text concludes (Sūtrasthāna 21,49):

> *tasmād dhitā-hitaṃ svapnaṃ buddhvā svapyāt sukhaṃ budhaḥ*
> Therefore, a wise man may sleep [in the daytime in summer] happily, discriminating between the wholesome sort of sleep and the unwholesome sort of sleep.[27]

*Vi-nidra, un-nidra (= prajāgara)*

As *pāna* (alcoholic drink) and *adhva-krama* (fatigue)[28] induce one to *nidrā*, so there are several factors which keep one awake (*un-nidra, vi-nidra*). Emotional tension and mental anguish prevent one from feeling drowsy, but keep one awake.[29] In reply to Dhr̥tarāṣṭra who complains of the lack of sleep, Vid-

---

[25] Cf. CS, Sūtrasthāna 21,39-42 (MITTWEDE 1993: 140f.) and SS, Sūtrasthāna 35,39 (ROŞU 1978: 174)

[26] Sūtrasthāna 21,44-48: *saṃrodhaḥ srotasāṃ jvaraḥ indriyāṇām a-sāmarthyaṃ viṣa-vega-pravartanam.*

[27] Cf. also 21,61:
*yebhyo yadā hitā nidrā yebhyaś cāpy a-hitā yadā*
*ati-nidrāyā-nidrāya bheṣajaṃ yad-bhavā ca sā*

[28] Cf. CS, Sūtrasthāna 21,35:
*yadā tu manasi klānte karmātmānaḥ klamānvitāḥ*
*viṣayebhyo nivartante tadā svapiti mānavaḥ*
and 21,58:
*tamo-bhavā śleṣma-samudbhavā ca manaḥ-śarīra-śrama-saṃbhavā ca*
*āgantukī vyādhy-anuvartinī ca rātri-svabhāva-prabhavā ca nidrā*
We note that in 35 *svapiti* appears in the place of *nidrā* in 58.

[29] But *vi-nidra* is not always used in the negative sense of 'sleepless'. A refreshed feeling after a sound sleep is also expressed by the word. Thus, when Satyavat awoke after a sound

ura enumerates five causes of sleeplessness (*prajāgara*) (MBH 5,33,13 = BÖHTLINGK 1966, 500):

*abhiyuktaṃ balavatā dur-balaṃ hīna-sādhanam*
*hr̥ta-svaṃ kāminaṃ coram āviśanti prajāgarāḥ*
Sleeplessness (*prajāgara*) takes place in him who is attacked by the powerful, who is weak, who is bereft of the proper means [to defend himself], who has lost his wealth (*hr̥ta-sva*), who is in love (*kāmin*) and who is a thief (*cora*).

Furthermore, three sorts of people are never liable to sleepiness (BÖHTLINGK 1966, 3720):

*nidrā bhadre kutas teṣāṃ ye guru-vyādhi-pīḍitāḥ*
*a-svādhīna-kalatrā ye yair jitāś ca na vairiṇaḥ*
Oh beautiful lady!, how is it possible for those to feel sleepy who are annoyed by heavy illness, whose wives are not obedient and whose enemies are not conquered?

Sleepless persons are annoyed by some sort of emotional tension and mental anguish. Below, we shall see them in the actual contexts.
— *Ati-manyu* (anger): An honourable warrior who has been humiliated cannot find sleep, ever thinking of revenge. Thus, Aśvatthāman can hardly get sleep, being ever revengeful (MBH 10,1,32-33ab):

sleep for a long time (*su-ciram*), Sāvitrī said to him (MBH 3,281,65) (with the translation of BROUGH 1951: 53):

*vi-śrānto 'si mahā-bhāga vi-nidraś ca nr̥pātma-ja*
*yadi śakyaṃ samuttiṣṭha vigāḍhāṃ paśya śarvarīm*
You are well-rested, highly fortunate one, and are no longer sleepy, prince. If you are able, stand up. See how deep the night is.

Arjuna suggested to the warriors to take a rest for a moment, so that they might fight again refreshed (MBH 7,159,25):

*tato vi-nidrā vi-śrāntāś candramasy udite punaḥ*
*saṃsādhayiṣyathānyon-'yaṃ svargāya kuru-pāṇḍavāḥ*
When the moon arises, being free from drowsiness (*vi-nidra*) and fatigue (*vi-śrānta*), you will kill each other again for [attaining] heaven, Kurus and Pāṇḍavas.

Note that here *vi-nidra* is used together with *vi-śrānta*.

*krodhāmarṣa-vaśaṃ prāpto droṇa-putras tu bhārata*
*naiva sma sa jagāmātha nidrāṃ sarpa iva śvasan (32)*
*na lebhe sa tu nidrāṃ vai dahyamāno 'ti-manyunā*
Being possessed by anger and impatience, o Bhārata!, the son of Droṇa did not feel drowsiness, breathing like a snake. He did not feel drowsiness, burnt by an excessive anger.[30]

— *Śoka* and *duḥkha* (grief and surrow): Sītā in confinement could not find *nidrā*, being plagued by sorrow (R 5,30,5ab):

*svapno 'pi nāyaṃ na hi me 'sti nidrā śokena duḥkhena ca pīḍitāyāḥ*
It cannot be a dream, for I never feel sleepy when oppressed by grief and sorrow.

— *Kāmin* (Love-sick) (AŚ 6,5ab) (with Emeneau's translation):

*ramyaṃ dveṣṭi yathā purā prakṛtibhir na praty-ahaṃ sevyate*
*śayyopānta-vivartanair vigamayaty un-nidrā eva kṣapāḥ*
He hates what he enjoyed; he is not waited upon daily by his ministers as he was before; just sleepless he passes his nights tossing back and forth upon the bed.[31]

---

[30] For revenge, cf. also MBH 7,157,38:
*phalgunasya hi tāṃ mṛtyum avagamya yuyutsataḥ*
*na nidrā na ca me harṣo manaso 'sti yudhāṃ vara*
As long as I can[not] ascertain the death of Arjuna who is ever willing to fight, I have neither sleep, nor joy in my heart, o foremost of warriors!

[31] Cf. also KSS 72,286f.:
*sā tasyenduyaśā nāma māra-vallīva mohinī*
*vaṇik-putrasya dṛṣṭvaiva viveśa hṛdi kanyakā*
*tataḥ sa gṛham āgatya vinidro niśi pāṇḍuraḥ*
*divā sañkucitas tat-sthāv ālambya kumuda-vratam*
That maiden Induyaśas by name, like a bewildering creeper of love, entered the heart of the young merchant as soon as he saw her. Then he returned home, and remained in a state of pallor, sleepless at night, and during the day cowering with contracted limbs, having taken upon himself the kumuda vow.
Sleeplessness is described as follows in VD 67 (p.153) (with Gray's translation, p. 63): *(kanyām) apaśyat svapne. atha tāṃ prīti-visphāritena cakṣuṣā pibann iva janiterṣyayeva nidrayā*

— *Caura* (thief): A thief who is active at night is expected not to be drowsy (CD 4,1) (with Woolner's translation):

*kr̥tvā niśāyāṃ vacanīya-dośaṃ nidrāṃ ca hitvā timiraṃ bhayaṃ ca*
*sa eva sūryodaya-manda-vīryaḥ śanair divā-candra ivāsmi bhītaḥ*
By night I did a famous wrong, overcoming sleep and darkling fear. But with the rising of the sun my valour grows gradually fainter like the moon in daylight, and I am frightened.

— *Daridra* (poor) (STERNBACH 1987, 10654) (with Sternbach's translation):

*kuto nidrā daridrasya para-preṣya-karasya ca*
*para-nārī-prasaktasya para-dravya-harasya ca*
How can there be sleep to a poor man, to one who is at the beck and call of another, to one who is attached to another's wife, and to one who robs another of his wealth?[32]

— *Bhinna* (separated [from kinsmen]) (MBH 5,36,53) (with van Buitenen's translation):

*sv-āstīrṇāni śayanāni prapannā na ca bhinnā jātu nidrāṃ labhante*
*na strīṣu rājan ratim āpnuvanti na māgadhaiḥ stūyamānā na sūtaiḥ*
Those who have separated from their kinsmen never find sleep, well-made though their beds may be; they get no pleasure from women, king, or from the praises of minstrels and bards.[33]

---

*cira-sevitayā (sa) mumuce* 'Then, while he drank her in, as it were, with eyes dilated with joy, sleep, which he had long served, became jealous and deserted him.'

[32] BÖHTLINGK 1966, 7503 reads: *kuto vyasanino nidrā* … .

[33] Cf. MD 84 (with Edgerton's translation):
*sa-vyāpārām ahani na tathā pīḍayen mad-viyogaḥ*
*śaṅke rātrau gurutara-śucaṃ nirvinodāṃ sakhīṃ te*
*mat-sandeśaiḥ sukhayitum alaṃ paśya sādhvīṃ niśīthe*
*tām un-nidrām avani-śayanāṃ sadma-vātāyana-sthaḥ*
Occupied by day, she may not be so dispirited by sunderance from me;
Without diversion, I fear thy friend's wife may grieve more sorely by night.
Visit the faithful girl at midnight with my tidings – enough to cheer her!
Standing in the window of her room, while she lies sleepless on the ground.

— *Cintayat* (worrying): When Kṛṣṇa failed to persuade the Kurus, Vidura worried about the future (MBH 5,142,9):

> *tataḥ kurūṇām anayo bhavitā vīra-nāśanaḥ*
> *cintayan na labhe nidrām ahaḥsu ca niśāsu ca*
> The bad policy of the Kurus will destroy heroes: ever worrying (*cintayan*), I find no sleep either by day or night.[34]

— King: As we shall see presently, kings are supposed to be ever-vigilant, watching over what is going on in their kingdom. In Kṛṣṇa's discourse to Sātyaki, we read as follows (H 3,75,2):

> *tiṣṭha yatnena rakṣasva purīṃ bahu-nṛpāśrayām*
> *na ca nidrā tvayā kāryā rātrau yadu-vṛṣa prabho*
> Stand up, by all means protect the town to which many kings resort. Do not slumber at night, o bull of the Yadu-people.[35]

Thus, kings are always awake. When the righteous king Kekaya was seized by a dreadful Rākṣasa, he said (MBH 12,78,23cd) (with Fitzgerald's translation):

> *rāṣṭre svapiti jāgarmi māmakāntaram āviśaḥ*
> When the country is asleep, I am awake. Why have you invaded my territory?[36]

— The words *vi-nidra* and *un-nidra* are also applied to flowers which are coming into bloom (*vikasita*) (*Kumārasambhava* 5,80):

> *a-saṃpadas tasya vṛṣeṇa gacchataḥ prabhinna-dig-vāraṇa-vāhano vṛṣā*
> *karoti pādāv upagamya maulinā vi-nidra-mandāra-rajo- 'ruṇāṅgulī*
> [Indra,] having the rutting [Eastern] quarter elephant for his mount, approached respectfully with the crown of his head the feet of the penniless one (= Śiva),

---

[34] Cf. *cittāturāṇāṃ na sukhaṃ na nidrā, kṣudhāturaṇāṃ na balaṃ na buddhiḥ* (BÖHTLINGK 1966, 601cd) 'Those who are afflicted by anxiety have no pleasure and sleep; those who are afflicted by hunger have no power and judgement.'

[35] Cf. H 3,75,26: *na pramādas tvayā kāryaḥ sarvadā yatnavān bhava*. Cf. also *Raghuvaṃśa* 5,66 (*tava gurur vinidras ...*) and COUTURE 1999: 41-43.

[36] Cf. *rājānaṃ kāminaṃ cauraṃ praviśanti prajāgarāḥ* (Mallinātha on *Raghuvaṃśa 5,64)* 'Wakefulness (*prajāgara*) enters king (*rājan*), lover (*kāmin*) and thief (*caura*) ...'.

riding the bull, and rendered the toes red with the pollen of the full-blown flowers of the coral trees.[37]

### Yoga-nidrā

Finally, a mention must be made of *yoga-nidrā* (yogic sleep).

— King's sleep: As we have just seen above, a king should not sleep deeply, but be always prepared to wake up in case of need. But this king's sleep (*svapna*) is often compared to *yoga-nidrā* (BÖHTLINGK 1966, 6524 = *Hitopadeśa* 3,73):

> *śaileṣu dur-ga-mārgeṣu vidheyaṃ nr̥pa-rakṣaṇam*
> *su-yodhair rakṣitasyāpi svapanaṃ yoga-nidrayā*
> A king should be protected in mountains which are hard to walk in. But, even when a king is protected by good soldiers, his sleep (*svapana*) should be *yoga-nidrā*.

Here we notice that *svapana* is distinguished from *nidrā*.

*Nītisāra* 15,44 too says that a king's sleep should be light and improvised:

> *mārge ca dur-ge viniviṣṭa-sainyo vidhāya rakṣāṃ vidhi-vad vidhi-jñaḥ*
> *sannaddha-pārśva-sthita-vīra-yodhaḥ seveta sādhvīṃ sukha-yoga-nidrām*
> Protecting himself properly with his army on the road which is hard to walk on, and having armed brave warriors at his side, a king who is versed in [military] rules should enjoy the proper and pleasant *yoga-nidrā*.[38]

In the *Pañcatantra*, we twice meet a king in *yoga-nidrā* (the state of being half-awake and half-asleep).[39] Here the king in *yoga-nidrā* happens to hear his sweeper's monologue, referring to the infamous stories about himself. Frightened by his muttering, the king suddenly springs up. This indicates that in *yo-*

---

[37] Cf. also *un-nidra-puṣpākṣi-sahasra-bhājā* (4,13b), and *un-nidra-priyaka-manoramaṃ* of *Śiśupālavadha* 8,28a.

[38] Cf. COUTURE 1999, who takes *yoga* in the sense of 'stratagem', and says that the king's sleep is intended to deceive his enemy. For this meaning of the word *yoga*, cf. MEHENDALE 1995: 25ff. (Kr̥ṣṇa as the *yogeśvara*).

[39] PT 1,132 (prose, p. 22,12f.) (*atha kadācit pratyūṣe yoga-nidrāṃ gatasya rājñaḥ śayyānte mārjanaṃ kurvann idam āha*) and 1,150 (prose, p. 24,27f.) (*atha gorambhas tatraiva gatvā yoga-nidrāṃ gatasya rājñaḥ sammārjana-kriyāṃ kurvan idam āha*). See p. 133 above.

*ga-nidrā* the king is conscious and attentive.

In fact, we do have it referred to together with the act of pondering (*vi* √*cint*). In PT 2,94 (prose, p. 21,8-10), we read on the rat Hiraṇyaka who lost all his friends:

> *te ca mām ekākinaṃ dṛṣṭvā viḍambanāṃ kurvanti. atha mayaikakinā yoga-nidrāṃ gatena bhūyo vicintitam*
> Seeing me alone, they began to ridicule me. Then I, by myself alone, pondered further in *yoga-nidrā*.

— Yogin's contemplation: This state of being half-awake and half-asleep is the object of Yogic contemplation (*Śukasaptati* 323,25-28):

> *deha-bhāvaṃ parityajya nir-ālambanam āśritaḥ*
> *ānanda-pada-saṃyogī sa yogī modate sukham*
> *nidrādau jāgarasyānte yo bhāva upajāyate*
> *taṃ bhāvaṃ bhāvayed yogī dvi-vidhā-bhāva-varjitam*
> Having abandoned attachment to one's body, resorting to self-sufficiency and attaining the state of [perfect] delight, a Yogin enjoys happiness. A Yogin should contemplate the state devoid of duality, which is produced at the beginning of sleep and at the end of awaking.

This state (*bhāva*) is apparently that of the religious ideal, as is sung by Bhartṛhari (Böhtlingk 1966, 2054 = *Śṛṅgāraśataka* 98):

> *gaṅgā-tīre himagiri-śilā-baddha-padmāsanasya*
> *brahma-dhyānābhyasana-vidhinā yoga-nidrāṃ gatasya*
> *kiṃ tair bhāvyaṃ mama su-divasair yeṣu te nir-viśaṅkāḥ*
> *kaṇḍūyante jaṭhara-hariṇāḥ śṛṅgam aṅge madīye*
> When would they come to me, the happy days, when old deer fearlessly rub their horns against my body, me who, on the bank of the river Ganges, resorts to *yoga-nidrā* with constant meditation on Brahman[40], sitting in the lotus-posture on the rocks of the Himālayas?

— Viṣṇu's sleep (cf. Coburn 1988: 194): This yogin's sleep at the beginning

---

[40] When reference clearly is to the god, the nominative *Brahmā* is used in this essay.

of sleep and at the end of awaking corresponds to Viṣṇu's sleep at the beginning and at the end of aeons (MBH 1,19,13) (with van Buitenen's translation):

> *adhyātma-yoga-nidrāṃ ca padmanābhasya sevataḥ*
> *yugādi-kāla-śayanaṃ viṣṇor a-mita-tejasaḥ*
> It is the bed of the boundlessly powerful Viṣṇu at the beginning of a new Eon, when the God of the lotus-navel sleeps the sleep of Yoga within the self.[41]

*Raghuvaṃśa* 13,6:

> *nābhi-prarūḍhāmbu-ruhāsanena saṃstūyamānaḥ prathamena dhātrā*
> *amuṃ yugāntocita-yoga-nidraḥ saṃhṛtya lokān puruṣo 'dhiśete*
> The primordial being (*puruṣa*) takes his repose upon it (the sea), while enjoying *yoga-nidrā* which is suited to the end of each Yuga after having annihilated the worlds, being praised by the Prime Creator who is seated on a lotus grown from [his own] navel.[42]

---

[41] Apparently, the god enjoys his *yoga-nidrā* on the hood of a snake. When two Asuras, Madhu and Kaiṭabha, tried to take the Vedas back again from the hands of the the gods, they saw the god in *nidrā-yoga* (MBH 12,335,57):

> *śvetaṃ candra-viśuddhābham aniruddha-tanau sthitam*
> *bhūyo 'py a-mita-vikrāntaṃ nidrā-yogam upāgatam*
> [They saw him who was] of fair complexion like the bright moon, taking the form of Aniruddha, of immeasurable prowess, and resorting to slumber (*nidrā*).

They awakened Hari (Viṣṇu) in order to fight with him, but were killed by him instead. (For the story of Madhu-Kaiṭabha, cf. H 40,8; 15; 26; 37; 44.)

[42] For further references to Viṣṇu's *yoga-nidrā*, cf. also MBH 12,47,39 (with Fitzgerald's translation):

> *sahasra-śirase tasmai puruṣāyā-mitātmane*
> *catuḥ-samudra-paryāya-yoganidrātmane namaḥ*
> I bow to him who has a thousand heads, the Measureless Person, who is embodied as the sleep of yoga meditation upon each of the four oceans in turn.

*Raghuvaṃśa* 10,14:

> *yoga-nidrānta-viśadaiḥ pāvanair avalokanaiḥ*
> *bhṛgv-ādīn anugṛhṇantaṃ saukhaśāyanikān ṛṣīn*
> Him (Viṣṇu) who was favouring with his purifying glances, bright at the end of yogic sleep, Bhṛgu and other sages who had asked him whether he had slept well.

In *Bhāgavatapurāṇa* 3,9,21, the god Brahmā offers homage to him who opens his eyes at the interval of *yoga-nidrā* like a lotus-petal:

All these examples show that the person who is in charge of the care of others should not sleep profoundly in his defenceless state, but always be conscious and prepared to wake up in case of need, as in the case of the king and Viṣṇu.

— *Yoga-nidrā* personified: In the *Devīmāhātmya* the same story of Madhu-Kaiṭabha as in note 41 is told, but there the goddess (*devī*) herself is called *yoga-nidrā* (1,49). At the end of the Kalpa, when the world was made into the single ocean, Viṣṇu enjoys *yoga-nidrā.* Then the two Asuras try to kill Brahmā. Being afraid, he resorts to Yoganidrā, who resides in Viṣṇu's eyes, and requests her to wake him up (MP 81,52f. = DM 1,52f.) (with Pargiter's translation):

> *tuṣṭāva yoga-nidrāṃ tām ekāgra-hṛdaya-sthitaḥ*
> *vibodhan-arthāya harer hari-netra-kṛtālayām*
> *viśveśvarīṃ jagad-dhātrīṃ sthiti-saṃhāra-kāriṇīm*
> *nidrāṃ bhagavatīṃ viṣṇor a-tulām tejasaḥ prabhuḥ*
>
> Standing with heart solely thereon intent, in order to awaken Hari, extolled that Sleep of contemplation which had made its dwelling in Hari's eyes – the lord of splendour extolled Viṣṇu's Sleep, which is Queen of the universe, the supporter of the world, the cause of permanence and dissolution, full of reverence, incomparable.

She is the goddess through whom even the god Viṣṇu is brought under the dominion of sleep (*nidrā-vaśaṃ nītaḥ*).[43] Not to mention Viṣṇu, all beings are deluded by her. Yet she favours them when they resort to her whole-heartedly.[44] Otherwise, she is called *viṣṇu-māyā* in DM 5,6, 5,12 and 13,2, who re-

---

*yan-nābhi-padma-bhavanād aham āsam īḍya lokatrayopakaraṇo yad-anugraheṇa*
*tasmai namas ta udarastha-bhavāya yoga-nidrāvasāna-vikasan-nalinekṣaṇāya*

[43] MP 81, 64 = DM 1,64:
*yayā tvayā jagat-sraṣṭā jagat pāty atti* (Pargieter's emendation for *pātātti*) *yo jagat*
*so 'pi nidrā-vaśaṃ nītaḥ kas tvāṃ stotum iheśvaraḥ*

[44] MP 93,2f. = DM 13,2f.:
*vidyā tathaiva kriyate bhagavad-viṣṇu-māyayā*
*tayā tvam eṣa vaiśyaś ca tathaivāne vivekinaḥ*
*mohyante mahitāś caiva moham eṣyanti cāpare*

sides in all beings in the form of *nidrā* (*sarva-bhūteṣu nidrā-rūpeṇa saṃsthitā*: 5,15).[45] In Sāṅkhyaic terminology, she is also called *prakr̥ti*, the primordial, highest, undifferentiated origin (of the world) in 4,6d (*a-vyākr̥tā hi paramā prakr̥tis tvam ādyā*).

### *Svapna*

Unlike *nidrā*, *svapna* means 'sleep' in general and 'dream' in particular.[46] Thus in this section we shall investigate first *svapna* in the sense of sleep, and then proceed to examine it as 'dream'. However, since we have discussed the ancient Indian concept of sleep as reflected in *nidrā* extensively, and in order to avoid repetition, our discussion below shall be brief, pointing out only aspects which are different from those of *nidrā*.

<u>*Svapna* in the sense of sleep</u>

— Conscious: Unlike *nidrā*, which approaches a man unnoticed and irresistibly, *svapna* is a conscious and intentional action. Like in the case of *svaptum icchāmy aham* in MBH 13,52,29c (p. 131 above), in the Sāvitryupākhyāna Satyavat has a severe headache and wishes to sleep (*svaptum icche*). He then says to his wife (MBH 3.281.5) (with the translation of BROUGH 1951: 43):

> *śūlair iva śiro viddham idaṃ saṃlakṣayāmy aham*
> *tat svaptum icche kalyāṇi na sthātuṃ śaktir asti me*
> I feel that this head of mine is being pierced with sharp stakes, as it were. I wish to sleep, sweet one, I have no power to stand.

As the object of the verb √*iṣ* 'desire', it is obvious that *svapna* is an intentional action.[47]

---

*tām upaihi mahā-rāja śaraṇaṃ parameśvarīṃ*
*ārādhitā saiva nr̥ṇāṃ bhoga-svargāpavarga-dā*

[45] Cf. also FILLIOZAT 1974: 216f.

[46] As FILLIOZAT 1974: 330 note 1 pointed out, people often confuse 'sommeil' and 'rêve' in translating *svapna*.

[47] Hence its optative usage. One should not sleep again (*na ... punaḥ svapet*), even if tired

— Intentional (*alīka-supta*): In the story of the fickle Vasudattā we read (KSS 77,56cd-57ab):

*mātrānupreṣitā bheje śayyāsthāpi na taṃ patim*
*prārthitā tena cālīka-suptaṃ cakre 'nya-mānasā*
Though ordered by her mother and already herself in bed, she did not make love with her husband. When requested by him, she pretended to be asleep, as her heart was fixed on another man.[48]

Controllable *svapna* can be pretended, but one cannot expect this in the case of uncontrollable *nidrā*.
— *Supta* as *a-vadhya*: Anyone apprehensive of danger would not wish to sleep, i.e. not indulge in the conscious and intentional act of *svapna*. Under such circumstances, when one wishes to sleep, one has to be certain about the security around oneself and entirely free from fear, for once asleep (*supta*), one becomes unconscious and thus completely defenceless.[49] It is because of this defencelessness that in war-ethics, an honourable warrior would not attack his enemy while asleep, hence the sleeping man's inclusion in a list of the *a-vadhya* (people not to be killed) in MS 7,92[50] (with Bühler's translation):

*na suptaṃ na vi-sannāhaṃ na nagnaṃ na nir-āyudham*
*nā-yudhyamānaṃ paśyantaṃ na pareṇa samāgatam*
Nor one who sleeps, nor one who has lost his coat of mail, nor one who is naked, nor one who is disarmed, nor one who looks on without taking part in the fight, nor one who is fighting with another (foe).[51]

— Arjuna did not attack such persons (MBH 10,8,18).

---

(*pariśrānta*), after reciting the Veda (*brahmādhītya*). MS 4,99.

[48] This is also called *lakṣya-supta* in MK 3,17 (prose, p. 86,3f.) (*idānīṃ parīkṣe kiṃ lakṣya-suptam, uta paramārtha-suptam idaṃ dvayam*). On *lakṣya-supta* cf. also MK 3,18d.

[49] For seminal discharge during sleep, cf. MS 2,181 (*svapne siktvā brahmacārī ...*).

[50] According to Bühler, this rule goes back to *Āpastambadharmasūtra* 2,20, *Gautamadharmasūtra* 10,18, *Baudhāyanadharmasūtra* 1,18,115. Cf. also *Yājñavalkyasmṛti* 1,325.

[51] Similarly, it is condemned as the lowest sort of marriage (*paiśāca vivāha*), if a man has intercourse with a girl who is asleep (MS 3,34).

*na ca suptaṃ pramattaṃ vā nyasta-śastraṃ kṛtāñjalim*
*dhāvantaṃ mukta-keśaṃ ca hanti pārtho dhanañjayaḥ*
Pārtha-Dhanañjaya never kills one who is asleep (*supta*), or one who is out of his mind, or one who has thrown away his weapon, or one who joins his hand for protection, or one who is retreating, or one whose hair has been dishevelled.[52]

— By contrast, Aśvatthāman violated the rule and adopted the path of the Rakṣas or Rākṣasas.[53] In the Sauptikaparvan, we read (MBH 10,6,20):

*śāstra-dṛṣṭān a-vadhyān yaḥ samatītya jighāṃsati*
*sa pathaḥ pracyuto dharmyāt ku-pathaṃ pratipadyate*
Transgressing [the rules] prescribed in scripture [with regard to] those who are not to be killed, he kills them. He falls from the path of righteousness and proceeds to the evil path.

— Sleep well (*sukhaṃ svapihi*): People wish their friends a sound sleep, restful, free from danger. In the story of the *parivrājaka* Tāmracūḍa, whose sleep had been disturbed by the rat Hiraṇyaka, his friend Bṛhatsphik succeeded in obtaining the treasure of the rat. Having eliminated the disturbing rat, Bṛhatsphik bade Tāmracūḍa in PT 2,81 (prose, p. 19,7f.): *bho bhagavan idānīṃ svapihi niḥśaṅkaḥ* 'Dear sir, now sleep fearlessly.'[54]

We have a similar expression in MBH 6,94,18:

*sukhaṃ svapihi gāndhāre śvo 'smi kartā mahā-raṇam*
*yaj janāḥ kathayiṣyanti yāvat sthāsyati medinī*
Sleep happily, o Gāndharī, I shall fight a great battle tomorrow that people will speak of as long as the earth continues.[55]

---

[52] Cf. also MBH 10,6,21-22ab),
*go-brāhmaṇa-nṛpa-strīṣu sakhyur mātur guros tathā*
*vṛddha-bāla-jaḍāndheṣu supta-bhītotthiteṣu ca*
*mattonmatta-pramatteṣu na śastrāṇy upadhārayet*

[53] For the violation of the rules of war, cf. MEHENDALE 1995: 15, 22.

[54] Cf. PT 2,83, line 1 of which reads: *tat svapihi tvaṃ gata-śaṅkaḥ.*

[55] For the construction of √*svap* with *sukham, nir-āśa, nirviṇṇa*, cf. also: *lakṣaṇaṃ tu prasādasya yathā tṛptaḥ sukhaṃ svapet* (MBH 3,203,36ab),

— *Svapna* is not a vice: Unlike *nidrā* which is condemned as one of the *yoga-doṣas, svapna* stands outside moral assessment, unless it is used synonymously with *nidrā*. According to the empirical observer of CS, *svapna* is indispensable to the proper maintainance of the body (*deha-vr̥tti*) and is the foundation of health, together with food (*āhāra*) (Sūtrasthāna 21,51):

> *deha-vr̥ttau yathāhāras tathā svapnaḥ sukho mataḥ*
> *svapnāhāra-samutthe ca sthaulya-kārśyaṃ viśeṣataḥ*
> As food is desirable for the maintenance of the body, so sound sleep (*sukha svapna*) is considered [necessary].[56] Fatness and slimness [of the body] are dependent upon sleep and food particularly.

It is further said that it enhances the growth (*upacaya*) of the human body (21, 29-34), as delight (*harṣa*), mental tranquility (*śama*), and other pleasant activities do.

It is also said that sound sleep (*svapna*) promises good health (*ārogya*) (*Kāvyamīmāṃsā* 52,25-27):

> *dvitīya-tr̥tīyau sādhu śayīta. saṃyak-svapno vapuṣaḥ paramārogyāya. caturthe sa-prayatnaṃ pratibudhyeta*
> For the period of the second and third [parts of the night] he should sleep well. Good sleep promises the highest healthiness (*ārogya*) of the body. In the fourth period, he should awake with an effort.[57]

— *Svapna-sthāna*: It is *svapna*, but not *nidrā*, which led Upaniṣadic thinkers to the well-known philosophical analysis of sleep. The most systematic pre-

---

*sukhaṃ nir-āśaḥ svapiti nairāśyaṃ paramaṃ sukham* (MBH 12,168,52),
*sukhaṃ svapiti nirviṇṇo nir-āśaś cārtha-sādhane* (MBH 12,171,14),
*na nityaṃ paribhūyārīn sukhaṃ svapiti vāsava*
*jāgarty eva ca duṣṭātmā saṅkare 'gnir ivotthitaḥ* (MBH 12,104,11),
*agnihotram an-ādr̥tya sukhaṃ svapatu sa dvijaḥ*
*parivrāṭ-kāma-vr̥tto 'stu yas te harati puṣkaram* (MBH 13,96,40).

[56] Cf. the compound *āhāra-svapna-ceṣṭādi*, SS, Sūtrasthāna 35,45.

[57] Cf. THIEME 1952: 17 : 'Der Schlaf ist "Lebenskraft enthaltend", wegen seiner erquickenden, verjungenden Wirkung.'

sentation of *jāgarita-sthāna* (the waking state), *svapna-sthāna* (the dream state), *suṣupta-sthāna* (the state of deep [dreamless] sleep) and *turīya* (the fourth, highest state) is met with in MU 3-7 and 9-12 (cf. also *Maitryupaniṣad* 7,7f.) but it was Yājñavalkya who used the expressions *svapnānta* (the dream state) and *buddhānta* (the waking state) (BAU 4,3,18), and described the dreamless state (BAU 4,3,19: *na kaṃ cana svapnaṃ paśyati*). Also, Uddālaka considered that, in *svapna*, one reaches one's own self (*svaṃ hy āpīto bhavati*), while giving an etymological explanation of *svapna* (CHU 6,8,1). According to what these philosophers say, in a dream the *ātman* creates a new world by itself, with streets, carriages, ponds with lotus flowers etc., as if in reality, though in a dream a blind man is not blind, and the hunchback is no more a hunchback. The movement of the *ātman* from reality to dream, and from dream back to reality, is compared to that of a large fish (*mahā-matsya*) touching this side (*kūla*) of a river and then the other (BAU 4,3,18).[58] Yet it is in the dreamless state (*suṣupti*) that the *ātman* attains perfection.[59]

Manu in one of the concluding passages also refers to *svapna-dhī,* which enables one to know *puruṣa* (the soul) (MS 12,122) (with Bühler's translation):

*praśāsitāraṃ sarveṣām aṇīyāṃsam aṇor api*

---

[58] Cf. also Roşu 1978: 69 and 158 (*Praśnopaniṣad* 4,5).

[59] Yet in *Gauḍapādakārikā* 1,14 we read:
*svapna-nidrā-yutāv ādyau prājñas tv a-svapna-nidrayā*
*na nidrāṃ naiva ca svapnaṃ turye paśyanti niścitāḥ*
The first two [states] (*vaiśvānara* and *taijasa*) are accompanied by *nidrā* and *svapna*, but the intellectual [state] is accompanied by *nidrā* (sleep) without *svapna* (dream). In the fourth [state] the determined ones see neither *nidrā* (sleep) nor *svapna* (dream).
Here the first two correspond to the waking state (*jāgarita*) and the dreaming state (*svapna*) respectively, while the third corresponds to dreamless sleep (*suṣupti*) and the fourth to the highest one (*turīya*). It is apparent that here *svapna* means 'dream', but *nidrā* may indicate 'the waking [state]' *jāgarita* as well as 'the sleeping [state]'. Apparently, here Gauḍapāda was not seriously concerned with the usage of these words. Cf. also *Paramārthasāra* 34f. (Silburn 1957: 37-39 and 75 note 1). Śaṅkara comments on the third stage, *prājña: prājñas tu svapna-varjita-kevalayaiva nidrayā yuta iti.*

*rukmābhaṃ svapna-dhī-gamyaṃ vidyāt taṃ puruṣaṃ param*
Let him know the supreme Male (Purusha, to be) the sovereign ruler of them all, smaller even than small, bright like gold, and perceptible by the intellect (only when) in (a state of) sleep(like-abstraction).

Kullūka comments:

*svapna-dhīś cakṣur-ādi-bāhyendriyoparame mano-mātreṇa janyata evam ātma-dhīr api*
Sleep-insight: When all the outer sense-organs such as eyes, etc. cease to function, insight pertaining to the self (*ātma-dhī*) is produced by means of the mind (*manas*) only.

Rāghavānanda says

*svapna-dhī-gamyaṃ tat tvam asy-ādi-vākyottha-nirvikalpaka-dhī-grāhyam iti*
'To be understood through sleep-insight' is that it can be grasped by the non-sensual knowledge, as is seen in the sentence 'you are that' and others.

*Svapna* in the sense of dream

This discussion of *svapna-sthāna* (dream and dreamless sleep) naturally leads us to another sense of the word. As a matter of fact, beyond the semantic field which *svapna* shares with *nidrā*, *svapna* has a further extension of its own to the meaning of 'dream'. In this sense of the word, the best-known title of a drama is *Svapnavāsavadatta* ascribed to Bhāsa, and the best-known story among Buddhist circles is Māyā's dream when she conceived the Buddha.

Though a dream is akin to an illusion (*bhrama*) on the one hand,[60] it has a relevance to reality (*satya*) on the other.[61] It is believed that a dream which one

---

[60] Cf. KSS 72,185: *svapnaḥ kiṃ nu bhramo vāyaṃ devatānugraho 'tha me | iti tad vīkṣya vīkṣyaiṣa yāvac citrīyate nṛpaḥ*; AS 6,11ab: *svapno nu māyā nu mati-bhramo nu kḷptaṃ nu tāvat phalam eva puṇyaiḥ*; KSS 17,112cd: *kiṃ svapno 'yam uta bhrāntir dhig etad atha vā dvayam.*

[61] In the well-known scene in Bhāsa's drama *Svapnavāsavadatta* (6,17ab) we read: *kiṃ nu satyam idaṃ svapnaḥ sā bhūyo dṛśyate mayā.* In the Sāvitryupākhyāna we find (MBH 3,281, 70):

*tad yadi tvaṃ vijānāsi kiṃ tad brūhi su-madhyame*
*svapno me yadi vā dṛṣṭo yadi vā satyam eva tat*

sees at the end of the night becomes true (*satya, a-vitatha*). Often a god appears in a dream and gives advice (KSS 6,91). The *sūcaka* element in a dream (*svapna*) relevant to reality (*satya*) is termed *gandha* by Śaṅkara.[62]

The relation between a dream and reality gave rise to the ancient belief in prophetic oneirocriticism.[63] It is said that to see a white elephant (cf. Pischel 1886: 114ff.) in a dream is a good sign (*su-svapna*),[64] and, according to Śaṅkara on BS 3,2,4, riding upon an elephant is lucky (*dhanya*) and riding on a donkey unlucky (*a-dhanya*) (p. 626,12f.).[65] CS also speaks of *dāruṇa* and *a-śubha* sorts of *svapna* as symptomatic of approaching death (Indriyasthāna 5, 40-46),[66] and further classifies dreams into seven types.[67] Anxiety pertaining to the dream[68] was responsible for the rise of the *svapna-vid* (decipherer of dreams).[69] There was also a belief in a *svapna-māṇavaka* (dream-mannequin), as we see in KSS 6,137-140 and 72,103,[70] and it is said that unconscious somniloquence (*svapna-vākya*) reveals one's mind's desire, even when it is consciously concealed while awake.[71]

---

[62] Śaṅkara on BS 3,2,4: *paramārtha-gandha* (p. 626,9), *satyārtha-gandha* (p. 626,14).

[63] Cf. FILLIOZAT 1974: 332-334. For *satya-svapna*, cf. also HAYASHI 2001.

[64] Cf. WINDISCH 1908: 153ff., especially pp. 160 and 175.

[65] For *su-svapna* and *duḥ-svapna* cf. MP 92,16.

[66] Cf. FILLIOZAT 1974: 332ff. and ROŞU 1978: 121.

[67] Cf. MEULENBELD 1999-2000, 1A: 49. For SS see pp. 219f.

[68] For the method of averting a bad dream by means of a *śānti* in general cf. KANE 1930-1962, 5: 728-732 and 775.

[69] Cf. 'Zeichendeuter' (WINDISCH 1908: 164). As for *svapna-vid* (*dvija*) cf. *Saundarananda* 2,51, for *supina-pāṭhaka* cf. Kuṇālajātaka (J 5,443,4), for *svapnādhyāyī-pāṭhaka Lalitavistara* 58,4 and for *svapnādhyāya-vid Saṅghabhedavastu* 40,20-22. According to *Lalitavistara* 156,17, *svapnādhyāya* is enumerated in a list of arts to be learnt by the Bodhisattva.

[70] Cf. MEULENBELD 1999-2000, 1B: 188.

[71] Cf. PT 1,134:
*śubhaṃ vā yadi vā pāpaṃ yan nṝṇāṃ hṛdi saṃsthitam*
*su-gūḍham api taj jñeyaṃ svapna-vākyāt tathā madāt*
Whether it be good or evil, what men have in their heart can be known, even when

However, since this dream-aspect of *svapna* requires another lengthy paper to be written, and here in this study it has no relevance to *nidrā*, we dispense with further detailed discussion.

### *Nidrā* and *svapna* in classical Indian dramatury

However, it is in the treatises of classical Indian dramaturgy that we meet clear definitions of *nidrā* and *svapna*. In Bharata's *Nāṭyaśāstra* 7,28ff., where the so-called thirty-three transitory states (*vyabhicāri-bhāva*) are enumerated, *supta* and *nidrā* are defined separately as the eighteenth and nineteenth. We shall quote the relevant passages from the *Nāṭyaśāstra*, *Sāhityadarpaṇa* and *Daśarūpa* below.

*Nidrā*

— NS 7,71f.:

*ālasyād daurbalyāt klamāc chramāc cintanāt sva-bhāvāc ca*
*rātrau jāgaraṇād api nidrā puruṣasya sambhavati*
*tāṃ mukha-gaurava-gātra-pratilolana-nayana-mīlana-jaḍatvaiḥ*
*jṛmbhaṇa-gātra-vimardair anubhāvair abhinayet prājñaḥ*

Drowsiness takes place at night, or even in the daytime for a man beset by sloth, weakness, fatigue, exhaustion, worry and his own [human] nature. The expert should display it on the stage by weariness of face, shaking of the body, closing of the eyes, dullness, with the gestures of yawning and weariness of limbs.[72]

— SD 3,157:

*atha nidrā –*
*cetaḥ-sammīlanaṃ nidrā śrama-klama-madādi-jā*
*jṛmbhākṣi-mīlanocchvāsa-gātra-bhaṅgādi-kāraṇam*

---

well-concealed, from somniloquence and intoxication as well.

[72] Cf. also the preceding prose: *nidrā nāma – daurbalya-śrama-klama-madālasya-cintāty-āhāra-sva-bhāvādibhir vibhāvaiḥ samutpadyate. tām abhinayed vadana-gaurava-śarīrāvalokana-netra-ghūrṇana-gātra-vijṛmbhaṇa-māndyocchvasita-sanna-gātratākṣi-nimīlanādibhir anubhāvaiḥ.*

Then, drowsiness: Drowsiness is a contraction of the mental facuties, occasioned by fatigue, exhaustion, introxication and so forth, and causes yawning, closing of the eyes, out-breathing (= snoring), relaxation of the body.[73]

— DR 4,28 (with Haas's translation):

*manaḥ-sammīlanaṃ nidrā cintālasya-klamādibhiḥ*
*tatra jṛmbhāṅga-bhaṅgākṣi-mīlanotsvapnatādayaḥ*
Sleeping (*nidrā*) is a cessation of the activity of the mind, induced by anxiety, indolence, fatigue, and the like; in it (may be observed) yawning, stretching the limbs, closing the eyes, starting up out of sleep, and so on.

Apparently, *nidrā* here is drowsiness, which is accompanied by *manaḥ-sammīlana*, and clearly distinguished from *svapna* (sleep or dream).

*Svapna*
— NS 7,75f.:

*nidrābhibhavendriyoparamaṇa-mohanair bhavet suptam*
*akṣi-nimīlocchvasanaiḥ svapnāyita-jalpitaiḥ kāryaḥ*
*socchvāsair niḥśvāsair mandākṣi-nimīlanena niś-ceṣṭaḥ*
*sarvendriya-sammohāt suptaṃ svapnaiś ca yuñjīta*
Sleep takes place as a result of the cessation and stupefaction of the sense-organs, overpowered by drowsiness (*nidrābhibhava*). It is to be presented [on stage] by [such gestures as] closing of the eyes, snoring and somniloquism. Being actionless due to the stupefaction of all the sense-organs, in order to indicate a sleeping man, one must use [such gestures as] in-breathings and out-breathings (= snoring), closing of one's dull eyes, and dreams.[74]

— SD 3,152:

[73] Cf. SD 3,151:
*atha vibodhaḥ –*
*nidrāpagama-hetubhyo vibodhaś cetanāgamaḥ*
*jṛmbhāṅga-bhaṅga-nayana-mīlanāṅgāvaloka-kṛt*

[74] Cf. the prose passage preceding these Āryās: *suptaṃ nāma – nidrābhibhava-viṣayopagamana-mohana-kṣiti-tala-śayana-prasāraṇānukarṣaṇādibhir vibhāvaiḥ samutpadyate nidrāsamuttham. tad ucchvāsita-sanna-gātrākṣi-nimīlana-sarvendriya-sammohanotsvapnāyitādibhir anubhāvair abhinayet.*

*atha svapnaḥ –*
*svapno nidrām upetasya viṣayānubhavas tu yaḥ*
*kopāvega-bhaya-glāni-sukha-duḥkhādi-kārakaḥ*
Then, the dream: The dream is an apprehension of the objects [of the senses] that a sleepy man experiences. It brings about anger, agitation, fear, fatigue, pleasure, sorrow and so forth.

— DR 4,27 (with Haas's translation):

*suptaṃ nidrodbhavaṃ tatra śvāsocchvāsa-kriyā-param*
Dreaming (*supta*) is (a state) originating in sleep; in it the action of heaving sighs and drawing sighs is the chief thing.

Here, *supta* is preceded by *nidrodbhava*, and the word *nidrā* should be translated as 'drowsiness or sleepiness'. The precedence of *nidrā* to *svapna*, particularly in the sense of dream, is well-testified to by Kālidāsa (MD 86) (with Edgerton's translation):[75]

*niḥśvāsenādhara-kisalaya-kleśināvikṣipantīṃ*
*śuddha-snānāt paruṣam alakaṃ nūnam āgaṇḍa-lambam*
*mat-saṃyogaḥ katham upanamet svapna-jo 'pīti nidrām*
*ākāṅkṣantīṃ nayana-salilotpīḍa-ruddhāvakāśām*
With a sigh that burns the bud of her lip, she tosses aside her hair hanging, surely, down to her cheek, and rough from washing in plain water;
In the hope that union with me might be won even in dreams she longs for sleep, but the way is blocked by the torrent of her tears.[76]

## Conclusion

Scholars who have studied sleep in ancient India (FILLIOZAT 1974, MITTWEDE 1993, COUTURE 1999) have been aware of the fact that sleep has two aspects, negative as well as positive. The negative aspect is apparently dominat-

[75] For the precedence of *nidrā* to *svapna*, cf. also MBH 10,1,31, J 1,50,10f. and J 1,334, 28ff. In the first, *supta* is used in the sense of 'sleep', while in the latter two it is in the sense of 'dream'.

[76] *Vikramorvaśīya* 2,10b: *katham upalabhe nidrāṃ svapne samāgama-kāriṇīm.*

ed by the ethico-religious ideology of *tamas,* while the positive aspect is based upon a medico-empirical observation of sleep as indispensable to good health.

Admitting the confusion caused by treating *nidrā* and *svapna* as synonyms, we are inclined to conclude that, of them, the negative aspect of sleep is reckoned on the side of *nidrā*, whereas the positive aspect is reckoned on the side of *svapna*.

As is mentioned above, *nidrā* is drowsiness[77] (MEULENBELD 1999-2002, 2A: 50 and 62) and the state of being half-asleep and half-awake (*nidrāndha*) is responsible for carelessness (*pramāda*), preceded by stupefaction of fhe mind (*mohana*),[78] which deprives people of proper judgement (MBH 10,8,75: *naṣṭa-saṃjñā*). As such, it incurs the fault of *yoga-dośa*. Its natural association with night and darkness links it with *tamas*, the lowest of the *tri-guṇa*, which further results in the psychological disadvantage of *mohana* in circles oriented towards asceticism.[79]

But once fallen asleep (√*svap*), one is not disturbed by sleepiness any more, and thus completely immune to any accusations of *pramāda, ālasya* etc.[80] The empirical writers in medical literature describe this objectively, and recommend that one should sleep at the proper time (*kāle*), for sleep (*svapna*) is indispensable to the maintenance of one's body (*deha-vr̥tti*), and a sound sleep always promises good health (*ārogya*) and sound judgement. They simply warn one not to sleep in an untimely fashion (*a-hita, a-yukta*).

Its relation to reality (*satya*) further provided *svapna* with a positive meaning of *satyārtha-gandha* (smell of reality), and it is in *svapna* that gods appear and people receive a divine revelation. Philosophers considered the presence as a premonition of *brahmātmaikya* (the absolute oneness of self with Brahman) in dreamless sleep (*suṣupti* or *turīya*) in their serious pursuit of *svapna*-

[77] On 'drowsiness' and 'sleepiness' as translations for *nidrā* see p. 132 above.

[78] *nidrayāpahr̥ta manas* in MBH 3,282,69 and *nidrayā mohita* in MBH 7,159,21.

[79] Cf. MITTWEDE 1993: 140.

[80] It bears being reminded that *nidrā* in the *Yogasūtra* is one of the five *citta-vr̥ttis* (YS 1,6 and 1,10: *a-bhāva-pratyayālambanā vr̥ttir nidrā*). Cf. also MITTWEDE 1993: 137.

*sthānas*.

In sharp contrast to *nidrā* which is classified as a fault (*doṣa*), we notice in *svapna* not only a positive role in ancient Indian belief and philosophy, but also a physical and pathological interest in Āyurveda.[81] Yet, sovereigns, both human and divine, seem to stand outside this demarcation, enjoying their *yoga-nidrā*.[82]

### Abbreviations

AŚ: *Abhijñānaśākuntala*. – Translation by M.B. Emeneau (Berkeley/Los Angeles: University of California Press).

BAU: *Bṛhadāraṇyakopaniṣad*.

BHG: *Bhagavadgītā*. – Translation by Franklin Edgerton (Cambridge, Mass.: Harvard University Press 1944. Harvard Oriental Series 38-39).

BS: *Brahmasūtra* (*Vedāntasūtra*), ed. J.L. Shastri (Delhi/Varanasi/Patna: Motilal Banarsidass 1980). – Translation by George Thibaut (Oxford: Clarendon Press 1890-1904. Sacred Books of the East 34, 38, 48).

CD: *Cārudatta*. – Translation by A.C. Woolner and Lakshman Sarup (*Thirteen Trivandrum Plays Attributed to Bhāsa*. London: Oxford University Press 1930. Panjab University Oriental Publications 13).

CHU: *Chāndogyopaniṣad*.

CS: *Carakasaṃhitā*, ed. Jādavaji Trikamji Āchārya (Bombay: Nirṇaya Sāgar Press[3]1941).

DM: *Devīmāhātmya*.

DR: *Daśarūpa*. – Translation by George C.O. Haas (New York: Columbia University Press 1912. Columbia University Indo-Iranian Series 7).

H: *Harivaṃśa*, ed. Parashuram Lakshman Vaidya (Poona: Bhandarkar Oriental Research Institute 1969-1971).

J: *Jātaka*s, ed. V. Fausbøll (Reprint. Oxford: Pali Text Society 1990-1992).

KD: *Kādambarī*. – Translation by C.M. Ridding (London: The Royal Asiatic Society 1896).

KSS: *Kathāsaritsāgara*, ed. Durgāprasāda Dvivedin (Muṃbaī: Nirṇayasāgarayantrālaya [4]1930). – Translation by C.H. Tawney (Calcutta: Baptist Mission Press 1880-1884).

[81] We also notice the difference of prefixes which are used with both words: *un-nidra* and *vi-nidra* for *nidrā*, *prasupta, saṃsupta* and *suṣupta* for √*svap*. Another difference might also be observed in their counterparts, that is, *nidrā* is often contrasted to *jāgarita*, √*svap* to *pra*√*budh* and its derivatives.

[82] For *yoga-nidrā*, cf. also FILLIOZAT 1974: 330f. and MITTWEDE 1993: 138.

MBH *Mahābhārata*, ed. Vishnu S. Sukthankar et al. (Poona: Bhandarkar Oriental Research Institute 1933-1972). – Translation by Johannes A.B. van Buitenen and James L. Fitzgerald (Chicago: University of Chicago Press 1973-).

MD: *Meghadūta*. – Translated by Franklin Edgerton and Eleanor Edgerton (*The Cloud Messenger*. Ann Arbor: University of Michigan Press 1964. Ann Arbor Paperbacks AA87).

MK: *Mṛcchakaṭika*, ed. Nārāyaṇa Rāma Ācārya (Mumbaī: Nirṇayasāgara-Mudraṇālaya $^{8}$1950).

MP: *Mārkaṇḍeyapurāṇa*, ed. K.M. Banerjea (Calcutta: Bishop's College Press 1855-1862. Bibliotheca Indica 29). – Translation by F. Eden Pargiter (Calcutta: The Asiatic Society 1904. Bibliotheca Indica 125).

MS: *Manusmṛti*, ed. Nārāyaṇa Rāma Ācārya (Mumbaī: Nirṇayasāgaramudraṇayantrālaya $^{10}$1946). – Translation by Georg Bühler (*The Laws of Manu*. Oxford: Clarendon Press 1886. Sacred Books of the East 25).

MU: *Māṇḍūkyopaniṣad* with Śaṅkara's commentary, ed. Abājī Viṣṇu Kāthavaṭe (Poona: Ānandāśrama Press 1890. The Ānandāśrama Sanskrit Series 10).

NS: *Nāṭyaśāstra*, ed. M. Ramakrishna Kavi (Baroda: Oriental Institute 1926-1954. Gaekwad's Oriental Series 36, 68, 124).

PT: *Pañcatantra*, ed. Georg Bühler and Franz Kielhorn (Bombay: Government Central Book Depôt $^{6}$1896 (Book 1), $^{4}$1891 (Books 2-5). Bombay Sanskrit Series 1, 3, 4).

R: *Rāmāyaṇa*, ed. J.M. Mehta et al. (Baroda: Oriental Institute 1960-1975).

SD: *Sāhityadarpaṇa*

SS: *Suśrutasaṃhitā*, ed. Nārāyaṇ Rām Āchārya (Bombay: Nirṇaya Sāgar Press 1945).

VD: *Vāsavadattā*, ed. and translation by Louis H. Gray (New York: Columbia University Press 1913. Indo-Iranian Series, Columbia University 8).

YS: *Yogasūtra*

## Bibliography

BÖHTLINGK, Otto 1966: *Indische Sprüche. Sanskrit und Deutsch*. Neudruck. der Ausgabe St. Petersburg 1870-1873. 3 volumes. Osnabrück: Otto Zeller Verlagsbuchhandlung/Wiesbaden: Antiquariat Otto Harrassowitz.

BROUGH, John 1951: *Selections from Classical Sanskrit Literature. With English Translation and Notes*. London: Luzac & Co.

COBURN, Thomas B. 1988: *Devī-māhātmya. The Crystallization of the Goddess Tradition*. Reprint. Delhi etc.: Motilal Banarsidass.

COUTURE, André 1999: 'The Problem of the Meaning of Yoganidrā's Name', *Journal of Indian Philosophy* 27: 35-47.

FILLIOZAT, Jean 1974: 'Le sommeil et les rêves selon les médecins indiens et les physiologues grecs', in: Jean Filliozat, *Laghu-prabandhāḥ. Choix d'articles d'indologie*. Leiden: E.J. Brill, pp. 212-232.

HAYASHI, Keijin 2001: 'The Term "True Dream (*Satya-Svapna*)" in the Buddhist Epistemological Tradition', *Journal of Indian Philosophy* 29: 559-574.

HOPKINS, E. Washburn 1901: *The Great Epic of India. Its Character and Origin*. New York: C. Scribner's Sons. Yale Bicentennial Publications.

KANE, Pandurang Vaman 1930-1962: *History of Dharmaśāstra (Ancient and Mediaeval, Religious and Civil Law)*. 5 volumes in 7 parts. Poona : Bhandarkar Oriental Research Institute. Government Oriental Series, Class B 6.

LESLIE, I. Julia 1989: *The Perfect Wife. The Orthodox Hindu Woman According to the Strīdharmapaddhati of Tryambakayajvan*. New Delhi etc.: Oxford University Press. Oxford University South Asian Studies Series

MEHENDALE, M.A. 1995: *Reflections on the Mahābhārata War*. Shimla: Indian Institute of Advanced Study.

MEULENBELD, G. Jan 1999-2002: *A History of Indian Medical Literature*. 3 volumes in 5 parts. Groningen: Egbert Forsten. Groningen Oriental Studies 15.

MITTWEDE, Martin 1993: 'Der Schlaf bei Caraka', *Journal of the European Āyurvedic Society* 3: 137-144.

PISCHEL, Richard 1886: 'Vedica', *Zeitschrift der Deutschen Morgenländischen Gesellschaft* 40: 111-126.

ROȘU, Arion 1978: *Les Conceptions psychologiques dans les textes médicaux indiens*. Paris: Institut de Civilisation indienne. Publications de l'Institut de Civilisation indienne, Série in-8° 43.

STERNBACH, Ludwik 1987: *Mahā-subhāṣita-saṁgraha. An extensive collection of wise sayings and entertaining verses in Sanskrit ... . Volume VI. Subhāṣita-s Nos. 9980-11491 (kiṃ-kai°)*. Hoshiarpur: Vishveshvaranand Vedic Research Institute. Vishveshvaranand Vedic Research Institute publication 664. Vishveshvaranand indological series 80.

SILBURN, Liliane 1957: *Le Paramārthasāra. Texte sanskrit édité et traduit*. Paris: Institut de Civilisation indienne. Publications de l'Institut de Civilisation indienne, Série in-8° 5.

THIEME, Paul 1952: *Studien zur indogermanischen Wortkunde und Religionsgeschichte*. Berlin: Akademie-Verlag. Berichte über die Verhandlungen der Sächsischen Akademie der Wissenschaften, Philologisch-historische Klasse 98,5.

WINDISCH, Ernst 1908: *Buddha's Geburt und die Lehre von der Seelenwanderung*. Leipzig: B.G. Teubner. Abhandlungen der Philologisch-Historischen Klasse der Königlich-Sächsischen Gesellschaft der Wissenschaften 26,2. Abhandlungen der Königlich-Sächsischen Gesellschaft der Wissenschaften 55,2.

# Kalyāṇamallas *Anaṅgaraṅga* übersetzt und erläutert (III)*

Klaus Mylius

## VIII. Abschnitt

*Hinweise zur passenden Heirat*

1. Ein Mädchen, das aus einer Familie vom selben Rang stammt, einer klugen, tapferen, verständigen, standhaften, reinen, religiösen, berühmten, reichen, ausgezeichneten Familie, und das selbst frei von Fehlern ist, tugendhaft, Brüder besitzend, schön, und die entsprechend den Regeln des Lehrbuches zum Liebesspiel geeignet ist – eine solche ist immer zu heiraten.

*Günstige Kennzeichen eines Mädchens*

2. Ihr Liebreiz ist wie der eines Blattes des blauen Lotos bzw. so schön wie der Glanz des Goldes. Bienenschwarz sind ihre Haare. Ihr Antlitz gleicht dem Mond, ihr Blick dem der Antilope. Ihre Nase ähnelt einer Sesamblüte, und sie hat zwei Reihen schöner Zähne. Schön sind auch ihre Ohren. Ihre Stimme gleicht der des indischen Kuckuks. Ihr Hals ist wie eine Muschel, und die Lippen sind rot wie die Bimba-Frucht[320].
3. Hände und Füße sind rötlich und mit dem Rad und anderen glückverheißenden Zeichen versehen. Ihr Bauch ist mager, denn sie ißt wenig. Ihre beiden Schenkel sind schön wie zwei Pisangstämme. Die Hüften sind breit, der Nabel ist tiefliegend. Ihr Gang ist wie der eines Elefanten. Sie selbst ist friedfertig, wobei sie dennoch wenig schläft. Sie ist charaktervoll und jungfräulich. Ein solches Mädchen ist auch von den besten Männern unbedingt zu ehelichen.

*Nachteilige Kennzeichen eines Mädchens*

4. Von vernünftigen Leuten mit Heiratsabsichten ist ein Mädchen mit fol-

---

* Fortsetzung aus *TSAM* 6 (2001): 97-119 und 7 (2003): 114-143.

[320] Die rote Frucht von *Momordica monadelpha*.

genden Eigenschaften stets zu meiden: eine Ungehobelte mit gelblichen Haaren und Augen, eine Verkrüppelte, oder eine solche, die übermäßig groß und hager ist, deren Lippen herunterhängen und deren Hals dick ist, die übermäßig viel ißt, deren Unterlippe schwärzlich ist, und die zu lange Zähne hat. Eine solche ist geschwätzig, ihre Brüste sind ungleich groß, ihr Gang ist hastig, sie hat Ohren wie Getreideschwingen und neigt zu Wutanfällen. Sie ist rauh; ihr Zunge schaut heraus; sie hat ein überaus grobes Wesen, einen Schnurrbart und ist behaart.

5. Sie schläft unmäßig viel. Beim Sprechen zittern ihre Lippen, während sich auf den Wangen Lachgrübchen zeigen. Die zweite Zehe ist größer als die große Zehe, während sie mit der kleinen Zehe den Erdboden nicht berührt; die mittlere Zehe wiederum besitzt keine Kuppe.
6. Sie hat einen unüblichen Namen, etwa den eines Berges, Vogels, Baumes, Flusses oder Gestirns. Sie wirkt alt und wird ständig von Krankheiten heimgesucht. Ihre Augenbrauen sind schnurgerade. Sie selbst ist ohne Scham. Ihre Wangen haben tiefe Gruben. Sie hat zu viele oder zu wenig Glieder. Außerdem hat sie einen schlechten Charakter.

*Günstige Kennzeichen eines Schwiegersohnes*

7. Wie das Gold auf vierfache Weise geprüft wird, nämlich durch Reiben, Schneiden, Erhitzen und Hämmern, so wird auf vierfache Weise der Mann geprüft, nämlich in Bezug auf Gelehrsamkeit, Charakter, Eigenschaften und Tätigkeit.
8. Ein Schwiegersohn mit den folgenden Eigenschaften wird von den größten Weisen als der beste beschrieben: Er ist ein Hort des Wissens, der Standhaftigkeit und des Reichtums, als Tugendschatz bekannt, dazu jung und schön. Er führt einen guten Wandel, stammt aus einer ebensolchen Familie, hat eine angenehme Stimme, ist gebefreudig, voller Mitleid und empfindsam. Er entstammt einer vielköpfigen Familie. In seinen Ansichten ist er beständig. Kräftig ist er, von Übel und Schmerzen frei.

*Nachteilige Kennzeichen eines Schwiegersohnes*

9. Von den Verständigen ist ein solcher niemals auszuwählen: der in un-

heilvolle Leidenschaften verstrickt ist, der Mitleidlose, der Kranke, der Bösewicht, der Impotente, der aus einer schlechten Familie Stammende, der Verleumder, der Spielwütige, der Arme, der Elende, einer, dessen Ansichten ständig wechseln, einer, der andauernd unterwegs ist, der Verschuldete, der Bettler und der Lieblose.

*Über chiromantische Zeichen bei Mann und Frau*

10. Jetzt werde ich die chiromantische Lehre verkünden, die als höchstes Kennzeichen über das Glück von Mann und Frau Auskunft gibt.
11. Dabei ist zunächst gemäß den Merkmalen die Lebensdauer zu untersuchen. Bei Männern und Frauen, die der Lebenskraft verlustig gegangen sind – was nutzen da schon andere Merkmale?

*Chiromantische Kennzeichen beim Mann*

12. Wenn eine Linie von der Basis des kleinen Fingers bis zum Zeigefinger verläuft, weist sie auf eine Lebenszeit von ununterbrochenen hundert Jahren.
13. Wenn eine Linie von der Basis des kleinen Fingers bis zum Mittelfinger verläuft, weist sie auf eine Lebenszeit von ununterbrochenen achtzig Jahren.
14. Wenn eine Linie von der Basis des kleinen Fingers bis zum Ringfinger verläuft, weist sie auf eine Lebenszeit von ununterbrochenen sechzig Jahren.
15. Sind viele Linien vorhanden, so wird dadurch Mühsal angezeigt; gibt es nur wenige, bedeutet dies Armut; das Vorhandensein von vier Linien bedeutet Glück, eine Vielzahl von Linien Armut.
16. Ein Mann, der am Unterglied des Daumens ein Zeichen trägt, das wie ein Gerstenkorn aussieht, ist hervorragend: er verdient stets sein Brot und lebt glücklich.
17. Die Schönheit verläßt nicht den Rotäugigen, das Geld nicht den mit goldgetöntem Teint, die Herrschaft nicht den Langarmigen, das Glück nicht den Fleischigen.
18. Wer eine breite Brust hat, wird stets Reichtum genießen; wer einen großen Kopf hat, wird ein hoher Herr oder gar König; wer breite Hüften

hat, bekommt viele Frauen und Söhne; wer große Füße hat, wird immer glücklich sein.

19. Wer rauhe Hände hat, obwohl er damit nicht arbeitet, wer zarte Füße hat, obwohl er viel reist: dessen Hände und Füße und der ganze Mann werden immer glücklich sein.
20. Aus dem Besitz eines langen Penis ergibt sich Armut; ein dicker Penis weist auf Besitzlosigkeit; ein dünner Penis bedeutet Glück; und mit einem kurzen Penis wird man sogar König.[321]

*Allgemeine günstige Kennzeichen*

21. Liebliche Augen bedeuten Wohlergehen, schöne Zähne das Vorhandensein von Nahrung, glatte Haut eine gute Lagerstatt, glatte Füße ein gutes Fahrzeug.

*Chiromantische Kennzeichen bei der Frau*

22. Eine Frau ohne glückverheißende Kennzeichen würde unbedingt Mutter und Vater, Bruder und Schwager[322] und den eigenen Mann zugrunde richten.
23. Die Frau, auf deren Füßen man ein Rad, einen Lotos, eine Flagge, einen Sonnenschirm, eine Kreuzfigur, einen Donnerkeil erblickt, wird gewiß eine Königin.
24. Die Frau, auf deren Fußsohle eine Linie auf die große Zehe zuläuft, wird bald einen Mann finden und sich der Liebe des Gatten erfreuen.
25. Eine Frau, deren kleine Zehe nicht den Erdboden berührt, wird ihren Mann überleben und sich später einen Hausfreund halten.
26. Eine, deren zweite Zehe an Größe die große Zehe übertrifft, treibt sich schon als Mädchen herum. Was soll man dann von ihr als junger Frau sagen?
27. Die Frau, deren Brüste strotzend sind und eng beieinander stehen,[323] de-

[321] Es scheint, als ob Kalyāṇamalla damit bestimmten Personengruppen Trost zusprechen wollte.

[322] Gemeint ist der Bruder des Gatten.

[323] Nach altindischer Schönheitsauffassung mußte die Busenfurche denkbar schmal sein.

ren Brust glatt und unbehaart ist, und deren Schenkel Elefantenrüsseln gleichen, wird glücklich werden.

28. Die auf der linken Brust ein schwarzes Mal trägt, ebenso an Ohr und am Hals: ein solches Mädchen wird dereinst treffliche Söhne haben und viel Glück spenden.

29. Eine Frau mit einem zu langen Hals ist grausam, aber auch arm. Bei einem zu kurzen Hals verhält es sich genauso. Eine Frau, deren Hals schön gerundet und mit den drei Linien versehen ist, die gewissermaßen nach rechts schauen, wird mehr als glücklich.

30. Eine Frau, auf deren Handteller sich ein Mal befindet, das wie eine Ringmauer oder ein Torbogen aussieht, wird, selbst wenn sie in einer Sklavenfamilie geboren sein sollte, einen König zum Gemahl bekommen.

31. Eine Frau, auf deren Handteller sich ein Mal befindet, das wie ein Stachel, ein Speer oder ein Rad aussieht, wird einen Sohn gebären und einen König zum Gemahl bekommen.

32. Ein Weiser heirate keine Ledige, die ihrer Kaste verlustig gegangen ist und günstiger Kennzeichen ermangelt; im übrigen handele er gemäß den Aussagen der Chiromantie.

33. Der Weise Nārada hat dargelegt, daß eine solche Frau Mutter und Vater, Bruder und Schwager[324] und den eigenen Mann töten und die ganze Familie zugrunde richten würde.

*Verbot des Umgangs mit fremden Ehefrauen*

34. Wer mit der Frau eines anderen fremdgeht, leidet Schaden an seiner Lebenskraft, wird elend und Gegenstand des Gespötts und Tadels; er verliert sein Geld und wird leichtsinnig. Selbst im Jenseits setzt sich sein Leiden fort. Doch sagt man, daß es unter bestimmten Bedingungen auch Verhältnisse gibt, die frei von Sünde sind.

35. Der Fürst von Laṅkā[325] ist durch den Raub der Tochter des Janaka,[326]

[324] Siehe Anm. 322.

[325] Gemeint ist Rāvaṇa, der sagenhafte König von Ceylon, heute Sri Lanka.

[326] Gemeint ist Sītā, deren Raub und Befreiung zentrales Thema des Epos *Rāmāyaṇa* ist.

Vālin[327] durch den der Tārā[328], Kīcaka[329] durch den der Pāñcāla-Gattin[330] umgekommen. Daher sollte man an den Umgang mit einer fremden Ehefrau nicht einmal denken.

*Wann das Fremdgehen als sündenfrei gilt*

36. Die Gelehrten haben zehn Stufen des Liebesverlangens aufgestellt: zuerst Liebe mit den Augen, danach Unruhe im Geist, Aufkeimen einer Absicht, Schlaflosigkeit, Abmagerung des Körpers, Versiegen des Schamgefühls, Abwenden von den Sinnesobjekten,[331] Tollheit, Ohnmacht, Tod.
37. Da er nur an den Beischlaf mit Urvaśī[332] dachte, ging König Purūravas[333] zugrunde. Um des Schutzes des eigenen Lebens willen mag also ein Mann an einer fremden Ehegattin teilhaben, doch nicht unter dem Gesichtspunkt der Wollust.[334]
38. Wenn ein Mädchen in vollem Jugendalter den ersehnten Geliebten nicht bekommt, wird es, von der Liebe ganz betört, umnachtet und findet sogar den Tod. Wenn man als Verständiger dies bedenkt, mag man eine solche Liebe verlangende Frau nach Belieben aufsuchen, doch nur gelegentlich, nicht immer – so sprach Vātsyāyana.
39. Keine Sünde, auch nicht aus Liebe, soll ein Mann mit der Gattin eines Brahmanen, eines Vedagelehrten, eines Königs, eines Freundes oder eines Verwandten begehen, selbst wenn sie schon fünf andere Männer ge-

[327] Name eines Affenfürsten.

[328] Name einer Äffin, Gattin des jüngeren Bruders des Vālin; auch diese Geschichte wird im *Rāmāyaṇa* erzählt.

[329] Name eines Heerführers, der im Epos *Mahābhārata* erwähnt wird.

[330] Gemeint ist Draupadī, die in Polyandrie fünf Pāñcāla-Prinzen angehörte und im *Mahābhārata* eine große Rolle spielt.

[331] Nichts kann den Verliebten noch interessieren, sofern es nicht die geliebte Frau betrifft.

[332] Name einer Apsaras oder himmlischen Nymphe.

[333] Name eines mythischen Königs. Die Legende seiner Liebesbeziehungen zu Urvaśī findet sich in *Ṛgvedasaṃhitā* X,95, im Epos *Mahābhārata* und im Drama *Vikramorvaśīya* des Kālidāsa.

[334] Vgl. *Kāmasūtra* V,1,3.

habt haben sollte.

*Zu meidende Frauen*

40. Stets sind von den Weisen folgende Arten von Frauen zu meiden: eine Jungfrau, eine Wandernonne, eine treue Ehefrau, die Frau eines Feindes, die Frau eines Freundes, eine Kranke, eine Schülerin, die Geliebte eines Brahmanen, eine Heruntergekommene, eine Verrückte, eine Verwandte, eine Greisin, die Gattin des Lehrers, eine Schwangere, eine Unbekannte[335], eine große Sünderin, eine von gelblicher Farbe und eine ganz Schwarze.

*Über Liebesbotinnen*

41. Von gescheiten Männern sind folgende Arten von Frauen als Liebesbotinnen zu entsenden: die Frau eines Kranzbinders, eine Freundin, eine Witwe, die Amme, eine Tänzerin, eine Handwerkerin, eine Kammerzofe, eine Hausangestellte, eine Wäscherin, eine Sklavin, eine Verwandte, ein Mädchen, eine Bettelnonne, eine Bettlerin, eine Milchverkäuferin, die bekannte Frau eines Dichters.

*Leicht zu erobernde Frauen*

42. Leicht zu erobernde Frauen sind die folgenden: eine Schamlose, eine Witwe, eine in den Künsten[336] Geschickte, eine sich auf Gesellschaften Herumtreibende, eine Arme, eine, deren Gatte impotent, fett, grob, zwergenhaft, greisenhaft oder häßlich ist, eine, die immer in der Haustür steht, eine Ruhelose, eine Unfruchtbare, eine Eingebildete, eine Jugendliche, eine Kindliche, und eine, die immer allein gelassen wird.

*Zeichen für weibliche Zuneigung*

43. Sie zeigt keine Scham, wenn er ihr direkt ins Antlitz schaut. Sie ritzt mit dem Fuß den Erdboden auf und lächelt dazu. Lachend entblößt sie ihren Körper. Wenn sie den Geliebten sieht, wirft sie Seitenblicke auf ihn.

44. Nach etwas gefragt, gibt sie mit einem Lächeln ausführliche Antwort;

---

[335] Die Wortrennung *garbhasahitā jñāta* der benutzten Ausgabe ist aufzuheben.

[336] Hier ist wohl speziell die Liebeskunst gemeint.

wenn er geht, folgt sie ihm langsam nach; wenn sie ihn erblickt hat, nutzt sie die Gelegenheit und beginnt unter einem Vorwand mit lauter Stimme ein Gespräch, wobei sie ihn anschaut.

45. Zur Schar seiner Freunde faßt sie Zuneigung. Ständig fragt sie ihn nach Neuigkeiten. Sie möchte wissen, wieviele Frauen es in seinem Haus gibt, ob sie schön sind und welche er besonders liebt.

46. Wenn sie ihn erblickt hat, streichelt sie ihren Busen mit der Hand, läßt die Fingergelenke knacken und gähnt[337]. Niemals zeigt sie sich ihm ungeschminkt, auch wenn sie unaufhörlich darum gebeten wird.

47. Sie schlägt ihn mit Blumen usw., läßt sich oft sehen,[338] kratzt sich mit der Hand den Arm, begibt sich unter einem Vorwand in sein Haus und beginnt, sobald sie ihn erblickt hat, an Händen, Füßen und im Gesicht zu schwitzen.

48. Wenn man eine solche mit den Zeichen der Verliebtheit versehene Frau bemerkt, dann soll man, zum Liebesspiel geneigt, ungesäumt eine Botin zu dieser klugen Gazellenäugigen entsenden.

*Schwer zu erobernde Frauen*

49. Die Weisen erinnern daran, daß folgende Frauen nur mit großer Mühe zu einem Fehltritt zu bewegen sind: die ihren Gatten liebt, die stets von einem einzigen geliebt wird, die sich aus der Liebe überhaupt nichts macht, die Eifersüchtige, die Mutter vieler Kinder, die Schamhafte, die sich vor Respektspersonen fürchtet,[339] die Standhafte, die Wohlhabende,[340] die dem Schwatzen mit anderen Leuten Abholde und die von jedem Begehr Freie.

*Wo man den Beischlaf nicht vollziehen soll*

50. Der Verständige übt keinen Beischlaf aus: am Feuer, in Gegenwart eines

---

[337] Darunter ist ein kokettes Sichräkeln zu verstehen.

[338] Hier ist möglicherweise der Originaltext verderbt.

[339] Gatte und Eltern scheinen vorzugsweise gemeint.

[340] Weil sie fürchtet, daß sie nur ihres Geldes wegen umworben wird.

Brahmanen oder einer anderen verehrungswürdigen Person, in einem Fluß, einem Tempel, einer Festung, an einem Kreuzweg, in einem fremden Haus, im Wald, auf einem Friedhof, bei Tageslicht, beim Eintritt der Sonne in ein neues Sternbild, in der Neumondsnacht, im Herbst, im Sommer, wenn man fiebert, wenn man durch ein Gelübde gebunden ist, in der Dämmerung und wenn man ermüdet ist.

*Für den Beischlaf günstige Bedingungen*

51. In einer geräumigen, anmutigen, mit Kalk geweißten, mit Bildern usw. geschmückten, behaglichen Wohnung oder auf einer hochgelegenen Terrasse, blumengeschmückt, beim Duft des geräucherten Aloeholzes, dem Klang der Musik und dem Leuchten des Lampenscheins soll man mit der Geliebten, ohne zu zaudern, so, wie man es wünscht, der Liebe pflegen.

## IX. Abschnitt

*Mittel zum äußerlichen Genuß*[341]

1. Der Verständige betreibe mit der Geliebten vor dem eigentlichen Beischlaf ein Vorspiel. Als erster Teil desselben wird von den Gelehrten die Umarmung bezeichnet, die von achtfacher Art sein kann.
2. Diese acht Arten sind die ‘Baumerkletterung’, ‘Sesam und Reis’, die ‘Stirnumarmung’, die ‘Schamgegendumarmung’, das ‘Brustpressen’, die ‘Schenkelumarmung’, ‘Milch und Wasser’ und als achtes das ‘Lianenschlingen’.

*Die einzelnen Umarmungen*

3. Wenn die Frau mit ihrem lotosgleichen Fuß auf einen Fuß des Gatten tritt und mit dem anderen Lotosfuß auf seinen Schenkel steigt wie auf einen Baum, wobei sie ihn wie eine Liane umschlingt und mit aufgerichtetem Körper küßt, so wird dies von den Fürsten der Weisen als

[341] Darunter werden die den Koitus einleitenden bzw. begleitenden Handlungen verstanden: Umarmungen, Küsse, Kratzer, Bisse, Schläge, Ausstoßen wollüstiger Laute.

'Baumerkletterung' bezeichnet.

4. Wenn man Arme und Geschlechtsteile ineinander verschränkt wie zu einer unbeweglichen Vereinigung, so nennen die Weisen dies die 'Sesam und Reis'-Umarmung.

5. Wenn man gegenseitig Stirn, Augen, Wangen, Mund, Herz und die Armlianen innig aufeinanderpreßt, wobei man im Übermaß der Leidenschaft unbeweglich verharrt, nennt man dies die 'Stirnumarmung'.

6. Wenn die Frau ihre Schamgegend an die Hüfte ihres Gatten drängt und ihn mit beiden Armen aus Leidenschaft fest umschlingt, wobei sie ihn nach dem Lösen ihres Haares und Gewandes küßt, so nennt man diese deutliche[342] Umschlingung die 'Schamgegendumarmung'.

7. Wenn die Frau ihren mit geschlossenen Augen stehenden Mann von hinten mit beiden Brüsten gleichsam durchbohrt und dann seinerseits er sie packt, so wird dies von den Weisen als das 'Brustpressen' bezeichnet.

8. Wenn der Mann, von fesselloser Leidenschaft erregt, das Schenkelpaar der Frau mit seinem eigenen Schenkelpaar zusammendrückt, sie gewissermaßen einschließend, so ist dies die 'Schenkelumarmung'.

9. Wenn der Liebste auf dem Bett sitzt, die Frau auf dem Schoß, so daß er ihr ins Angesicht schaut, und wenn er dann mit seinen Gliedmaßen gewissermaßen in sie eindringt, so heißt diese Umarmung 'Milch und Wasser'.

10. Wenn die geradwüchsige Geliebte den Mann umschlingt wie eine Liane den Baum, und wenn sie ihn küßt, wobei sie aus Leidenschaft leise *sīt* macht, so wird von den Weisen dies das 'Lianenschlingen' genannt.

*Über die Arten der Küsse*

11. Die Lippen, die Augen, die Wangen, der Kopf, der Mund, die Busenfurche und der Hals sind die von den Gelehrten für Umarmungen und danach auch für Küsse bestimmten Stellen.

12. Die Bewohner von Lāṭa[343] küssen beim Liebesspiel auch beide Achsel-

---

[342] Die Position der Frau ist hierbei so, daß ihre Leidenschaft besonders deutlich wird.

[343] Siehe Anm. 80.

höhlen, den Tempel des Liebesgottes und die Nabelgrube. Sie tun dies nach der Sitte ihres Landes. Diese Art des Küssens gibt es anderwärts nicht.[344]

13. Wenn der Mann mit Gewalt die Lippen der Frau an seinen Mund heranzieht, die Frau aus Zorn darüber den Kuß aber nicht erwidert, so heißt dies der 'vereinte' Kuß.
14. Die Frau küßt die Unterlippe des Geliebten, der sie ihr dann in den Mund steckt; sie trinkt sie jedoch nicht.[345] Als 'zuckend' ist dieser Kuß bekannt.
15. Wenn die Frau mit der Hand die Augen des Geliebten zuhält und ihre Zunge in seinen Mund einführt, wobei sie ihn spielerisch küßt und selbst die Augen geschlossen hält, nennen die Weisen dies den Kuß 'der Gefangenen'[346].
16. Wenn der Mann, sich hinter der Frau befindend, mit der Hand das Kinn der Geliebten ergreift und sie in die Lippen beißt, so heißt bei den Fürsten der Weisen dies der 'schräge' Kuß.
17. Wollüstig spielend ergreift die Frau mit den Zähnen die Lippen des Gatten, küßt und beißt sie flink. Der Geliebte tut dasselbe. Die Fürsten der Weisen sprechen dann von einem 'Oberlippenkuß'.
18. Die Frau ergreift flink die Lippen des Gatten mit zwei tütenförmig gebogenen Fingern, reibt die Lippen mit der Zungenspitze und küßt sie; als 'pressender' Kuß ist dies bekannt.
19. Der Mann saugt mit tütenförmig gebogenen Lippen an den Lippen der Liebsten, und sie tut das gleiche bei ihrem Mann, was auf beiden Seiten ein Übermaß an Liebe verrät. Das ist der 'Tütenkuß'.
20. Wenn der Gatte zu seiner in Schlaf gesunkenen Liebsten kommt und sie insgeheim lange küßt, so ist dieser Kuß, der ein Übermaß an Leidenschaft ausdrückt, bei den Fürsten der Weisen als der 'erweckende' bekannt.
21. Die Geliebte drückt mit ihren beiden Lippen das Lippenpaar des Gatten

[344] Auch in Europa erfuhr sie erst nach dem I. Weltkrieg stärkere Verbreitung.

[345] D.h. sie zieht die Lippen nicht weiter in ihren Mund hinein, dem Mann also die Erfüllung des Küssens versagend.

[346] Nämlich der Zunge. Doch ist diese Stelle nicht ganz sicher überliefert. Im *Ratirahasya* ist VII,3 von einem berührenden Kuß die Rede.

zusammen und küßt es mit ihrer Zunge; danach tanzt sie. Dieser Kuß wird als 'Lippenkuß' bezeichnet.

*Regeln zur Anwendung der Nägel*

22. Der Hals, die Hände, die Schenkel, die Schamgegend, die Brüste, der Rücken, die Achselhöhlen, die Herzgegend, die Seiten und die Wangen sind die für den Gebrauch der Fingernägel geeigneten Stellen. Zu gebrauchen sind die Nägel beim Schmollen[347], beim ersten Beischlaf,[348] nach einer Trennung, auf einer Reise, beim Verlust des Vermögens, am Schluß[349] und im Rausch.
23. Die sechs von den Fingernägeln aufzuweisenden Eigenschaften sind von den Weisen in der Lehre der Liebeskunst wie folgt aufgezeigt worden: Freisein von Rillen und Schmutz, Glanz, Wuchsfreudigkeit, Reinheit und Glätte.
24. Eine von allen Nägeln hervorgebrachte Aktion, die auf Wangen, Brüsten und Lippen nur undeutliche, schwache Linien zeichnet, aber die Körperhärchen zum Sträuben bringt, nennt man Churita.
25. Ein an Hals und Busen angebrachtes krummes, deutlich hervorgetretenes Nägelmal ist der 'Halbmond'. Stehen zwei dieser Art einander gegenüber, so sprechen die Weisen vom 'Kreis'.
26. Eine an Länge zwei bis drei Finger übersteigende Nägelspur bringt man am Kopf, an den Schenkeln, an den Geschlechtsteilen, an den Brüsten an. Die in den Liebeskünsten Erfahrenen bezeichnen sie als 'Linie'. Diese gereicht einem Mädchen zur Zierde.
27. Wenn mit allen Nägeln die Brustwarzen umritzt werden, wobei der Daumen unterhalb derselben eindringt, entsteht der 'Pfauenfuß'. Das Kratzen mit allen Fingernägeln oberhalb des Busens bewirkt den 'Hasensprung'[350].

---

[347] Nämlich der Frau.

[348] Gemeint ist beim erstmaligen intimen Zusammensein mit der Frau.

[349] Nämlich des Geschlechtsverkehrs.

[350] Vgl. zur Deutung dieses Satzes die Anmerkung zu *Ratirahasya* VIII,6.

28. Drei Linien, angebracht auf dem Rücken, am Busen oder an den Geschlechtsteilen, können aussehen wie ein Lotosblatt und werden demgemäß bezeichnet. Es dient, wenn der Mann zu einer Reise aufbricht, zur Erinnerung.
29. Wenn die Nägel aus Zuneigung von liebeskundigen Männern zur Anwendung gebracht werden, sind sie die Ursache vollständigen, hohen Glücks für die Frauen, das von nichts anderem übertroffen wird.

*Regeln zur Anwendung der Zähne*

30. Mit Ausnahme der Lippen, der Mundhöhle und der Augen sind die Zähne an den gleichen Stellen wie die Nägel anzuwenden. Von den in den Regeln der Liebeskunst Erfahrenen wird auf die Bedeutung des Ausstoßens wollüstiger Laute[351] beim Gebrauch der Zähne hingewiesen.
31. Gerühmt werden Zähne, die farblich attraktiv, sehr glatt und gleichmäßig sind, dicht beieinander stehen, schmal, scharf und glänzend sind. Schadhafte, rauhe, klaffende, vorstehende und fleckige Zähne sind zu tadeln.
32. Ein leichter Biß in die Unterlippe, der nur eine Rötung zur Folge hat, heißt 'versteckter' Biß. Als 'geschwollener' Biß wird von den Weisen das Drücken der Zähne auf Lippen und Wangen bezeichnet.
33. Durch eine besondere Zusammenfügung[352] von Zahn und Lippe entsteht der 'Korallenstein'. Wiederholte Übung vorausgesetzt, gewährt er Eheleuten eine Befriedigung wie kein anderes Vergnügen.
34. Wenn der Geliebte auf der Unterlippe der Frau mit zwei Zähnen eine Spur hinterläßt, so ist dies der 'Punkt'. Mit allen Zähnen ausgeführt, entsteht die 'Punktgirlande'.
35. Mit den Zahnspitzen ritzt man in die Wangen, die Brust, den Hals und die Stirngegend den 'Wolkenriß' ein. Dieses Mal von der Form einer Kreisscheibe verleiht dem Körper der Frauen einen außerordentlich schönen Schmuck.
36. Wenn der Gatte auf dem Körper der Frau lückenlose, dichte Zahnspur-

351 Etwa *hiṅ* und *sīt*.

352 Vgl. die Anmerkung zu *Ratirahasya* IX,2.

streifen hervorruft, was besonders vor Antritt einer Reise zur Erinnerung geschieht, nenne die Kundigen dies das 'Eberknabbern'.

*Regeln für das Streicheln der Haare*[353]

37. Weiche, dichte, lockige und dunkelfarbige Haare bei jungen Frauen werden gepriesen. Zur Steigerung der Liebe sind sie gemäß dieser Regel vom Mann in angenehmer Weise zu ergreifen, wobei er der Frau gleichzeitig einen Kuß gibt.
38. Wenn der Gatte mit beiden Händen die Locken umfaßt und die Liebste dabei küßt, heißt dies 'Gleichhändigkeit'; greift er nur mit einer Hand zu, ist dies die 'Wellenbühne'.
39. Wenn der Mann, von Leidenschaft ergriffen, die Haare um seine Hand schlingt und die Geliebte so festhält, bezeichnen die der Gesamtheit des Liebesspiels Kundigen dies als 'Schlangenliane'.
40. Wenn Mann und Frau einander küssen und er ihre Haare über dem Ohr streichelt, ehe sie sich aus Leidenschaft zum Beischlaf niederlassen, wird dieses Haarestreicheln als 'Liebesstirnkranz' bezeichnet.
41. So sind der Reihe nach einige der bekanntesten Arten des vorbereitenden Liebesspiels von mir aufgeführt worden. Aus Sorge um den Umfang dieses Buches sind andere als die bekanntesten Arten nicht dargelegt worden.

## X. Abschnitt

*Über die Stellungen beim Geschlechtsverkehr*

1. Der kundige Mann soll die Frau entsprechend ihrer Wesensart[354] durch äußerliche Handlungen für den Verkehr vorbereiten. Ist dadurch ihre Scheide weit geworden, soll er ihr auf der Stätte des Liebesspiels beiwohnen.
2. Auch eine eng gebaute Frau wird locker, wenn sie ihr Schenkelpaar täglich spreizt. Umgekehrt wird eine Frau mit weiter Scheide eng, wenn sie

[353] Weder im *Kāmasūtra* noch im *Ratirahasya* finden sich die hier gegebenen Regeln.

[354] Gemeint sind Anlagen, Typ, Herkunft usw.

beim Verkehr ihr Schenkelpaar schließt.

3. Die Beischlafkundigen unterscheiden folgende Stellungen: liegend, seitlich, sitzend, stehend, geneigt. Die Unterarten dieser fünf Grundstellungen werde ich jetzt der Reihe nach besprechen.

*Die Rückenlage*

4. Wenn sich die Frau vergnügt, indem sie sich auf den Rücken und ihre Beine auf die Schultern des Mannes legt, dann nennen die in den Regeln des Beischlafs Erfahrenen dies die 'gleichfüßige' Stellung.
5. Wenn der Mann sich so im Liebestempel der auf dem Rücken liegenden Frau befindet, daß er ihre beiden Schenkel faßt, die sie außerhalb seiner Hüften hält, nennt man diese Stellung 'städtisch'.
6. Die Frau legt das eine Bein auf den Boden, das andere an ihren Kopf; der Mann vergnügt sich, während er beide Hände auf die Erde legt; dies wird die 'Stellung des Gottes Viṣṇu' genannt.[355]
7. Die auf dem Bett ruhende Schöne zieht mit beiden Händen ihre Füße an sich; der Mann beschläft sie, wobei er ihre Brüste ergreift. Diese Stellung heißt 'Himmelsspur'.[356]
8. Wenn der Mann sich zwischen den Schenkeln der Liebsten befindet und die Frau beschläft, während er die Hände auf den Boden legt,[357] so heißt diese Stellung das 'Rad der Liebe'; in der Welt der Liebesleute ist sie besonders beliebt.
9. Die Frau bringt ihre beiden Füße an die Brust des Gatten und umarmt ihn mit beiden Händen. er seinerseits beschläft die Frau mit leicht gebeugten Schenkeln. Von den Fürsten der Weisen wird dies als die 'herabgeführte' Stellung bezeichnet.
10. Der Geliebte befindet sich zwischen den gespreizten Schenkeln der auf dem Rücken liegenden Frau, wobei er sie während des Beischlafs fest

[355] In *Kāmasūtra* II,6,29 heißt diese Stellung das 'Speerdurchbohren' und gilt als schwer erlernbar.

[356] Die in den folgenden Versen 8-10 erwähnten Stellungen nennt das *Kāmasūtra* nicht.

[357] Wahrscheinlich liegen die Hände nicht schlechthin auf dem Boden, sondern unter den Gesäßbacken der Frau.

umarmt. Diese den Liebenden angenehme Stellung wird von den alten Weisen als die ‘Soma’[358]-Stellung bezeichnet.

11. Wenn die Lotosäugige ihren Gatten in der Weise genießt, daß sie beide Schenkel gekrümmt aufstellt, so ist diese als ‘klaffend’ bezeichnete Stellung ein Wonnespender für junge Leute.[359]

12. Wenn der Mann die verschränkten Schenkel der Geliebten, von Liebesgedanken erfüllt, zusammenpreßt und sie so beschläft, nennen die Weisen diese Stellung die ‘verschlungene’.

13. Wenn sich der Gatte den einen Schenkel der Frau auf die Schulter legt, den anderen aber weit abgespreizt nach unten hält und so in die Frau eindringt, ist dies das ‘Bambusspalten’.

14. Wenn der Gatte der Schönen die Schenkel zusammendrückt[360] und sie oberhalb davon umarmt, ist dies das ‘Zerbrechen’; wenn die beiden Füße der Frau an die Brust des Geliebten gehalten werden, heißt dies das ‘Bersten’.

*Die Seitenlage*

15. Wenn das eine Bein der Frau an der Herzgegend des Mannes zu liegen kommt, das andere aber auf dem Bett ruht, heißt dies die ‘Laute’. Sie ist Frauen im Alter zwischen 30 und 35 Jahren zu empfehlen.[361]

16. Der auf der Seite liegende Mann führt, die Frau umarmend, in höchster Erregung den Beischlaf aus. Von den alten Weisen ist diese Stellung als ‘Schachtel’ bezeichnet worden.

17. Wenn die Beine der Frau eingebogen sind und der Mann den Beischlaf ausführt, indem er sie an seine Nabelgegend bringt, wird von den Für-

---

[358] Trotz unzähliger Bemühungen ist noch keine botanische Identifizierung dieser im alten Iran und Indien kultisch stark genutzten Pflanze beweiskräftig geglückt. Viele vermuten eine *Ephedra*-Art.

[359] *Ratirahasya* X,22 beschreibt diese Stellung genauer.

[360] Nämlich nach der *immissio penis*.

[361] Sehr richtig beobachtet, wie denn überhaupt die Seitenlagen vorzugsweise für ältere bzw. gesundheitlich nicht ganz intakte Paare als “Schonstellungen” (insbesondere *a tergo*) in Betracht kommen.

sten der Weisen dies als 'Krebsstellung' bezeichnet.

*Stellungen im Sitzen*

18. Wenn die Frau in heftiger Leidenschaft ihre Schenkel kreuzt, so daß sie gleichsam eine Schaukel werden, ist dies der 'Lotossitz'. Wird nur ein Schenkel überkreuzt, ergibt sich der 'Halblotossitz'.
19. Wenn die Gazellenäugige ihre Arme innerhalb ihrer Knie hält und den Mann so umarmt, und wenn der Mann sich ebenso verhält, wird dies von den Weisen als 'Fesselung' bezeichnet.[362]
20. Wenn beide Partner in der eben beschriebenen Weise verfahren, die Arme aber jeweils unter den Knien durchziehen, ist dies als 'Schlangenfessel' bekannt.
21. Der Mann legt sich das Schenkelpaar der jungen Frau in seine Ellenbogen[363] und umfaßt mit beiden Armen ihren Hals; dies ist als 'Bändigung' bekannt.
22. Wenn der Mann so in die Frau eindringt, daß Mund auf Mund, Arme an Arme und Schenkel an Schenkel gepreßt sind, spricht man von der 'Schildkrötenstellung'; sind die beiden Schenkel emporgerichtet, ist es die 'umgewendete' Stellung.
23. Wenn der Mann in schräger Körperhaltung die Frau beschläft, wenn sie ihre Beine gekrümmt hat, sprechen die im Liebesspiel Erfahrenen von der 'Beinpaarstellung'.[364]
24. Wenn der Gatte sich zwischen den Knien der Schönen befindet, wobei er sich in den Hüften wiegt, gilt dies als 'Reibung'. Findet die Vereinigung so statt, daß sich beide dabei anschauen, ist dies die 'Affenstellung'.

*Stellungen im Stehen*

25. Wenn der Mann den Beischlaf ausübt, indem er mit dem Ellenbogen die

---

[362] In *Ratirahasya* X,26 ist dies die 'Schlangenfessel'. Überhaupt ordnet der *Anaṅgaraṅga* traditionelle Positionssnamen in abweichender Weise ein.

[363] *kūrpara-* kann allerdings sowohl 'Ellenbogen' als auch 'Knie' bedeuten.

[364] *Ratirahasya* X,31 beschreibt die Stellung anders.

Knie der Frau umfaßt, die ihrerseits den Hals niederbeugt, so ist das die 'Ellenbogen- bzw. Knie-Stellung'.

26. Wenn in der eben beschriebenen Stellung die Frau ein Bein hochhält, entsteht die mit 'Hari-Schritt' bezeichnete Stellung;[365] sie ist besonders bei jungen Frauen beliebt.

27. Wenn die Frau den Akt vollzieht, indem sie sich mit den Armen am Hals des Gatten festhält und seine Hüfte mit ihrem Schenkelpaar fest umklammert, wird dies von den Fürsten der Weisen als 'Ruhmesstellung' bezeichnet.[366]

### *Die gebeugte Stellung*[367]

28. Wenn die Frau beide Hände und Füße aufsetzt und auch das Gesicht nach unten neigt, so daß sie die Stellung einer Kuh einnimmt, und der Gatte sie liebt, indem er ihre Hüften besteigt, wird dies die 'Kuh-Stellung' genannt.

29. Wenn der Mann wie ein Elefant die mit dem Gesicht, dem Kopf, den Armen und den Brüsten auf dem Bauch liegende Frau besteigt, so gilt diese Art des Liebesspiels als 'Elefantenstellung'.

30. Der Mann kann noch zahlreiche andere Stellungen einnehmen: die des Antilopenmännchens, des Ebers, des Esels usw. Als wenig üblich und tadelnswert werden sie jedoch von mir nicht beschrieben.

### *Der* coitus inversus[368]

31. Wenn die Frau gewahrt, daß der Mann erschöpft ist, sie selbst aber vom Verkehr sich noch nicht befriedigt fühlt, weil sie noch von stürmischer Liebe erfüllt ist, mag sie aus eigenem Antrieb zur vollständigen Befriedigung sich ihrerseits auf den Mann legen.

---

[365] Vgl. *Ratirahasya* X,35.

[366] Diese Stellung, bei der die Frau sozusagen am Manne emporklettern muß, ist gewiß nicht weniger schwierig als die Erwerbung von Ruhm.

[367] Gemeint ist der *coitus a tergo*, vgl. die Anmerkung zu *Ratirahasya* X,37.

[368] Hierunter sind diejenigen Stellungen zu verststehen, bei denen die Frau auf dem Mann liegt.

32. Wenn die Frau, nachdem sie den Penis in ihre Scheide eingeführt hat, auf dem Mann liegt, indem sie ihn umarmt und mit ihrem Unterleib die Beischlafbewegungen ausführt, ist die die 'umgekehrte' Stellung.
33. Wenn die Frau, vom Penis des liegenden Mannes aufgespießt, sich mit angewinkelten Beinen so im Kreis dreht, daß sie ein Rad beschreibt, heißt dies die 'umherschweifende Stellung'[369].[370]
34. Nachdem die Frau den Penis des Gatten in ihr Liebesnest[371] eingeführt hat, bewegt sie wie eine Schaukel Hüften und Unterleib nach allen Seiten hin und her; das ist die 'aufgeblühte Stellung'.
35. Beim umgekehrten Beischlaf soll die Frau gurrend und mit entzücktem Antlitz lachend ausrufen: 'Du Schuft, jetzt bist du in meine Gewalt geraten! Von mir bist du im Liebeskampf besiegt worden!'
36. Nachdem sie dies anmutig hat verlauten lassen, werden ihr die Haare gestreichelt und die Lippen geküßt; vom Beischlaf ermattet, wird die Schönäugige dann zum Orgasmus gelangen.
37. Das Erschlaffen ihres lianenhaften Körpers, Ohnmacht, das Schließen der Lotosaugen, vollkommene Kraftlosigkeit – wenn dies der Mann gewahrt, nehme er es als Zeichen des Orgasmus bei der Frau.
38. Ein weiser Mann verwehre folgenden Typen von Frauen den umgekehrten Verkehr: der Elefantenkuh, der Gazelle, einer Schwangeren, einer Wöchnerin, einer Menstruierenden, einer Mageren, einer Fiebernden und einem ganz jungen Mädchen.
39. Ein in der Kunst des Liebesspiels Erfahrener soll auch die Stellungen der Antilope, des Esels als auch die des Hundes und des Büffels zur Anwendung bringen.[372]
40. Wenn die Frau bei den früher beschriebenen Arten des Beischlafs keine

---

[369] Oder auch: 'die "Bienenstellung"'.

[370] Das ist die berühmte 'Mühle', bei der sich die Frau, ohne sich vom Mann zu lösen, mit dem Penis als Achse im Kreis dreht. Das *Kāmasūtra* kennt diese Stellung nur bei der auf dem Rücken liegenden Frau.

[371] Hier übersetzen wir poetischer als Kalyāṇamalla, denn *smarayantra-* heißt wörtlich 'Liebesapparat, -instrument, -maschine'.

[372] Das ist allerdings ein Widerspruch zu der in Vers 30 geäußerten Ansicht.

Befriedigung erlangt, dann soll der Mann die 'umgekehrte' Stellung einnehmen.

41. Eine Frau, die das Glück des Orgasmus nicht erlangt hat, schlägt den Geliebten; sie schüttelt die Hand; sie läßt ihn nicht aufstehen, und sie übt Vergeltung.

42. Eine Jungfrau, eine Gazelle, eine Korpulente, eine Menstruierende, eine Entkräftete, eine Schwangere und eine Wöchnerin lasse man die umgekehrte Stellung nicht einnehmen.[373]

43. Eine in herrlicher Jugend Prangende, Schlanke, die keine Müdigkeit kennt, die ihre Schamhaftigkeit überwunden hat und verliebt ist, eine solche schöne Frau mag beim Beischlaf die Stellung des Mannes einnehmen.

44. Ein vernünftiger Mann aber wird, wenn er sieht, daß die Frau der Müdigkeit anheimfällt, sie auf das Bett legen und sie in der 'Schachtelstellung' zum Orgasmus bringen.[374]

45. Wenn die Frau mit dem Mund und der Schamgegend herandrückt, stöhnt, seufzt, schwitzt und alle Scham fahren läßt, dann sind dies die Anzeichen dafür, daß ihr Orgasmus gekommen ist.

46. Ohnmacht und ein Schließen der Augen sind weitere Anzeichen dafür, daß die Zeit ihres Ergusses gekommen ist. Sobald der Mann dies alles bemerkt hat, soll er die Frau zum höchsten Glück führen.[375]

47. Wenn der Frau das Glück des Orgasmus gekommen ist, bemächtigen sich Schweiß und Schlaffheit ihres Körpers. Sie bringt ihre Haare, Kleider usw. in Ordnung und hat nun den Wunsch nach Ruhe.

48. Ein kundiger Mann, der spürt, daß die Geliebte in ihren Beischlafbewegungen schneller wird, richte seinen Geist auf andere Dinge und werde in seinen eigenen Bewegungen für eine Weile langsamer.[376] Indem er die Frau umarmt und ihr leidenschaftliche Worte zuflüstert, soll er, wenn

---

[373] Die teilweise Wiederholung von Passagen aus Vers 38 deutet auf eine Unsicherheit in der Textüberlieferung.

[374] Vgl. Vers 16 und Anm. 361.

[375] D.h. er darf gerade jetzt seine Bewegungen nicht etwa verlangsamen.

[376] So soll die vorzeitige Ejakulation vermieden werden.

ihr der Orgasmus kommt, seinen Samen in sie ergießen.[377]

49. So ist das Wollustgefühl die Ursache dafür, daß eine Frau in die Gewalt des Mannes gerät. Bis zum Tode wird sie ihn selbst um des Geldes, der Familie und des Lebens willen nicht verlassen.[378] Andererseits wird der in der Glückserfüllung Erfahrene zur Gefügigmachung der Frau weder Zaubersprüche noch Liebestränke, Opfer, Schicksalsfügungen oder Besitztümer vonnöten haben.

*Anweisungen zum Schlagen mit der Hand und zum* sīt-*Laut*

50. Zum Liebeskampf der beiden Körper gehören auch das Schlagen mit der Hand und das Ausstoßen gurrender Laute. Dabei ist das Schlagen von vierfacher, das Gurren von fünffacher Art.

51. Das Schlagen geschieht mit der ausgestreckten Hand, mit dem Handrükken,[379] mit der Faust und mit der glatten Handfläche, also in vierfacher Weise.[380] Über die dafür geeigneten Stellen werde ich jetzt sprechen.

52. Mit der flachen Hand schlägt man auf die Seiten und die Geschlechtsteile, mit der Faust auf den Rücken und auf den Kopf, auf die Nasenflügel mit der ausgestreckten Hand, auf die Herzgegend mit dem Handrücken.

*Besondere Arten des Schlagens*

53. Wenn die Frau beim Beischlaf auf dem Mann liegt und ihn mit der Faust auf die Herzgegend schlägt, so wird dieser Schlag mit der Hand von den Weisen als 'ausgeführt' bezeichnet.

54. Wenn die Frau den Gatten während des Beischlafs mit der ausgebreiteten Hand schlägt, heißt diese Art 'beflaggt'; erfolgen die Schläge nur mit dem Daumen, sprechen die Kundigen von der 'Tropfengirlande'.

---

[377] Der Autor sieht also in der Gleichzeitigkeit der Spannungslösung ein Maximum an partnerschaftlicher Harmonie.

[378] D.h. selbst der Verlust der Habe, der Widerstand der Familie und die Bedrohung des eigenen Lebens könnten sie nicht dazu bringen, von dem Mann abzulassen.

[379] So nach *Ratirahasya* X,54 zu ergänzen.

[380] Es ist nicht an heftige Schläge, sondern eher an liebevolle und dabei aufmunternde Klapse zu denken.

55. Verabfolgt die Frau die Schläge mit Daumen und Mittelfinger, und zwar langsam, aber in großer Leidenschaft, so wird dies von den alten Weisen als 'wonnebereitender Ring' bezeichnet.

### Sīt *und andere Wollustlaute*

56. Jetzt werde ich die fünf Arten der Wollustlaute der Reihe nach darlegen; es sind der *hiṅ*-Laut, das 'Donnern', der *sīt*-, *ut*- und *phūt*-Laut.[381]
57. Der *hiṅ*-Laut entsteht als gleichzeitig aus Mund und Nase entweichender Laut. Das 'Donnern' erinnert an den tiefen Laut einer Gewitterwolke.[382]
58. Der *sīt*-Laut klingt wie das Zischen einer Schlange, und der *ut*-Laut verursacht ein Geräusch wie splitternder Bambus; der *phūt*-Laut dagegen
59. klingt wie Regentropfen, die auf eine Wasseroberfläche fallen. Damit sind die fünf Arten der Wollust- bzw. Schmerzlaute der Reihe nach abgehandelt.
60. Während des Liebesgenusses stößt die Schöne noch andere Laute wie *hiṅ* usw. aus, die wie die Schreie einer Wachtel, eines indischen Kuckucks, einer Taube, eines Schwans und eines Pfaus klingen.
61. Wenn der Gatte beim Beischlaf die Frau heftig in die Lippen beißt, dann macht diese sofort *sīt*, womit sie wiederum höchste Leidenschaft bewirkt.

### *Merkmale der acht Typen von Damen*[383]

62. Eine Dame, deren Mann morgens heimkommt, mit allen Merkmalen des Geschlechtsverkehrs mit einer Nebenbuhlerin gezeichnet, die Augen von Schlaflosigkeit gerötet und trübe, und der dann aus Befangenheit süße Worte zu ihr spricht – eine solche Dame bezeichnet man als 'hintergangen'.
63. Eine Frau, die zu Hause schön gekleidet nachts auf dem Bett lagert und ihren Blick auf den von einer Reise zurückkehrenden Gatten richtet, wird von den Weisen als 'am Schlafzimmer haftend' bezeichnet.
64. Eine Frau, die den ihr zu Füßen gesunkenen Gatten mit rauhen Worten in großem Zorn wegstößt, hinterher aber den Schmerz der Trennung be-

---

[381] Vgl. zu den einzelnen Lauten die Anmerkungen zu *Ratirahasya* X,55.

[382] Nach dem *Kāmasūtra* ein gutturaler *ham*-Laut.

[383] Diese sind im *Kāmasūtra* wie im *Ratirahasya* nicht aufgeführt.

klagt, nennen die Fürsten der Weisen eine 'Streitsüchtige'.

65. Eine Frau, die, von Wollust erfüllt und bar jeder Scham, mit angelegtem Schmuck nachts heimlich in ein fremdes Haus zum Beischlaf geht, nennen die Weisen eine 'Buhlerin'.

66. Eine Frau, die, um den Liebsten herbeizubringen, eine Botin ausgesandt hat und die nun, vom Geschlechtstrieb beherrscht, zum Ort des Rendezvous geht, dort aber die Botin ohne den Mann zurückkommen sieht, und die daraufhin in tiefste Bekümmernis verfällt, wird die 'Enttäuschte' genannt.

67. Eine Frau, deren Gatte im Ausland weilt und deren Schönheit trotz Mondschein, Lotos und Sandel leidet, wird von den Weisen als die 'Verlassene' bezeichnet.

68. Eine Frau, deren Mann allen Arten von Liebesspielen abhold ist und der sie nur wegen des bloßen Vorhandenseins des Geschlechtstriebes nicht verläßt, die aber durch den Beischlaf kein Wollustgefühl erfährt, wird von den Weisen als 'vom Gatten unabhängig' bezeichnet.

69. Eine schöne Frau, die ihren Körper mit mannigfaltigen Blumengewinden geschmückt hat, nach dem Beischlaf verlangt, von Zuneigung zu ihrem Geliebten erfüllt ist und beweglichen Blickes lange Zeit im Schlafzimmer wartet – eine solche Frau wird von den besten der Weisen als 'sehnsuchtsvoll' bezeichnet.

70. Damit sind die acht Typen von Damen geschildert: die am Schlafzimmer Haftende, die Sehnsuchtsvolle, die vom Gatten Unabhängige, die Streitsüchtige, die Enttäuschte, die Buhlerin, die Hintergangene und die Verlassene.

71. Als wohlbekanntes höchstes Ziel des Lehrbuches der Liebeskunst soll der Verständige durch mannigfaltige Liebesvergnügungen die Sinne der Frauen täglich aus Zuneigung erfreuen. Mit Leichtigkeit wird ein solcher Mann unvergängliches Glück erfahren.

72. Solange der göttliche Fluß[384] im Kopf des Heilbringers[385] und Gaurī[386]

[384] Der Ganges, als Gaṅgā weiblich vorgestellt. Dies und das Folgende ist mythologisch-symbolisch zu verstehen.

[385] Gemeint ist Śiva.

in dessen anderer Körperhälfte ihre Stätte haben, solange die Liebe der Meerestochter[387] zum Vaikuṇṭha[388]-Herren, zu Hari[389], währt, solange man am Vedastudium sich erfreut, und solange Erde, Sonne und Mond bestehen – solange möge der *Anaṅgaraṅga* stets den Verliebten zur Freude gereichen.

**Ende des *Anaṅgaraṅga***

386 Śivas Gattin.

387 Lakṣmī, Gattin des Gottes Viṣṇu.

388 Himmlischer Aufenthaltsort Viṣṇus.

389 'Der Falbe', Beiname Viṣṇus.

# Miraculous Maternity: A Gender Paradox in the Bengali *Rāmāyāṇa*[*]

MANDAKRANTA BOSE

Story-tellers can do wonders with their tales. They can take us to a make-believe world and convince us of the feasibility of extraordinary happenings. Especially when an author relates a miraculous event that turns out to have some basis in an older text of established authority, one is led to wonder what might be the proportions of veracity, realism and fancy behind its claims upon one's belief. At the same time, one also wonders what purpose is served by the invention of such an incredible event. Old myths and legends are of course full of miraculous happenings. But few can compare in fancifulness with an episode that we find in the 15th century Bengali version of the epic *Rāmāyaṇa* (*Rāmāẏaṇ* in Bengali) by Kr̥ttibās, which, I shall argue in this essay, celebrates devotional spirituality at the same time as it serves the ideals of a patriarchal society under Brahminical tutelage. The event I speak of is one of miraculous birth, one of several in the epic, that seems to have been invented by Kr̥ttibās to facilitate plot development. But it also carries an intriguing social subtext. This is the account of the birth of Bhagīratha, an ancestor of Rāma. How this account is skilfully woven into the narrative scheme of the epic tale to make it appealing and believable, and how it reinforces the epic's class and gender ideals, is the subject of the present discussion.

For centuries the *Rāmāyaṇa* remained perhaps the most widely known literary product of India, reaching both literate and sub-literate audiences and rendered in many languages and versions. In Bengali there have been many retellings of the *Rāmāyaṇa* from early to recent times, covering a wide range of narrative and sectarian choices, from renditions of the entire plot to selected episodes, and used to advance both Vaiṣṇava and Śākta messages. The version of

---

[*] Pronunciation with regard to the silent *a* is disregarded in the transliteration of the Bengali text passages quoted, and of the names of the *dramatis personae* common to Sanskrit and Bengali, but taken into account in the transliteration of the names of Bengali works and persons. – As the second part of a ligature (except after *b* and *r*) *b* is transliterated as *v*.

the epic that Bengali audiences knew – and still know – best is Kr̥ttibās's 15th century rendering of Vālmīki's original poem,[1] and its popularity depended to a large extent on Kr̥ttibās's supple verse form, a particularly suitable form for recitation. Because of the numerous editions that its popularity has brought forth, without, however, a definitive critical edition, one has to be cautious in commenting on details of the text, although all editions do agree on the main lines of the story and rarely vary in plot details.

Close to 1500 manuscripts of the *Kr̥ttibāsī Rāmāyaṇ* are extant, most from the 19th century.[2] The earliest dependable text is the one published in 1803 by the Serampore Mission Press, which was followed by others that rely largely upon it but sometimes introduce changes or interpolations, specially the editions known as Baṭ'talā or mass-market editions. But since they agree as to the bulk of Kr̥ttibās's departures from Vālmīki's original, and since they fit the narrative scheme of the *Kr̥ttibāsī Rāmāyaṇ* organically, it is reasonable to attribute these inventions to a single authorial imagination, that of Kr̥ttibās himself. The episode we are considering here, that of the supernatural birth of Bhagīratha, is a case in point. Included fully in the 1803 edition but removed by a later editor who brought out a 'cleaner' version of the *Kr̥ttibāsī Rāmāyaṇ* (MUKHOPĀDHYĀẎ 1957), it continues to appear unchanged in popular editions which clearly view the 1803 edition as the more reliable. In sum, the *Rāmāyaṇa* current in the Bengali market is the *Kr̥ttibāsī* one, a text entirely oriented to the Vaiṣṇava devotional line.

Kr̥ttibās wrote at a time when devotional Hinduism was sweeping through Eastern India. Not surprisingly, while he followed Vālmīki's text faithfully in its main lines and in the overwhelming majority of details, he consistently re-

1 While the exact date of Vālmīkī's *Rāmāyaṇa* is not known, scholars place it between the 2nd century BC and 2nd century AD.

2 Recently a catalogue of the late Professor Sukumar Sen's collection has appeared: *Catalogue for the Sukumar Sen (Barddhamān Sāhitya Sabhā) Manuscript Collection* compiled by Rebecca J. Manring with Hena Basu. Ann Arbor, Michigan: Association for Asian Studies 2006. It contains a large number of manuscript copies of the *Kr̥ttibāsī Rāmāyaṇ*, which, however, still lacks a definitive critical edition.

moulded the older story to emphasise Rāma's divinity, thereby placing Rāma firmly at the centre of devotional Vaiṣṇavism. In his hands the Rāma tale becomes solely an illustration of Viṣṇu's design for creation and his redemptive plan for earthly beings, both human and non-human. Thus, every event in the long story, beginning in heaven and evolving through eons before Rāma's actual life-span, is either a direct illustration or a necessary condition of his divinity, power and benevolence. Such seems to be the immediate point of the story of Bhagīratha's birth.

Kr̥ttibās's account of his birth greatly stretches credulity. The situation when the episode begins is a grave one comprising two crises, one originating in the past, the other looming over the future. The first occurs when a past ruler of the Raghu dynasty, King Sagara, loses his sixty thousand sons to the wrath of Kapilamuni whose angry gaze burns them to cinders, because of which they are ineligible for receiving proper funerary rites. But the sage tells Aṃśumān[3], Sagara's grandson, that Sagara's sons would be redeemed if one of their descendants could bring the holy Gaṅgā from heaven to wash over their ashes. Accordingly, beginning with Sagara himself, every Raghu king in each generation performs many austerities and penances to bring the Gaṅgā to earth but everyone fails to do so, leaving a taint on the family. The crisis deepens when Dilīpa, great-grandson of Sagara, dies without leaving any child to carry on the quest. But his death has other implications and brings about the second crisis, which is immediate and potentially catastrophic. Since Dilīpa has left behind two queens but no son, his line faces extinction, which causes great consternation among the gods, for unless the line continues, not only will there be none to bring Gaṅgā to earth but no Rāma will be born to rid the world of the Rākṣasa king Rāvaṇa. Requested by the gods, Śiva visits Dilīpa's queens and advises them to copulate with one another. Out of their union is born a son. But as the child is born without bones, the distraught queens take him to the river to drown him.

We must look at the text better to grasp the nuances of Kr̥ttibās's narration. Here is the first part of the story (SR, Ādikāṇḍa, p. 28):

[3] Nominative form, since in Bengali the stem form is, as a rule, the Sanskrit nominative.

*mariẏā dilīpa rājā gela brahmaloka* ||
*arājaka haïla rājya ayodhyā-nagara* |
*svargete cintita brahmā āra purandara* ||
*śuniẏāchi janmibena biṣṇu sūryakule* |
*kemane bāṙibe baṃśa nirmūla haïle* ||
*bhābiẏā sakala deba yukti kari mane* |
*ayodhyāẏa pāṭhāila prabhu trilocane* ||
*dilīpera dui jāẏā āchilena bāse* |
*bṛṣa ārohaṇe śiba gelena sakāśe* ||
*kahilena dõhākāra prati tripurāri* ||
*mama bare putrabatī habe eka nārī* |
*dui nārī kahe, śuni śibera bacana* ||
*bidhabā āmarā kise haïbe nandana* |
*śaṅkara balena, duijane kara rati* ||
*mama bare ekera haïbe susantati* |
*ei bara diẏā gela deba tripurāri* |
*snāna kari gela dui dilīpera nārī* ||
*samprītite āchilena se dui yubatī* |
*katadine ekajana haïla ṛtumatī* ||
*dõhete jānila yadi dõhāra sandarbha* |
*dõhe keli karite ekera haïla garbha* ||
*daśamāsa haïla garbha prasaba samaẏa* |
*māṃsapiṇḍa mātra putra haïla udaẏa* ||
*putra kole kariẏā kāndena duijana* |
*hena putra-bara kena dilā trilocana* ||
*asthi nāhi māṃsapiṇḍa calite nā pāre* |
*dekhiẏā hāsibe loka sakala saṃsāre* ||
*kole kari nila tāhā cupaṙi bhitare* |
*sarayūra tīre gela phelibāra tare* ||

King Dilīpa went to Brahmaloka when he died, and the kingdom Ayodhyā became lawless. In heaven, Brahmā[4] and Purandara became worried. [They said,]

---

[4] Cf. note 3.

> 'We have heard that Viṣṇu will take birth in the Sūrya dynasty, [but] how can that happen if the lineage is extinguished [lit: becomes rootless)?' Having thought [about this], the gods decided to send lord Trilocana (Śiva) to Ayodhyā. The two wives of Dilīpa were residing [there, and] Śiva went there riding on his bull. Tripurāri (Śiva) told the two women, 'By my boon one woman [of the two of you] will have a son.' Hearing these words of Śiva, the two women said, 'We are widows, how can we have a son?' Śaṅkara said, 'You two copulate, and one of you will have a fine son by my boon.' Having bestowed this boon Lord Tripurāri left. Dilīpa's two women left after taking their baths.[5] These two young women enjoyed a close friendship, and [when] after a while one of them entered the fertility cycle,[6] they understood their situation, and upon uniting sexually with one another, one conceived. The time of birth approached after the tenth month, [but] the son was born a lump of flesh. The two queens began to cry and lament, 'Why did Trilocana give us this boon? There is no bone, [only] a lump of flesh unable to walk, and everyone in the world will laugh [at him].' Putting [him] in a basket, [they] went to the banks of the Sarayū to drown him.

Before going on with the rest of the story, let us stop to take account of some important elements. First, the gods concerned are some of the chief deities in the Hindu pantheon and arbiters of human affairs, who are fulfilling their roles as guardians of history and human destiny. Second, they are themselves bound to a predetermined course of events and must exert themselves to keep those events on track. But why does their intervention opt for so outrageous a solution? On the human level the text becomes even more intriguing. Producing an offspring is usually not a problem for myths in general and the *Rāmāyaṇa* in particular: there are always convenient gods or holy sages to donate their seed, magic potions to ensure conception, and even rape (as in the birth of this same Bhagīratha's ancestor Hārīta). There is also the more prominent case of Sītā's birth in the furrow of King Janaka's plough, although that may be a sexual metaphor. With these precedents already set, the text had no need to opt for exclusively female progenitors, a solution utterly bizarre in its violation of human biology.

---

[5] They were obviously accosted at the bathing place.

[6] On *ṛtu-* cf. DAS 2003: 14-16.

In Kr̥ttibās's milieu, however, that solution may not have seemed quite so unnatural. His authority for this scientific marvel is no less than the legendary physician Suśruta, whose work, the *Suśrutasaṃhitā,* remains one of the pillars of Āyurvedic knowledge and practice. In the second chapter of the work, the Śārīrasthāna, occurs the following verse (2,47):[7]

> *yadā nāryāv upeyātāṃ vr̥ṣasyantyau kathañcana* |
> *muñcataḥ śukram anyo'nyam anasthis tatra jāyate* ||
> When two women, both in heat, approach one another somehow [and] release semen, the [offspring] is born without any bone.

To what extent this biological prodigy was an accepted part of Āyurvedic belief remains to be assessed, for Jejjaṭa, an authoritative early commentator on the *Suśrutasaṃhitā,* dismisses it summarily,[8] while the commentators Gayadāsa and Ḍalhaṇa do not (DAS 2003: 229). On his part, Kr̥ttibās follows this source closely in its two crucial elements, picking out for particular mention the women's erotic reciprocity – the queens are in a state of mutual *samprīti* and engage in *keli* or sexual play – and the birth of the offspring without bones. It is perhaps fruitless to speculate why he did so beyond saying that he lends the story credibility by implicitly drawing upon medical authority, even though his source need not have directly been Suśruta's text. More worth speculating are the social implications of his invention, particularly social attitudes about sexuality and gender status. Does the matter-of-fact reporting of a same-sex relationship indicate that it was common and sanctioned in contemporary society? Or does the context of marvellous happenings suggest that actions, no matter how extraordinary, are validated if ordained by the gods?

More questions arise as we move on to the rest of the story, which has reached a crisis: what good is a son so unnaturally deformed? But kindly fate in the shape of two holy men intervenes (SR, Ādikāṇḍa, p. 29):

---

7 ACHARYA/ACHARYA 1945: 343. – For drawing my attention to this information, I am grateful to Rahul Peter Das, who discusses the Āyurvedic belief system exhaustively in DAS 2003. Variants of the verse are noted by DAS 2003: 229, note 795.

8 Cited by DESHPANDE 1978: 43 (in this edition, the śloka in question is numbered 50).

*henakāle dekhila baśiṣṭha tapodhana* |
*dhyānete jānila tāra sakala lakṣaṇa* ||
*muni bale thuẏe jāo pathe śoẏāiẏā* |
*karuṇā karibe keha ātura dekhiẏā* ||
*putre pathe śoẏāiẏā dõhe gela bāse* |
*snāna karibāre muni aṣṭābakra āse* ||
*āṭa ṭhā̃i bā̃kā muni gamane kātara* |
*bālaka temani kare pathera upara* ||
*eka dr̥ṣṭe aṣṭābakra tāra pāne cāẏa* |
*mane bhābe āmāre e dekhiẏā bheṅāẏa* ||
*āmāre dekhiẏā yadi kara upahāsa* |
*mama brahmaśāpe habe śarīra bināśa* ||
*yadi taba deha haẏa svabhabe emana* |
*mama bare hao tumi madana-mohana* ||
*aṣṭābakra muni sei biṣṇura samāna* |
*yāre bara śāpa dena kabhu nahe āna* ||
*aṣṭābakra munira mahimā camatkāra* |
*dā̃ṙāila uṭhiẏā se rājāra kumāra* ||
*dhyāne jānilena aṣṭābakra tapodhana* |
*baṭe mahāpuruṣa e dilīpanandana* ||
*ubhaẏa rāṇīke ḍāki āne munibara* |
*putra peẏe harasita dõhe gela ghara* ||
*āsiẏā sakala muni karila kalyāṇa* |
*bhage bhage janma hetu bhagīratha nāma* ||
*mahākabi kr̥ttibāsa paṇḍita parama* |
*ādikāṇḍe gāna bhagīrathera janama* ||

At this time the great sage Vaśiṣṭha saw [them and] learned of all aspects of the matter through meditation. The sage said, 'Place [the deformed baby] by the roadside and someone will take pity on seeing such a helpless one.' The two [queens] went home leaving their son by the roadside. The sage Aṣṭāvakra, walking painfully as his body was bent in eight places, came [along the same road] to take a bath. The boy looked similarly [deformed to the sage as he lay] by the road. Aṣṭāvakra looked at him and thought that [the boy] was mocking him. [He cursed him, saying,] 'If you are making fun as you look at me, your body will be destroyed by the Brahman-curse (Brahmin's curse). [But] if your body is naturally [deformed] like this, become beautiful, as pleasing as Cupid.' The sage Aṣṭāvakra is like Viṣṇu himself and his curse or boon can never be otherwise. Marvellous was Aṣṭāvakra's glory: the son of the king rose up [on his feet]! The sage Aṣṭāvakra came to know through his meditation that this was a great man, son of Dilīpa, and called the two queens. Ecstatic at getting a son, the two went home and all the sages came to bless them. Since the son was born from two *bhaga*s (female organs), [he] was named Bhagīratha. The great poet Kr̥ttibās, a great scholar, [thus] sings of Bhagīratha's birth in the opening chapter [of his *Rāmāyaṇ*].

The female agency intimated earlier in the course of the story, where the two young women are said to be in a continuing relationship (*samprītite āchilena se dui yubati*) and enjoy sexual play (*keli*), seems further emphasised in the conclusion. Here the narrator goes out of his way to derive the name *Bhagīratha* from the word *bhaga* (vulva), a forced construction not warranted by Sanskrit usage.[9] This is indeed a great departure from the Vālmīki version, from which Kr̥ttibās's work was derived, and also from any other version. But to infer that the poet is thereby identifying women's innate power as the key to the resolution of the crisis would be a serious error of interpretation. The bulk of the story actually proves quite the opposite. As we trace its course, we find that the two women seem in fact no more than biological receptacles of destiny and governed wholly by male authority. The story can indeed be taken to be a clear illustration of the old dictum *putrārthe kriyate bhāryā* 'a wife is made (= taken) for the purpose of [begetting] a son'.

It is hardly without significance that the queens, of all the characters in the episode, remain unnamed. It is a male deity, Śiva, who devises the solution to their childlessness and dictates it to them, reassuring them as they lament their widowhood. Their sexuality is released only under male guidance and is in itself ineffectual as a creative act. Though one of them does conceive, she produces only an incomplete human being. For the process to be completed, the

[9] On the classification and linguistic history of the compound *bhagin* + *ratha* = *bhagīratha* see WACKERNAGEL 1957: 133 (§ 56c).

women have to be guided step by step by yet another male authority figure, this time the sage Vaśiṣṭha, the Raghu dynasty's preceptor. Clearly, women may produce offspring on their own without male intervention but not perfect ones, the biological assumption here situated not too far from the Aristotelian thesis that females are unrealised males. But the final demonstration of male potency comes when the boneless lump of flesh that is the product of two women's bodies is viewed by Aṣṭāvakra, who completes the task half done by the women by transforming the lump of flesh into a properly constituted male child, handsome and strong.[10] Instead of celebrating female capability and far from suggesting female self-sufficiency, the story would thus seem actually to assert female insufficiency and dependency, indeed, history's dependency, on male authority. Femaleness itself becomes ambiguous at least for one of the two queens, the one who does not conceive and presumably plays the male role by contributing what Suśruta's śloka calls semen. The paradox of the story is that women in it are at once potent and impotent. They can impregnate other women but cannot engender a complete child, which only a male can. Both in strategic planning (the gods and Vaśiṣṭha) and physical performance (Aṣṭāvakra), masculine ability saves the world.

Let us not forget that the lesbian relationship Kr̥ttibās describes is devised by the gods and blessed by the sages. Divine sanction being so ready, Kr̥ttibās could have ended the episode with the birth of a healthy and normal child. But he did not. Is it because so immediately happy an outcome would be a threat to masculinity by rendering male participation in procreation irrelevant? For we can safely assume that no male would be pleased to see that women are capable of creating life independently, even if it be by divine intervention or total surrender to God. The *Suśrutasaṃhitā* too, on whose authority Kr̥ttibās may ultimately be drawing, keeps the ethos and the power structure of patriarchy intact by asserting the supremacy of the masculine physique.

But even if it would thus be an error to simply interpret the location of the

[10] Note that the child can stand, whereas according to the passage previously quoted it was being carried in a basket by the queens, seemingly just after its birth. That it can now stand indicates that the queens wanted to drown a child already old enough to potentially stand, or else that the boon has given a younger child this power.

resolution of the crisis (i.e., the saving of the dynasty and ensuring Rāma's birth) in the female womb as a testament to feminine power, the devaluation of the female that is traced above as a possible interpretation need not be a piece of deliberately designed misogyny particular to Kr̥ttibās. In fact, his *Rām-āyaṇ*, like the *Rāmāyaṇa* versions of Tul'sīdās and a host of other post-Vālmīki narrators, exalts female characters[11] – most prominently Sītā, but also several forest dwelling and many Rākṣasa women, including Rāvaṇa's chief queen Mandodarī. This attitude is in fact essential to the ethos of *bhakti*, or devotional Hinduism, particularly of the Vaiṣṇava variety to which Kr̥ttibās subscribes and which promotes tolerance, gentleness, forgiveness and non-violence as indispensable to spiritual elevation. A degree of feminisation of the individual is inescapable within the Vaiṣṇava metaphysic which regards God in the form of Viṣṇu as the ultimate male (*puruṣa*) in the sense that He is the one and indivisible source of all potency, to whom all creatures must surrender. Necessarily then, the devotee has to be in a position of submission, for which the socially dictated meekness of the female persona is an apt metaphor.[12]

The controlling impulse of the Bhagīratha episode is of course *bhakti*, for it proves the loving care with which the gods keep watch over human life and ensure the incarnation of Viṣṇu as Rāma, and this can be requited only by human devotion. Kr̥ttibās's entire work is aimed at asserting that *bhakti* is at the root of all action, and underneath appearances sometimes to the contrary, all creatures are actually in a situation of yearning for and submission (*prapatti*) to the Divine. The Bhagīratha story and all such deviations from Vālmīki's original seem unvaryingly designed to orient the epic to a devotional matrix. The devotional impulse is so strong that Kr̥ttibās adds twists in the story that reveal almost every notable Rākṣasa ultimately as a true devotee of Rāma, although they may not always seem to be so, as we see in the stories of Ahirāvaṇa, Mahirāvaṇa, Vīrabāhu and Taraṇīsena. Even Rāvaṇa may have chosen his evil

---

[11] See AKLUJKAR 2000. One must, however, bear in mind that the exaltation of women as personifications of virtue and moral purity is a common means of marginalising them.

[12] For a discussion of the devotee's relationship with the Lord see, e.g., GONDA 1970, chapter 3, particularly pp. 60f.

ways as a sure method of fast-tracking to liberation by inviting death at Rāma's hands. Rāma knows in his heart that *āmāra parama bhakta rājā daśānana* 'King Daśānana (= Rāvaṇa) is an unsurpassed devotee of mine' (SR, Laṅkākāṇda, p. 343), and the dying Rāvaṇa confesses to Rāma: *ciradina āmi dāsa caraṇe tomāra* 'I am a servant at your feet forever' (SR, Laṅkākāṇḍa, p. 344).

Within this ethos of submission to a higher authority the subjugation of King Dilīpa's two queens to the dynastic agenda fits perfectly. Devotion is a necessary condition for the Bhagīratha episode to flow smoothly, but it is the crisis of lineage that is foregrounded in the narrative. That the primary concern is social becomes even more evident as we consider the follow-up to the story, where the connection between birth, social status and service to the establishment receives careful attention. Still harping on Bhagīratha's birth, Kṛttibās says that at the age of five the child was taunted as a bastard by another boy. But his mother reassured him by divulging the truth about his divinely ordained birth and his high destiny, that of redeeming his forefathers by bringing Gaṅgā to earth. So predestined, Bhagīratha accomplishes his task and lives on in public memory as a model of resolute virtue. In thus setting aside an origin that would be evidently considered ignominious in the narrator's own society, Kṛttibās is surely placing the integrity of a power establishment over birth. A parallel occurs earlier in the same part of his *Rāmāyaṇ*, where the great sage Śukra's daughter Abjā is violently raped by his pupil, King Daṇḍa of the Sūrya dynasty. The sage's wrathful gaze burns the king into ashes and the dynasty is threatened with extinction, but is saved when Abjā's illegitimate son Hārīta is acknowledged as the rightful heir to the throne. Taken together, these stories pragmatically place perpetuation above purity where the survival of lineage is concerned; the much advertised value of women's sexual immaculateness becomes secondary.

The compromise of standardised female chastity also raises the question of reception. How might its sensational lesbianism have been received by Kṛttibās's audience? Would they have been offended by this seeming valorisation of a sexuality that had no public sanction as far as we know? If they were not offended, what would be the grounds for exemption?

The explanation frequently offered of the marvellous and the supernatural is that they are symbolic expressions of some deep truth. The readiness to discover symbols, however, characterises an academic rather than a mass audience. An ordinary reader or listener, whether he or she believed in the biological reality of same-sex conception or not, might simply have accepted it as a literary necessity in a tale of divine beings and supernatural heroes located in an unimaginably distant past, the truth value of which is so completely unverifiable as to be irrelevant.

On the other hand, AZIZ/MALONEY 1985: 109, 190, mention a general belief in Bangladesh that the offspring of homosexual women are unhealthy. The reason for this can be deduced from other statements in the work cited. According to these, the result of female masturbation[13] is that 'they lose the strength of the semen' (p. 105), which parallels the same result due to male masturbation (pp. 106, 190) and male homosexuality (p. 108). The linkage between wastage of semen, be it due to excessive intercourse or 'unnatural' semen emission, and weakness of the semen is a common topos (pp. 115ff.).

On the strength of this evidence and the clear parallels between the male and the female, it seems self-evident that 'semen' of women has, like male semen, a role to play in the procreatory process in the belief system underlying the statements above. Thus, though this source has no clear statement on the possibility of two women copulating with each other to produce a child, the parallels between male and female mentioned do not make such a belief *a priori* impossible. Unfortunately, this is all that can be said at this stage due to a seeming dearth of further studies on such matters.

If such a birth was indeed deemed possible by Kr̥ttibās's audience, but considered unhealthy and undesirable, then the invention of the Bhagīratha story was a particularly effective tactic to demonstrate the transformative potency of divine intervention and – not just any, but – Brahminical masculinity.

In any case, the story seems an integral part of Kr̥ttibās's work for narrative as much as ideological reasons. On the narrative level, Kr̥ttibās makes Bhagīratha's birth a precondition to Rāma's redemptive appearance on earth; on the ideological front, he makes it – if our interpretation be correct – the validation of an idealised governance system based on hierarchies of social station and gen-

[13] Using fingers, eggplants, cucumbers or candles.

der: power emanates from the gods and channels to ordinary mortals through holy and learned men's knowledge, and arms men to perform heroic deeds all through history. While the gods can overrule nature, the sages can guide mortals by their insights into the true meaning of events, as we see in Vaśiṣṭha's felicitous counsel to the distraught queens and Aṣṭāvakra's acuity. All of this is the frame in which Rāma's prefiguration in the person of Bhagīratha receives the power to purify the earth by bringing the Gaṅgā down from heaven.

In this grand scheme for upholding *dharma*, the two queens are nameless instruments, passed over as soon as their bodies have performed their required functions. Even though unprovable, it seems probable that there is also the implicit reassurance as to the validation of those functions by the knowledge of another sage, the great Suśruta. But though essential to this crucial birth, these women are thereafter irrelevant to its outcomes and therefore to the epic. One is tempted to see in them the prefiguration of Sītā herself, the woman for whom the war of the *Rāmāyaṇa* is fought, but who is rejected by Rāma at the very moment of her rescue. Kr̥ttibās softens Vālmīki's original, in which Rāma tells Sītā that his reason for waging the war was to reclaim his dynasty's prestige, and that she is in herself irrelevant to him. But even Kr̥ttibās's Rāma, heartbroken though he is by the cruel duty he has to perform, invokes family prestige as his reason both for rescuing Sītā and for later casting her off. Such seems to be the paradoxical position of women in the epic: essential to the story, they are irrelevant to its world.[14]

## Bibliography


ACHARYA, Narayana Ram; ACHARYA Jadavji Trikamji (eds.) 1945: *The Suśrutasaṃhitā of Suśruta*. Bombay: Nirṇaya Sāgar Press.

AZIZ, K.M. Ashraful; MALONEY, Clarence 1985: *Life Stages, Gender and Fertility in Bangladesh*. Dhaka: International Centre for Diarrhoeal Disease Research, Bangladesh. Monograph 3.

AKLUJKAR, Vidyut 2000. 'Anasūyā: A Pativratā with Panache', in: Mandakranta Bose (ed.), *Faces of the Feminine in Ancient, Medieval and Modern India*. New York: Oxford University Press, pp. 56-68.


---

[14] I am grateful to Rahul Peter Das for his comments and suggestions.

DAS, Rahul Peter 2003: *The Origin of the Life of a Human Being. Conception and the Female According to Ancient Indian Medical and Sexological Literature*. Delhi: Motilal Banarsidass Publishers. Indian Medical Tradition 6.

DESHPANDE, Nilkanth D. (ed.) 1978: *Suśruta Saṃhitā. Śārīrasthāna*, Varanasi: Chowkhamba Sanskrit Series

GONDA, Jan 1970: *Viṣṇuism and Śivaism. A Comparison*. London: The Athlone Press, University of London. Jordan Lectures in Comparative Religion 9.

MUKHOPĀDHYĀẎ, Harekr̥ṣṇa (ed.) 1957: *Rāmāẏaṇ. Kr̥ttibās biracita*. Kalikātā: Sāhitya Saṃsad.

SR: *Saptakāṇḍa Rāmāẏaṇ*. Kalikātā: Akṣaẏ Lāibrerī Beng. era 1361 (= 1954).

WACKERNAGEL, Jakob 1957: *Altindische Grammatik. Band II,1. Einleitung zur Wortlehre. Nominalkompositon*. 2. unveränderte Auflage. Göttingen: Vandenhoeck & Ruprecht.

# Dogs in a Rare Zoological Book in Sanskrit

WILLEM B. BOLLÉE

In 1993, the Mahārāṣṭra Rājya Sāhitya āṇi Saṃskr̥tī Maṇḍal (Muṃbaī) published Haṃsadeva's *Mr̥gapakṣiśāstra*, edited, with a Marathi translation, by [the ornithologist] Mārutī Citam'pallī and [the late Sanskrit scholar] Kai.Pa. Narasiṃha Bhāt'khaṇḍe (CITAMAPALLĪ/BHĀTAKHAṆḌE 1993)

According to the introduction, vv.[1] 1 and 27ff., and the colophon, Haṃsadeva was a poet living in the village of Maṇḍaka in the *Jīyāj-janapada* of King Śauḍadeva.[2] On the order of his master, the wazir Tārananda asked Haṃsadeva in the durbar to compose a treatise on mammals and birds. As stated in VELANKAR 1944: 313, there is a manuscript of it in the palace library in Trivandrum. Originally, as JAIN 2004 tells us, it 'was available to Shri Raghavacharya of Madras, who presented it to the Maharaja of Travancore'.[3] T. Srinivasaraghavacharlu[4] specifies this in that he makes the epigraphist 'Pandit Sreeman Vijayaraghavachariar' supply 'copies of the original text (in manuscript) to His Highness The Maharaja of Travancore for the use of the State Museum, and to Dr. Caseywood[5] of McGill University of Montreal city (in N. America.)'.

Probably due to the deprivation of the power of royalty – culture is usually not in good hands in a republic –, 'it was in the early Eighties that the Museum library took shape, with hundreds of books lying in various Government offices

---

[1] Abbreviations: v. = verse, vv. = verses.

[2] Cf. also v. 3: *jīyāj-janapura-*.

[3] JAIN 2004: 478 note 200.

[4] In the 'Note' before the 'Preface' of SUNDARACHARYA 1927. – Incidentally, this English rendering, or better paraphrase, of the *Mr̥gapakṣiśāstra*, which omits unclear words, is found in Europe only in the British Library, where £ 75 are charged for photocopies of the 166 pages. Dr. (Ms.) Sunanda Shastri, who read a so far unpublished paper on the *Mr̥gapakṣiśāstra* at the *Seminar on Kalās and Vidyās in Indian Tradition* at the Institute of Oriental Study, Thane, on the 28th of December, 2002, was kind enough to copy her original for the present author, together with her paper. The book has extensive indices.

[5] Thus read for 'K.C. Wood'.

and other places getting deposited there. ... Most of the books are, however, in bad shape as the Museum does not have adequate funds for the upkeep of the library. ... Plans are also afoot to ensure that the rare and old books are properly preserved.' Thus G. Mahadevan in an article in the newspapaer *The Hindu* of May 28, 2002, where he further states that 'one of the treasures of this [Trivandrum] library is the Sanskrit and English version, written by hand, of the 13th century Botanical work "Hamsadeva".' These may be the copies brought out 'in Manuscript for the first time by well-known Pandit V. Vijayaraghavacharya Epigraphist, and published later on by Mr V. Krish[n]aswamy.'[6] Otto Schrader, the then director of the Adyar library, may have known this epigrapher and his manuscript, because he wanted to edit the latter with an English or German translation, but was hindered from this plan by his internment in Ahmednagar during World War I .[7]

The 'Foreword' to CHITAMPALLI 2001[8] states that Mārutī Citam'pallī found that 'the original manuscript of this famous treatise is with the Tirupati temple library'. There he copied the entire book though he was not conversant with Sanskrit. In order to read it he then learnt Sanskrit, probably with the help of his later co-editor, Kai.Pa. Narasiṃha Bhāt'khaṇḍe, and was apparently unaware of the manuscript and translation in the Trivandrum library. An indication that this manuscript sometimes differs from the one in the Tirupati temple may be the rendering of v. 965 in CITAMAPALLĪ/BHĀTAKHAṆḌE 1993 by SUNDARACHARYA 1927: 75.

Srinivasaraghavacharlu characterises Haṃsadeva as a famous Jain poet; his *Mr̥gapakṣiśāstra* is inserted in VELANKAR 1944, and CITAMAPALLĪ/BHĀTAKHAṆḌE 1993 has a wrapper with a Śvetāmbara monk. However, as Dr. Sunanda Shastri stresses in her paper mentioned in note 4, 'the poet does not tell anything about himself, his place or date'; neither do we know his king Śauḍadeva or the place which SUNDARACHARYA 1927 calls Jinapura in the Author's Intro-

---

[6] 'Preface' by T.V. Lakshmi Nrisimhacharya to SUNDARACHARYA 1927.

[7] In the 'Preface' cited above.

[8] An English version by Virag Pachpore of the Marathi introduction to CITAMAPALLĪ/BHĀTAKHAṆḌE 1993.

duction (p. 1),[9] and CHITAMPALLI 2001: 9 Jinapuri. According to VELANKAR 1944: 313, 'the author [of the *Mṛgapakṣiśāstra*] is said to have lived in the 13th century', which is adopted by JAIN 2004: 458, but without citing any source.

CHITAMPALLI 2001: 1, however, says that 'this treatise is believed to have been written ... nearly in 800 B.C.', though on p. 3 he opines that 'Hansadev has chosen this name [*Mṛgapakṣiśāstra*] for his treatise according to definition in the *Amarkosha* …'. His co-editor Bhāṭ'khaṇḍe, who died in June 1989, may not have seen this.

As can be expected, Haṃsadeva starts his treatise with lions, the kings of animals, and ends the mammals with dogs, the lowest among them.[10]

In view of this rare work being practically unknown, and as a kind of appendix to BOLLÉE 2006, dealing with dogs, vv. 941-973 are romanised and translated here as an example.[11] They describe the six canine races.[12]

1. The Śvan

941 *rakta-varṇa-yutāḥ śvānaḥ kiñ-cit tuṅga-śarīrakāḥ*
Śvans are of a red[dish][13] colour and somewhat tall.
942 *grāma-vāsâika-niratāḥ śāntâtmānaś*[14] *ca te matāḥ*
*kṣut-kāle kopa-śīlāś ca vīthī-dravyâdi-bhakṣakāḥ*
They prefer living in villages, are friendly, but irritable and eating things on the street,[15] etc., when hungry.

---

[9] Dr. Sunanda Shastri conjectures to read *jīyājjinapurādhīśaḥ* for *jīyājjanapurā°* of v. 3.

[10] BOLLÉE 2006: 5 note 2.

[11] The translation is not fully literal in that words like *tathā*, *mata-*, *ca*, *te*, *tu* etc. are not translated when clearly used as *pādapūrakas*. Also, words like 'but', 'and' etc. have been added when the meaning requires them.

[12] In texts on canines this distinction seems actually irrelevant. See also BOLLÉE 2006: 13ff.

[13] See BOLLÉE 2006: 17.

[14] Text: *śāntatmānaś*.

[15] Cf. v. 964.

943 *sadā sañcāra-śīlāś ca cchāyā-nidrā-parāyaṇāḥ*
*sva-yūtha-kalahâsaktāḥ pūrṇa-kāmāś ca te matāḥ*

Always straying, they like to sleep in the shadow; they are intent on fighting in their own pack and lustful.

944 *sthūlôdarāḥ puṣṭa-kāyās tīkṣṇa-karṇa-puṭās tathā*
*dīrgha-pucchā vakra-nakhā manuṣya-vaśa-vartinaḥ*

They are big-bellied, fat, prick-eared, and have a long tail and curved nails; they obey man.

945 *nātha-vātsalya-vantaś ca kraurya-hīnāś ca te matāḥ*
*sv-alpa-saundarya-yuktāś ca niśāyāṃ bhīravaś ca te*

Affectionate towards their owner, they are not savage, with little prettiness and fearful at night.

2. The Kukkura

946 *kukkurās te tu vijñeyāḥ prāyaḥ kṛṣṇa-śarīrakāḥ*
*dīrgha-pucchāḥ sv-alpa-balā nitarāṃ kopa-śīlakāḥ*

The Kukkuras are to be known as mostly black, with a long tail, not very strong, yet highly irritable.

947 *santataṃ krūra-nādāś ca te paraṃ mārga-rodhakāḥ*
*sva-yūtha-kalahâsaktāḥ niśāyāṃ sv-alpa-nidrakāḥ*

They constantly bark fiercely, are frequently in people's way, intent on fighting in their own pack, hardly sleeping at night.

948 *śara-vad-vega*[16]*-pādāś ca sāntva-vākya-parāś ca te*
*bṛhan-mastaka-saṃyuktāḥ sv-alpa-kāma-javā matāḥ*

Swift on their feet as an arrow, they are fond of kind words. They have a large head and are not impetuous lovers.

949 *dur-gandha-dehāḥ satataṃ ātape lamba-jihvakāḥ*
*dṛḍha-smṛti-yutāś câiva kārya-dakṣāś ca te matāḥ*

They are of evil smell, always panting in the heat, have a strong memory and can execute orders.

---

[16] Thus read for °*vetha*°.

3. The Śunaka

950 *śunakā hrasva-kāyāś ca hrasva-pādāḥ prakīrtikāḥ*
*nānā-varṇa-yutāḥ prāyaś câika-varṇa-yutās tu vā*
The Sunakas are said to be of small size and feet, mostly multihued or plain.
951 *nitānta-vegāḥ satataṃ te bṛhan-mastakā matāḥ*
*śānta-sva-bhāvāḥ satataṃ*[17] *nātha-cittânuvartinaḥ*
They always run fast, have a big head, are friendly … and follow the thoughts of their master.
952 *sv-alpa-kāmāḥ pūrṇa-balāḥ sūkṣma-buddhi-kalāś ca te*
*kṣut-tṛṭ-śītâtapa-sahāḥ moha-kāryâdi-varjitāḥ*
They are not very passionate, but full of strength, keenly intelligent[18] and canorous (*kala-*)[19] and bearing hunger, thirst, cold and heat without bewilderment of any kind/much ado.
953 *kope tu krūra-nādās te vaktra-pucchāś ca te matāḥ*
However, when angry they bark fiercely. They have a curved tail.

4. The Hound (*mṛga-daṃśaka*)

953 *mṛga-daṃśās te tu paraṃ tuṅga-kāyā balânvitāḥ*
Hounds are very tall and strong.
954 *dhūmra-varṇāḥ kṛṣṇa-varṇā hrasva-pucchāś ca te matāḥ*
*ajānāṃ hariṇānāṃ ca dhenūnāṃ ca gavām api*
955 *pāda-grahaṇa-lolāś ca tan-māṃsâdāś ca te matāḥ*
*santataṃ krūra-nādāś ca kṣudra-prāṇi-vihiṃsakāḥ*
They are grey or black and have a short tail, like to seize goats, deer, cows and even oxen by the leg and eat their flesh. They always bark fiercely and harm small animals.
956 *bhṛśa-karkaśa-româḍhyāḥ durdharṣā rudhira-priyāḥ*

---

[17] Cf. 90: *śānta-sva-bhāvāḥ śaurye 'pi.*

[18] This translation of *sūkṣma-buddhi-* accords with its use in late Sanskrit and modern South Asian languages.

[19] Or: 'of keen intellect and skill (*kalā-*)'.

*sāntva-vāg-vimukhāś câiva krūra-cittāś ca te matāḥ*

Their fur is very rough; they are dangerous, bloodthirsty, inaccessible to friendly words and vicious.

957 *daṃṣṭrā-karāla-vadanā bālānāṃ bhīti-dāyakāḥ*

Their mouth has dreadful canine teeth; they frighten children.

5. The Sārameya

957 *sārameyāḥ śānta-cittā nānā-varṇa-samanvitāḥ*

Sārameyas are tranquil-minded and of different colours.

958 *nānā-varṇâṅkanôpetāḥ kiñ-cit tuṅga-śarīrakāḥ*
*nātha-vātsalya-vantaś ca kopa-mohâdi-varjitāḥ*

They are variegated/with multicoloured patches, somewhat tall, affectionate towards their owner, and lack anger, bewilderment etc.

959 *dr̥ḍha-smaraṇa-yuktāś ca nānā-kārya-vicakṣaṇāḥ*
*mr̥gayâsakta-cittāś ca sv-alpa-kāma-javā matāḥ*

They have a strong memory and can perform various tasks; their thoughts are always with hunting and they are not impetuous lovers.

960 *nitarāṃ ramya-dehāś ca dīrgha-vālāḥ prakīrtitāḥ*
*grāma-vāsâika-niratāḥ nānā-līlā-vidaś ca te*

With their long tails they are very nice to see, prefer living in a village and know various plays.

961 *yauvane mada-yuktāś ca coditā vega-gāminaḥ*
*kiñ-cit kr̥śa-śarīrāś ca niśāyām alpa-nidrakāḥ*

In their youth they are unrestrained, excited and [therefore] running fast. They are somewhat slim and do not sleep much at night.

6. The Grāmyamr̥ga

962 *kṣudra-kāyā grāmya-mr̥gā nīca-kāryâika-tat-parāḥ*
*nānā-varṇā dhūmra-varṇā hrasva-karṇāś ca te matāḥ*

Grāmyamr̥gas (literally.: tame animals) are small, [and thus] only engaged in low activities.[20] They are multihued and grey, with small ears.

[20] 'Low activities' could refer to activities near the ground, such as sniffing or eating things

963 *kopa-yuktā manda-javāḥ sva-yūtha-kalahôtsukāḥ*
*santata-bhramaṇāḥ prāyo nitarāṃ manda-buddhayaḥ*

When angry they are slow;[21] they like to fight in their own pack, as a rule are always straying and quite dull-minded.

964 *varāha-gardabha-gaṇaiḥ prāyo yuddhâbhilāṣiṇaḥ*[22]
*rakta-māṃsâsthi-durgandha-dravya-bhakṣaṇa-tat-parāḥ*

Usually they are keen on fighting families of wild boars[23] and herds of asses, and eagerly eat blood, meat, bones and evil-smelling substances.[24]

965 *prāyeṇa te vyartha-śikṣā nindyās te '-hita-karmabhiḥ*[25]

Generally, teaching them is of no use. They should be blamed/punished [only?] when they misbehave/cause damage.[26]

*evaṃ bahu-vidhāḥ śvānaḥ nānā-varṇa-śarīrakāḥ*

Thus there are dogs of many kinds and colours.[27]

966 *grāmeṣv ābhīra-pallīṣu*[28] *tatra tatra viśeṣataḥ*

---

on the street (cf. v. 942). Or 'low' could have the connotation 'lowly', referring to activities considered repugnant by humans, such as public sex, eating faeces, licking of the anus etc.

21 For the reverse cf., e.g., v. 517: *kope made vega-pādāḥ* (said of buffaloes).

22 Thus read for °*lasinaḥ*.

23 The wild boar is a loner – cf. French *sanglier* < *singularis* (*porcus*) –, but can have a family, as is shown, e.g., on the picture by Johann E. Ridinger in TYLINEK/TYLINEK/TEICHMANN 1974: 191.

24 Dogs feel attracted by spoilt foodstuffs because their organism needs the ammonia contained in these (TYLINEK/TYLINEK/TEICHMANN 1974: 36f.).

25 Reading *'hita-°* for *hita-°*.

26 The second half of this stanza does not fit the first one because of *evaṃ* and perhaps *śvānaḥ*. The two halves are therefore separated. It is unclear whether *śvānaḥ* refers to dogs in general or the Śvan class again.

27 The version of SUNDARACHARYA 1927: 147 is so much different that it may be based on another text: 'They have ugly bodies and very unpleasant bark especially during nights. They are very harmful to minor animals.'

28 Thus read for *vallīṣu*.

*pāpiṣṭhā nīca-janmānaḥ paraṃ te sūkṣma-buddhayaḥ*

In villages [with/and] abodes of Ābhīra cowherds[29] they are particularly wicked everywhere and of low breed, but keen understanding.

967 *saṅgrāhyā bālya-vayasi nānā-śikṣaṇa-yogyakāḥ*
*mṛgayā-gamane rakṣā-nayanâdiṣu kovidāḥ*

They must be caught as pups. [Then] they can be taught various things [so as to be] good at hunting and guarding.

968 *sad-dravye bhojinas te tu rakṣaṇīyāś ca bhūmipaiḥ*
*te paraṃ dīrgha-suratāḥ lajjā-hīnāś ca kīrtitāḥ*

As to a titbit, they like it, but should be kept [only] by the nobility.[30] They are very long sexually active, and shameless.

969 *varṣā-kāle viśeṣeṇa kāma-yuktāś ca kīrtitāḥ*
*śunyaḥ śunaka-tulyās tāḥ śāntâtmānaś ca niścitāḥ*

Especially in the monsoon bitches and dogs are said to be lustful,[31] [but] calm-minded and determined.[32]

970 *kiñ-cin manda-javāḥ prāyaḥ tāḥ paraṃ sūkṣma-buddhayaḥ*
*su-vṛtta-jaghanôpetāḥ krorya*[33]*-hīnā balânvitāḥ*

They are a little slow, but usually of keen understanding, quite curved from behind, not vicious, but strong.

971 *yauvane ramya-dehāś ca rakṣaṇīyāś ca bhūmipaiḥ*
*sapta-varṣâvadhi śunāṃ yauvanaṃ parikīrtitam*

---

[29] Dogs of the Ābhīras (in Northwest India) are also mentioned in the *Mānasollāsa* (see BOLLÉE 2006: 13).

[30] Cf. v. 971. The gerundive seems to make sense here only with a restriction. For √*rakṣ* the dictionaries do not give the meaning 'raise'.

[31] The monsoon excites not only humans (for whom see e.g., BOCCALI 1996, with older literature on p. 449 note 1), but also animals.

[32] Or: 'Especially in the monsoon they are said to be lustful. Bitches are like dogs, but calm-minded and determined.'

[33] Thus read for *krorya*°.

They are attractive when young, and should be kept [only] by the nobility.[34] Dogs are young up to seven years.

972 *tataḥ paraṃ te jarayā pīḍitâṅgā viniścitāḥ*
*śunakānāṃ paraṃ câyur-daśa-varṣāṇi kīrtitam*

After that they have age problems. The life of a dog is known as ten years at the most.[35]

973 *jāti-kriyâdi-bhedena te matās tāmasôttamāḥ*

By the difference in race, acts, etc., they are taken to be extremely affected by *tamas* (i.e. dull?).[36]

## Bibliography

BOCCALI, Giuliano 1996: 'Les images de la saison des pluies chez Aśvaghoṣa', in: Nalini Balbir, Georges-Jean Pinault and Jean Fezas (eds.), *Langue, style et structure dans le monde indien. Centenaire de Louis Renou. Actes du Colloque international (Paris, 25-27 janvier 1996)*. Paris: Librairie Honoré Champion. Bibliothèque de l'École des Hautes Études, Sciences historiques et philologiques 334, pp. 449-466.

BOLLÉE, Willem 2006: *Gone to the Dogs in Ancient India*. München: Verlag der Bayerischen Akademie der Wissenschaften. Sitzungsberichte der Bayerischen Akademie der Wissenschaften, Philosophisch-Historische Klasse 2006, 2.

CHITAMPALLI, Maruti: 2001: *An introduction to Mrigpakshishastra of Hansadev*. New Delhi: Samskrita Bharati. Indian Heritage of Science & Technology.

CITAMAPALLĪ, Mārutī; BHĀTAKHAṆḌE, Kai.Pa. Narasiṃhaśāstrī (eds.) 1993: *Haṃsadevaviracita Mr̥gapakṣiśāstra (mūḷa saṃskr̥tāsaha)*. Muṃbaī: Mahārāṣṭra Rājya Sāhitya āṇi Saṃskr̥tī Maṇḍala.[37]

JAIN, J. C. 2004: *History and Development of Prakrit Literature*. Delhi: Manohar Publishers & Distriubutors.

SUNDARACHARYA, M. 1927: *English Translation of the Sanskrit Text of Mriga-Pakshi-Sastra.*

[34] Cf. v. 968.

[35] *Param* can also mean 'thereafter', i.e. after the seven years of youth. – The age of Yudhiṣṭhira's dog, when at the gate of heaven, is not indicated in the *Mahābhārata*. This could otherwise have been relevant for a comparison with the maximum canine age supposed here.

[36] I do not understand this line, which seems to be illogical and to contradict vv. 966 and 970, though agreeing with v. 963.

[37] Marathi is transliterated here like Sanskrit, i.e. without regard to unpronounced *a*.

*Or Science of Animals and Birds (Zoology in India) by Haṃsadeva, a Jain Author of 13th Century A.D.* Kalahasti: V. Krishnaswamy.

TYLINEK, Erich; TYLINEK, Isabella; TEICHMANN, Peter 1974: *Unsere Hunde*. Bonn: Hörnemann Verlag.

VELANKAR, Hari Damodar 1944: *Jinaratnakośa. An Alphabetical Register of Jain Works and Authors. Vol. 1. Works*. Poona: Bhandarkar Oriental Research Institute. Government Oriental Series, Class C 4.

# Reviews and Notices

Ḍāliẏā Bā̃duṙī, *Carak'saṃhitār dārśanik bhābanā-samīkṣā*. Kal'kā-tā: Di Eśiẏāṭik Sosāiṭi 2006. *bāro*;253 pp. Rs 220.–/US-$ 22.–.

It is a well-known fact that the *Carakasaṃhitā* (= CA) contains passages with philosophical content. The philosophical theories presented in these passages show parallelisms or affinities to Nyāya, Vaiśeṣika or Sāṃkhya.[1] These passages have attracted the interest of many researchers of the history of Indian philosophy, as Arion Roşu states.[2] Roşu then points to S.N. Dasgupta's view that the art of logical debating was first developed in the medical sphere, seeming to adhere to this view,[3] while also pointing out that 'les premiers manuels indiens de logique ont pu être le fruit de spéculations philosophiques'. He then goes on to state:

> L'analyse des moyens de jugement (*Sūtra* XI, 17-27; *Vimāna* IV, 3-5) aussi bien que les définitions de termes techniques et les procédés de controverse (*saṃbhāṣā-vidhi*) dans les assemblées de specialistes (*Vimāna* VIII, 15-66 et 152-153) attestent la démarche logique des médecins. Leur souci de rationalité, manifesté dans la théorie du raisonnement et la technique de l'argumentation, justifie un exposé des règles de la logique dans un corpus médical, ce qui constitue une exception dans toute l'histoire générale de la médecine.[4]

The study in Bengali by Ḍāliẏā Bā̃duṙī being reviewed here deals with this matter. CA contains technical terms of philosophy such as *padārtha-*, *mahābhūta-*, *indriya-* and *indriyabuddhi-*, *manas-* and *ātman-*, and refers to reincar-

---

[1] Cf., e.g., pp. 39-42 of Antonella Comba, 'Carakasaṃhitā, Śārīrasthāna I and Vaiśeṣika Philosophy', in: G. Jan Meulenbeld, Dominik Wujastyk (eds.), *Studies on Indian Medical History*, Reprint edition, Indian Medical Tradition 5, Delhi (Motilal Banarsidass Publishers) 2001, pp. 39-55.

[2] Arion Roşu, *Les conceptions psychologiques dans les textes médicaux indiens*, Publications de l'Institut de Civilisation Indienne, Série in-8° 43, Paris (Institut de Civilisation Indienne) 1978, p. 77: 'Appliqué aux conditions de validité des observations et des jugements étiologiques, ce traité offre un terrain de comparaison avec les *Nyāyasūtra* et les textes de logique des bouddhistes et de jinistes.'

[3] I reserve comment upon this.

[4] Roşu refers to some articles on this topic in note 2 on p. 77.

nation, liberation (*mokṣa-*), time (*kāla-*), *puruṣa-* and *prakṛti-*. The author devotes one chapter to each of these terms, first explaining its usage in CA, then referring to its definitions and illustrations in philosophical texts. The philosophical texts consulted by the author, who is a specialist for Nyāya, are very often Nyāya texts such as *Nyāyasūtra*, *Nyāyabhāṣya* etc. But she does include parallels from Vaiśeṣika, Sāṅkhya, or Buddhist logical texts (e.g. Śāntarakṣita) and Jaina logical works (e.g. Vādidevasūri's *Pramāṇanayatattvālokālaṅkāra*), where they are relevant. The *Suśrutasaṃhitā* (= SU) is also often consulted by her, although the philosophical statements contained in SU are usually very brief and terse. This other medical authority clearly has less philosophical character than CA.

Besides these philosophical terms listed above, Bā̃duṛī deals with terms which are proper to Āyurveda, namely the human body (*śarīra-*), morbific entities (*doṣa-*), body-elements (*dhātu-*), impurities (*mala-*), and *tantrayukti-*.[5] All these passages from medical and philosophical works are quoted in the original Sanskrit in footnotes. Therefore, this study is also of use to all those who have knowledge of the Bengali alphabet, but do not necessarily understand the Bengali language itself.

Each topic has a relatively small section and a brief headline in bold style, so that readers can utilise the work as a reference book for philosophical terms occurring in CA.

Sometimes Bā̃duṛī goes further than solely quoting parallel passages, and tries to illuminate their background: in those cases where the parallels deviate between CA and the philosophical schools, she analyses this discrepancy and tries to elucidate its cause. For instance, in CA the number of the attributes (*guṇa-*) is given as 41, which is far more than the 24 cited by the Nyāya-Vaiśeṣika. Bā̃duṛī (p. 9), surmising the cause of this discrepancy, states that the CA theory keeps up with the necessity of clinical practice. In other words, physicians needed additional expressions or technical terms to describe their clinical

[5] For *tantrayukti-*, Bā̃duṛī only refers to medical texts. However, *tantrayukti-* has parallels in Kauṭilya's *Arthaśāstra*, the *Yuktidīpikā* of the Sāṅkhya school, the Pali grammatical work *Saddanīti*, and grammatical works in Tamil. Cf. Roşu, p. 84f.

cases in an adequate manner.[6]

Bāduṙī thus presents instances in which the definitions of technical terms are based on clinical practice; therefore such definitions, properly belonging to medical science, are found only in CA and not in philosophical texts. I may point to another instance: CA first defines the notion of action (*karman-*) as in the Vaiśeṣika school; Sūtrasthāna 1,52 defines it as being the cause of union and separation, which seems to recapture the definition of the Vaiśeṣika.[7] However, for *pravṛtti-*, a term included under the actions (*karman-*), CA makes a unique definition that a performance/effort to produce a result is *pravṛtti-*, which is called activity (*kriyā-*), action (*karman-*), effort (*yatna-*) and undertaking for [achieving] a result (*kāryasamārambha-*).[8] The term *pravṛtti-* is also found in the *Nyāyasūtra*, but the definition made by CA looks very different from that made by the *Nyāyasūtra*, which states that an undertaking of speech, mind/intellect (*buddhi-*) and body is *pravṛtti-*.[9] Bāduṙī believes (p. 20) it to be possible that this definition of CA might have originated in the clinical practice of Āyurveda. According to her opinion (pp. 19f.), it might refer to or have to do with CA, Sūtrasthāna 26,13, which defines the term *karman-* as an act of treatment which brings forth an expected result.[10] She also remarks that it might reflect the five remedial methods such as vomiting (*vamana-*) etc. called *pañcakarman-*.[11]

The fact that the number of the means of proof (*pramāṇa-*) varies within CA could suggest that this is not a homogeneous text, but a patchwork containing

[6] For instance, the terms describing the qualities of a material such as *picchila-, ślakṣṇa-, khara-, sāndra-:* cf. Bāduṙī, p.9, note 2.

[7] Sūtrasthāna 1,52: *saṃyoge ca vibhāge ca kāraṇaṃ dravyam āśitam. – Vaiśeṣikasūtra* 1,1, 17: *ekadravyam aguṇaṃ saṃyogavibhāgeṣv anapekṣakāraṇam iti karmalakṣaṇam.*

[8] Vimānasthāna 8,77: *pravṛttis tu khalu ceṣṭā kāryārthā: saiva kriyā karma yatnaḥ kārya-samārambhaś ca.*

[9] *Nyāyasūtra* 1,1,17: *pravṛttir vāgbuddhiśarīrārambhaḥ.*

[10] *dravyāṇi hi dravyaprabhāvād guṇaprabhāvād dravyaguṇaprabhāvāc ca tasmiṃs tasmin kāle tat tad adhikaraṇam āsādya tāṃ tāṃ ca yuktim arthaṃ ca taṃ tam abhipretya yat kurvanti tat karma.*

[11] Cf. Sūtrasthāna 26,10: *karma pañcavidham uktaṃ vamanādi.*

contradictory statements. Thus, in Vimānasthāna 4,5 and 8,83, the *pramāṇa-* is said to be twofold, i.e. direct perception (*pratyakṣa-*) and inference (*anumāna-*),[12] which is in accordance with the Cārvāka school. But immediately after this statement, CA also mentions the number three, adding as a third the statements of authorities (*upadeśa-* or *āpta-*).[13] Furthermore, Vimānasthāna 8,33 mentions the number four, i.e. *āgama-, pratyakṣa-, anumāna-,* and *upamāna-*, which is in accordance with the *Nyāyasūtra* (Bāduṙī, p. 71, note 2) and the Buddhist text *Upāyahṛdaya* (Bāduṙī, p. 72). In CA, Sūtrasthāna 11,17, the number is also four, but with *yukti-* instead of *upamāna-*.[14] The term *yukti-* is unique to CA; it is not found in any other text, either medical or philosophical.

On this point, Bāduṙī (pp. 69-73) proposes an intriguing interpretation: the number varies according to the context, i.e. according to the necessity of clinical practice. For instance, CA, Vimānasthāna 4,9, which mentions the number three, i.e. *pramāṇa-, anumāna-* and *upadeśa-*, is interpreted by her[15] as showing that the physician only needs these three in order to know about (i.e. recognise) the disease.[16] By contrast, for diagnosis the physician needs a fourth *pramāṇa-* called *yukti-* or synthetic judgment. For in diagnosis, the physician identifies a disease by observing various symptoms on a patient, and reasoning inductively; adopting synthetic judgment (*yukti-*) based on these symptoms which are perceptible, the physician comes to identify the disease which is in itself imperceptible.[17]

---

[12] Vimānasthāna 4,5: *tasmād dvividhā parīkṣā jñānavatāṃ pratyakṣam anumānaṃ ca*. Vimānasthāna 8,83: *dvividhā tu khalu parīkṣā jñānavatāṃ pratyakṣam anumānaṃ ca*.

[13] Vimānasthāna 4,5 and 8,83: *trividhā vā sahopadeśena*. 4,5 also: *trividhe tv asmin jñānasamudaye pūrvam āptopadeśāj jñānam*. See too 4,9 in note 15.

[14] *caturvidhā parīkṣā āptopadeśaḥ pratyakṣam anumānaṃ yuktiś ceti*.

[15] Cf. Bāduṙī, p. 70. CA, Vimānasthāna 4,9:
*āptataś copadeśena pratyakṣakaraṇena ca*
*anumānena ca vyādhīn samyag vidyād vicakṣaṇaḥ*.

[16] CA in this context considers the synonym of *pramāṇa-* to be *vijñāna-* 'knowledge/knowing', cf. Bāduṙī, p. 70.

[17] On *yukti-* cf. Pierre-Sylvain Filliozat: '*Yukti,* le quatrième *pramāṇa* des médecins (Cara-

Thus the reciprocal inconsistency of the theories contained in the CA is not only due to the heterogeneity of the text, but also due to the effort of keeping up with the necessity of clinical practice, if we may take these interpretations by Bā̃duṙī to be correct. The physicians, according to this, chose different philosophical theories to suit different occasions, using what was practically needed and ignoring what was not.

However, the problem is how to interpret in the cases where CA and philosophical texts have technical terms in common, but their definition or usage deviates from one to another. For instance, in CA, some philosophical terms such as *padārtha-*, *pramāṇa-* etc. are not defined, but only illustrated with concrete examples,[18] in contrast to the philosophical texts in which every term, including its characteristics (*lakṣaṇa-*), is defined precisely. Bā̃duṙī seems to believe that the cause for this condition is that the general definition of such a term is explicit in the 'ancient tradition' (*prācīn'kāler dhārā*); thus the author(s)[19] of CA did not need to mention it specifically. I.e., Bā̃duṙī appears to assume philosophical notions commonly spreading among the intellectual elite at the time in which the philosophical statements in CA originate.[20] She seems to consider this common philosophical way of thinking as being the breeding ground for philosophical schools such as Nyāya, Vaiśeṣika and Sāṅkhya.

Indeed, Bā̃duṙī often writes things which imply that she thinks that the philosophical passages contained in CA preserve an earlier stage of philosophical

kasaṃhitā, Sūtrasthāna XI, 25)', *Journal of the European Āyurvedic Society* 1 (1990): 33-46.

[18] Bā̃duṙī, p.1 and 67. The term *vākchala-*, one of the *padārtha*-s, is not defined, but explained by illustrations; cf. Bā̃duṙī, p. 51.

[19] Bā̃duṙī (p. ix) discusses the CA being composed by plural authors. But one gains the impression that she does not pay attention to this point minutely enough in her interpretation of the text.

[20] See e.g. p. 11, note 1: *carak o suśruter ei lakṣan'ṭi tat'kāle pracalita dārśanik paribeśer dbārā prabhābita bale dhare neoẏā yete pare* 'One may assume that this characteristic of Caraka and Suśruta is influenced by the philosophical milieus which were current in that period'. Actually, 'that period' is too vague an expression, as these two medical works could have been composed in completely different periods distant from each other. I thus wonder which age 'that period' exactly denotes.

thought than the philosophical texts.[21] Bãduṙī's interpretation thus appears to be contrary to that of, for instance, Bruns,[22] Comba[23] and Lyssenko,[24] who argue that CA borrowed terms and notions from the philosophical texts (or their archetypes) and not vice versa.[25] On the other hand, Bãduṙī, in several cases, thinks that the CA simplified a philosophical theory, suitably modifying it for clinical practice,[26] which actually is quite the opposite of her stated interpretation. Even leaving that aside, she does not develop her discussion in a sufficient manner. If there was indeed a philosophical milieu from which CA's philosophical statements originate (and not vice versa, as is also theoretically possible[27]), what is the distance in time or textual relationship between CA and such a given philosophical milieu? Are the two close enough to each other to have enabled this? Or, was the philosophical milieu situated somehow apart from CA after all, and did CA nevertheless borrow from it?

Thus, when CA and the philosophical texts deviate from each other, there

---

[21] E.g. on p. ix: *carak'saṃhitāẏ paribeśita dārśanik'tattber beś kichu aṃśa pariśīlita tattbarūpe paribartita ebaṃ paribardhita haẏe nabakalebar dhāraṇ kareche ei samasta subinyasta cintāsamr̥ddha darśan'śāstragulite*. The general idea is: a large portion of the philosophical thoughts contained in CA, being modified and enlarged in a sophisticated form, acquired a new shape/body in the philosophical texts/*śāstra*-s which were systematised and deliberated.

[22] Prudence F. Bruns, 'Philosophical Influence in Indian Medicine', *Sagar. A South Asia Graduate Research Journal* 13 (2004): 53-68.

[23] See note 1.

[24] Viktoria Lyssenko, 'The Human Body Composition in Statics and Dynamics: Āyurveda and the Philosophical Schools of Vaiśeṣika and Sāṃkhya', *Journal of Indian Philosophy* 32 (2004): 31-56.

[25] Criticism of such a-prioristic assumptions is found in Rahul Peter Das, *The Origin of the Life of a Human Being. Conception and the Female According to Ancient Indian Medical and Sexological Literature*, Indian Medical Tradition 6, Delhi (Motilal Banarsidass Publishers) 2003, pp. 1f.

[26] Bãduṙī., states on p. xi (translated from the original Bengali): 'What is necessary for the doctors to know on the ground of experience through logical argumentation is not that much required for the [properly] philosophical schools of Nyāya and Vaiśeṣika.'

[27] For instance by reasoning that it is medical science that developed a methodology of debate, and the philosophical schools imported the methodology of medical science.

are three possible presumptions: firstly, CA preserves an original, briefer version of philosophical thinking; the later philosophical schools elaborated it into a fuller form. Secondly, CA made an addition to the philosophical theory which was established at that time, in which case CA would have developed and elaborated the original terse theory. The final possibility is that CA reduced or simplified the philosophical theory. It is not very clear, on what criteria Bā̃duṙī bases her decision to side with one or the other of these three interpretative possibilities.

The matter is made more troublesome by the fact that the representation of CA available at present is merely an edited version by Dr̥ḍhabala, dating to approx. 900 AD, while the earliest version of CA is thought to date to the third or second century BC. We do not know exactly to what extent the present representation displays the original state of the text of the third or second century, or how large the portion of secondary additions by Dr̥ḍhabala is. Bā̃duṙī uses vague expressions like 'at that time' constantly.[28] It is unclear when exactly she considers 'at that time' to have been.

What is very intriguing and should not be forgotten is that other medical works contain very few parallels to the philosophical passages of CA. Except for very basic philosophical terms, the SU for example contains far less parallels, and no parallel at all to the CA passages dealing with debate (*vāda-*). The definitions of philosophical terms in SU are mostly very concise; therefore it would not be appropriate to declare that philosophy plays a great role in SU. Indeed, SU utilises the philosophical terms to a minimum, only as much as is practically necessary. Observed in this light, it turns out that CA's preference for logic and philosophy seems to be a unique exception among medical literature. If this is so, then Roşu's statement on p. 212 would have to be taken with some reservation.

Perhaps we are attaching too much importance to the philosophical passages of CA, maybe simply because it is considered to be old.[29] If we took SU

[28] E.g. on p. 25: *abhāb'ke pr̥thak padārtha hisābe sthān nā dileo abhāb cintaner sūtrapāt haẏechilo sekāle*. The gist of this is that at that time there was already a beginning of the notion of inexistence (*abhāva-*), though no place was given for inexistence among substances (*padārtha-*).

[29] On the other hand, at least some parts of SU might preserve an older version of the text than the redaction of CA by Dr̥ḍhabala.

instead of CA as the reference yardstick, we could definitely not say that philosophy is an essential component of Āyurveda. MAKOTO KITADA

Lallanji Gopal, *Vṛkṣāyurveda in Ancient India. (With Original Texts and Translation)*. New Delhi: Sundeep Prakashan 2000. vi;246 pp. ISBN 81-7574-085-X. Rs 1200.–.

In this volume Lallanji Gopal (1934-1999) has collected the fruits of his studies on Vṛkṣāyurveda. Those who are conversant with his various writings on this subject will obviously find much material already published elsewhere. But even though one does sporadically come across passages that are nearly verbatim reproductions of parts of earlier studies – e.g. pp. 11 and 13f. of Chapter 2 ('Emergence of *Vṛkṣāyurveda* as a Science: Kauṭilya and Varāhamihira', pp. 7-17), which correspond respectively to pp. 168f. and 170f. of Lallanji Gopal, 'Emergence of Vṛkṣāyurveda', *Indian Journal of History of Science* 31 (1996): 167-172 –, this book is neither a reprint collection of older articles, nor a simple rehash of what was written in these. In fact, it is a testimony to the fact that right until the end of his life Lallanji Gopal, not content to rest upon previous laurels, was applying his formidable acumen and open mind to gaining ever new insights into this subject so fascinating and at the same time still relatively unknown.

Neither a sentimentalist nor an apologist, he regarded historical research as the quest to find out what actually was, and not what should have been. This made him impatient with tendencies running contrary to this principle, and he could be rather blunt in his criticism, as in his dismissal, in Chapter 5 ('Vṛkṣāyurveda of Parāśara: A Modern eponymous text', pp. 29-37), of the claims to ancientness of the *Vṛkṣāyurveda* attributed to Parāśara.[30]

A source of irritation upto this day are articles on Vṛkṣāyurveda, by various authors, which clearly are based on unclear notions of what Vṛkṣāyurveda actually is. In view of this, Chapter 1 ('Meaning and scope of Vṛkṣāyurveda', pp. 3-6) cannot be highlighted enough. Though very brief, it gives a good overview on the problems of defining Vṛkṣāyurveda, on what it is and is not, and

[30] On this issue see also Rahul Peter Das, 'On the *Vṛkṣāyurveda* of Parāśara', *Journal of the European Āyurvedic Society* 5 (1997): 196-215.

on its relations to other branches of knowledge.

Lallanji Gopal has attempted to comprehensively garner and sift what is known on Vr̥kṣāyurveda, and then to present this to the interested general public in a manner giving a good overview on the subject without delving into details or listing secondary sources inappropriate to the context. On the other hand, he presents information on a large mass of primary texts which, even though South Asian in origin, are hardly known in modern South Asia itself, and in doing so he even does not fail to make appropriate use of this reviewer's edition (and annotated German translation) of Surapāla's *Vr̥kṣāyurveda* and several other minor texts. This latter is something which is still rare in publications emanating from India, including the facsimile edition (with English translation) of Surapāla's text.[31]

All the above refers to the first, descriptive, part of the book, consisting of eight chapters. The following and larger part (pp. 87-235) consists of English translations of major primary sources on Vr̥kṣāyurveda, including a complete translation of Surapāla's *Vr̥kṣāyurveda*. This part is bilingual, with the Sanskrit original and the English translation facing each other. The end of the work is made up of an appendix in which Sanskrit plant names are explained, overwhelmingly according to the binomial classification system.

The book is well printed and well made up. Unfortunately, it is marred by some misprints. Most of these are not serious, even though one does wince at chapter headings like 'In Kāśyapasaṁhitā Vr̥kṣāyurveda' (Chapter 3) and 'Ancient Authorities or Vr̥kṣāyurveda' (Chapter 4).[32] What could, however, seriously annoy a Sanskritist is the treatment often meted out to the Sanskrit text in Nāgarī. Unfortunately, this is nothing uncommon in today's South Asia; compositors often clearly do not understand what they are typesetting.

But these are, on the whole, minor quibbles that cannot detract from the fact

---

[31] *Surapala's Vrikshayurveda (The Science of Plant Life by Surapala)*, Translated by Nalini Sadhale. With Commentaries by K.L. Mehra, S.M. Virmani, and Y.L. Nene, Agri-History Bulletin 1, Secunderabad (Asian Agri-History Foundation) 1996. Cf. the review by Sreeramula Rajeswara Sarma in *Traditional South Asian Medicine* 6 (2001): 171-173.

[32] It also pains this reviewer personally that his *Das Wissen von der Lebensspanne der Bäume* has been transformed into *Das Wissen vonder debensspanneder Bauma* on p. 68.

that this book is and will for a long time remain a must-read for all seriously interested in Vr̥kṣāyurveda. RAHUL PETER DAS

*Traditional Medicine in Asia*. Edited by Ranjit Roy Chaudhury, Uton Muchtar Rafei. New Delhi: World Health Organization, Regional Office for South-East Asia 2002. SEARO Regional Publications 39. vii;309 pp. ISBN 92 9022 2247. Swiss Fr 20.–.

The preface of this WHO-publication that deals with traditional medicine in Asian countries such as China, India, Sri Lanka, Nepal, Bangladesh, Indonesia, Thailand, North and South Korea states that the WHO Regional Office for South-East Asia has published this book 'in order to present to the governments, policy makers, clinical investigators, regulatory authorities, doctors, practitioners of the traditional systems of medicine and the public the state of the art in these wide and many-faceted fields. It is felt that the information in this publication, presented by some of the most eminent international authorities, would help not only in our understanding of these systems but also in making better use of them' (p. iv). Have the objectives, informing and inviting better usage of Traditional Asian Medicine, been met by this book?

While going into these matters, I shall also give a brief overview of its contents. The first part, called 'Systems', contains seven articles in which basic principles and issues like pathogenesis, diagnosis and therapeutic measures, as well as the contemporary state of the art in fields such as education and application, are described. The section respectively discusses: Āyurveda, Traditional Chinese Medicine (TCM), Yūnānī (Greek-Islamic) medicine, and the medical traditions of Indonesia and North Korea, Chinese Acupuncture-Moxibustion, and Yoga therapy.

The second part of the book, named 'Policy Issues' contains four articles. Prof. Zhu-fan Xie, honorary director of the Institute of Integrated Chinese and Western Medicine, Peking University, discusses the way in which traditional and modern medicine are "harmonised" in the People's Republic of China. In the second article of this section the secretary of the Department of Indian Systems of Medicine and Homoeopathy, New Delhi, gives us an insight into the way the Government of India tries to integrate its medical traditions in national health care. Gerry Bodeker of Oxford University and GIFTS for Health (an NGO) develops an outline for comparing the costs of traditional and conventional medical interventions. To my knowledge this contribution is quite unique in the way it takes the cost factor seriously and develops a model for actually comparing traditional medicines and biomedicine. The last article in this section, written by two WHO-consultants (Palitha Abeykoon, O. Akerele), informs us about training programmes for Asian medical traditions. Together with the book's third part, called 'Technical Issues', this second section is the best this WHO publication has to offer.

'Technical Issues' also consists of four articles in which regulation of traditional medical systems, the accredition of practitioners, the quality of medical products, laboratory and clinical research on standardisation, toxicity and efficacy, Intellectual Property Rights, patenting, the protection of medical plants, drug development and drug manufacturing are discussed. Ranjit Roy Chaudhury and Mandakini Roy Chaudhury, two Indian pharmacologists, have written the best article in this section. Their conclusions are grim when they state that: 'Inadequate standardization of medical plants, unacceptable preclinical toxicology studies and inappropriate uncontrolled and badly designed clinical trials form the triad of constraining factors which have held back the use of medical plants for health development and belied the longstanding hopes that research on medical plants would lead to a host of new drugs' (p. 209). The authors obviously know what they are talking about, and indeed good modern pharmacological research is necessary for the acceptance of traditional medicines among policy makers. What is equally important is the fact that patients, consumers and traditional practitioners are entitled to have genuine, safe and effective medications. However, the authors do not show sensitivity towards differences between traditional pharmacology and its modern counterpart. Therefore they do not answer the question whether the paradigm of logical positivism is suitable for defining and researching the content and efficacy of traditional medicines based on systematic correspondences between the human body and its natural and social environment. Indeed, humoral pharmacology with its anthropocentric approach offers a different way of looking at the interactions between natural substances and human biology and physiology. This is seldom acknowledged, because modern scientists do not appreciate the ontology, epistemology and phenomenological concepts of humoral pathology. Such a cultural insensitivity will rob us of an alternative to modern pharmacology.

The fourth part of the book contains eleven short monographs discussing the current status of traditional medicines in respectively Bangladesh, Bhutan, North Korea, India, the Maldives, Burma (Myanmar), Nepal, Sri Lanka and Thailand. These short descriptions suffer most from one the book's main shortcomings, which is the gap between policy measures and their effects in real life. There is too much talk about what should be, whereas a real insight into the actual state of medical traditions in Asian countries is often missing. For example, the WHO proclaims that 80% of the Asians depend upon traditional medicine. My own discussions in India with people professionally involved in traditional medicine, and the fact that biomedical drugs and, to a lesser extent, biomedical diagnostic practices have penetrated deeply into the Indian subcontinent and have made their inroads into, for example, Āyurvedic education and practice, make this figure seem too high. We need better knowledge of what is actually happening on the ground.

The edited volume also lacks sensitivity towards the consequences of the dominance of biomedicine in Asian countries for the status and form of contemporary Asian medical traditions. Nevertheless, *Traditional Medicine in Asia* contains a lot of information about the medical traditions themselves, and with good articles on cost evaluation and the shortcomings of modern pharmacological research on standardisation, toxicity and efficacy, the book makes good reading for those with an interest in the status of traditional medicine in Asia. Relative newcomers to the field will also benefit from the articles on basic principles and the integration between Asian medical traditions and biomedicine.

MAARTEN BODE

Rahul Peter Das, *The Origin of the Life of a Human Being. Conception and the Female according to Ancient Indian Medical and Sexological Literature*. Delhi: Motilal Banarsidass Publishers 2003. Indian Medical Tradition 6. xvi;729 pp. ISBN 81-208-1998-5. Rs 1250.–.

The main title of this voluminous work, which is a revised version of the author's post-doctoral thesis, is slightly misleading. It does not comprehensively deal with the origin of a human being according to the ancient Indian medical and sexological (the author's approximation to *kāmaśāstra*) tradition, but rather, as the subtitle indicates, with one important aspect of it, namely the role and contribution of the female in conception. While describing conception and the generation of a human being, ancient Indian medical theory postulates that 'procreatory fluids' of man and woman combine to produce a new human being. A varying number of other factors (e.g. self, mind, suitable nutrition of the pregnant woman etc., see e. g. *Carakasaṃhitā*, Śārīrasthāna 3) may also contribute to conception. In the case of the man the identity of the procreatory fluid is usually undisputed, while in the case of the female the exact identity of the procreatory fluid presents problems. As the terms employed in ancient Indian medical literature for naming this female procreatory fluid are synonyms for blood (*rakta-, asr̥j-, śoṇita-* etc.) or menstrual blood (*ārtava-*), the relationship between blood, menstrual blood and the female procreatory fluid in ancient Indian medicine is a matter of discussion. The largest part of this book is devoted to studying this problem in ancient Indian medical literature. The author analyses relevant passages in the four classical works (*Carakasaṃhitā, Suśrutasaṃhitā, Aṣṭāṅgasaṅgraha, Aṣṭāṅgahr̥daya*) ascribed to the 'ancient triad' of Āyurveda. A large number of commentaries to the classical works (some of them existing in manuscript form only) have also been studied carefully. In contrast to most authors in this field, Das has also considered interpretations of modern Āyurvedic authors writing in modern Indian languages or English. Other ancient literature (especially the *Bhelasaṃhitā* and *Kāśyapasaṃhitā*) and later medical works (especially, though not only, the *Śārṅgadharasaṃhitā*) are dealt with in separate chapters. The importance of the parents having an orgasm in order to conceive a child, a notion referred to in medical works, brings the author to studying classical Indian sexological literature. This part of the book provides insights into procreatory fluids, female orgasm and the anatomy of the female genital tract as understood by classical Indian sexology; Vātsyāyana's *Kāmasūtra* and its classical commentary are studied as well as other sexological works. A chapter on tubular structures and vital fluids discusses special problems arising from some remarks in sexological as well as medical works.

The first of two appendices discusses parallels in Greek and Yūnānī medicine. The second appendix presents extremely useful discussions of selected technical terms in ancient Indian medical literature. Three indices (index rerum, index verborum, index locorum) complete the work.

The general approach of this work, namely taking up a specific question and studying it through the ancient medical literature, bringing to bear upon the study the whole range of philological methods and insights, is original and commendable. It is hoped that other studies will follow this model. The analysis of the original texts is detailed and discursive, reminding one often of discussions in a Sanskrit class. These discussions, tiring as they sometimes are, serve a purpose, if one bears in mind that many extant translations and interpretations of ancient Sanskrit medical literature are often superficial and sometimes even misleading (the author refers to such works). However, one wonders if it would not have sufficed to discuss only a few passages at length and summarise the results in other cases. The author's criticism of other works and authors seems at times out of place in style and wording. The biggest drawback of the work, however, is the author's prose style, an English version of what has jestingly been called *Indologendeutsch*. He seems to delight in long hypotactical sentences which are sometimes nearly unreadable and barely intelligible. One example, found on p. 35 and referring to the *Carakasaṃhitā*, may illustrate this point: 'The procreatory fluid (uniting with semen from the male) is called *ārtava-* in Śā 2,14 and 4,7 and one of the common words for "blood" (see §2.1) in all other clear cases I could find, without our being able to gain any more relevant information from this apart from the fact that the nomenclature used could suggest that the procreatory fluid was viewed as being blood or maybe like blood (which are two different notions), though this need not necessarily be the case, for there could be other reasons – reasons which to us may not be obvious and not having to do with its colour – for calling this fluid "blood".'

It would be highly regrettable if the style should deter prospective readers, as this work is a mine of information and well-grounded discussion not only for the specific question dealt with, but also for ancient Indian medicine in general. Especially Appendix II, titled 'Discussion of Selected Technical Terms', should become a standard point of reference in studies on Āyurveda.

Anyone wondering about the possible meaning of terms like *agni-* or *rasa-* in classical Āyurveda is strongly advised to look up the thorough discussion of these terms in this book. The reviewer's recommendation for readers would thus be to read the conclusion first and then work through the discussion of individual texts as necessary. The three indices will help to make this work a useful reference work for anyone working on ancient Indian medical literature.[33]

ANANDA SAMIR CHOPRA

Joseph S. Alter, *Yoga in Modern India. The Body between Science and Philosophy.* Princeton/Oxford: Princeton University Press 2004. xxiii;326 pp. ISBN 0-691-11873-6 (cloth), 0-691-11874-4 (paper). US-$ 65.–/£ 41.95 (cloth), US-$ 19.95/£ 12.95 (paper).

Yoga ist innerhalb der letzten 50 Jahre ein solch bekanntes, allseits akzeptiertes Phänomen im Westen geworden, daß man kaum eine Zeitschrift aufschlagen kann, ohne auf ihn in irgendeiner Form zu stoßen. Die Eingeweihten pflegen dann zu seufzen, daß er ja eigentlich gar nicht so populär, und vor allem nicht so körperbezogen gemeint sei, "ursprünglich", sondern zu Höherem wie etwa Erleuchtung führen solle. Aber natürlich wäre ja vom materiellen Westen nichts anderes als ein solches Mißverständnis zu erwarten. Die meisten Beobachter vergessen darüber, einen Blick auf Indien zu werfen, um zu sehen, was sich dort auf dem Yogamarkt tut. Man würde sich wundern – wie auch etwa, wenn man J.S. Alters Buch liest, in dem gezeigt wird, daß sich dort seit ca. 80 Jahren ein Yoga etabliert hat, der dem im Westen außerordentlich ähnlich sieht. Nicht nur das, auch die wissenschaftliche Erforschung des Yoga, die so erzwestlich und materialistisch aussieht, wurde insbesondere von Swami Kuvalayanda (Kap. 3) seit den zwanziger Jahren des letzten Jahrhunderts vorangetrieben. Es war sein Bestreben, den Yoga aus seiner okkulten Ecke zu holen, d.h., 'the approach the antimystics took to the body was in terms of physical fitness, applied medical research, and pragmatic popularism rather than arcane philosophy and spiritualism' (S. 7f.).

Alter stellt diese Verwendung des Yoga in den Zusammenhang der indi-

[33] Cf. also the review by Claus Vogel in *Indo-Iranian Journal* 48 (2005): 127-132.

schen Freiheitsbewegung, innerhalb derer 'körperliche Ertüchtigung' durch indigene Methoden die nationale Stärke und Identität fördern sollte. So fügten sich yoga-artige Übungen auch gut in das Ausbildungsprogramm nationalistischer Bewegungen wie RSS, wobei allerdings die universale Verwendbarkeit des Yoga einer ausschließlich nationalistischen Interpretation entgegensteht. Parallel zur indischen Freiheitsbewegung entwickelten sich unter staatlicher Förderung Kliniken für Naturheilverfahren (Kap. 4), deren Verfechter nun ebenso wie die des Yoga die Idee vertreten, daß der Körper aus sich selbst heraus, wenn er nur richtig angeleitet ist, Krankheiten und Mängel ausgleichen bzw. heilen kann. Als ähnlich verwandt dem indischen Streben nach 'Selbstbezogenheit' beschreibt Alter die Eigenurintherapie (Kap. 6), die zwar seit 1918 durch die Schriften J.W. Armstrongs in Indien bekannt wurde, aber im *Śivāmbukalpa* des *Ḍāmaratantra* wiedergefunden werden, und einige Popularität erlangen konnte.

Großen Raum (Kap. 2) innerhalb des Werks nimmt die Frage nach der Wissenschaftlichkeit der Yogaforschung ein, die zwar bei den empirischen Untersuchungen durchaus in westlichem Sinne gegeben ist, jedoch in der Interpretation der Fakten häufig einmündet in die vom Sāṅkhya vorgegebene Ontologie und die 'yogische' Physiologie der *nāḍī*-s und *cakra*-s. Ähnlich verhält es sich mit *prāṇa*-, der einerseits als Atem auf der Ebene der Gesundheit betrachtet wird, aber andererseits als 'Lebenskraft' dem Bereich der Metaphysik angehört (S. 36). D.h., die moderne westliche Medizin wird von Propagandisten des Yoga häufig dazu benutzt, indische Philosophie zu rechtfertigen – zweifelsohne ein zum großen Teil dem Kolonialismus geschuldetes Unterfangen. Allerdings ist die Ansiedlung des Körpers in einem Raum, in dem sich Transzendenz und Materie treffen, zumindest dem Haṭhayoga nicht fremd, dem, anders als dem klassischen Sāṅkhya, die letztendliche Einheit von Śiva und Śakti, Geist und Materie, zugrundeliegt. Eine rein körperliche Erklärung des Herzlotus als nach unten hängendem Fleischklumpen findet man übrigens bemerkenswerterweise bereits im Śaṅkara zugeschriebenen Kommentar der *Yogasūtras* zu 2,34, was man kontrastierend im Zusammenhang der Diskussion von Yogeshwaranands Lokalisationen der *cakra*-s im Körper (S. 46-51) noch erwähnen könnte. Was allerdings nicht in den *Yogasūtras* erwähnt wird, sind *nāḍī*-s und *cakra*-s, bzw.

*suṣumnā-*, die Alter (S. 100) dort gesichtet hat (wohl versehentlich aus einem Kommentar herangezogen). Dies, wie seine häufig unkorrekte Schreibung von Wörtern indischen Ursprungs, oder daß Jñāneśvarī statt Jñāneśvar als Autor einer Textpassage zur Umwandlung des Körpers bezeichnet wird (fälschlicherweise im Zusammenhang mit der Urintherapie, was aber nicht Alters, sondern Karlekars Fehler ist), können sein Verdienst um die Darstellung der Geschichte und des Verständnisses von Yoga innerhalb der letzten 100 Jahre in Indien nicht wirklich schmälern. Vor einer Neuauflage des Buches wird sich sicherlich ein Indologe finden lassen, welcher Derartiges beseitigt.

Alter hat einen wichtigen Beitrag zur Ideengeschichte geleistet, der zweifelsohne den ihm verliehenen Coomaraswamy Book Prize verdient hat und zu weiteren Überlegungen anregen wird – besonders die theoriefreundlichen Anthropologen/Ethnologen, die sich am ersten und letzten Kapitel erfreuen werden, aber auch die 'Orientalists', die sicherlich aus ihren Texten heraus noch viel zum Verständnis des Körpers in Yoga und anderen indischen Systemen wie Āyurveda und Rasāyana beitragen können. CATHARINA KIEHNLE

*Du corps humain, au carrefour de plusiers savoirs en Inde. Mélanges offerts à Arion Roşu par ses collègues et ses amis à l'occasion de son 80e anniversaire. The Human Body, at the Crossroads of Multiple Indian Ways of Knowing. Papers Presented to Arion Roşu by his Colleagues and Friends on the Occasion of his Eightieth Birthday.* Sous la direction de Oscar Botto, Colette Caillat, Pierre Delaveau, Pierre-Sylvain Filliozat, Siegfried Lienhard, G. Jan Meulenbeld et Priya Vrat Sharma. Travaux réunis et édités par Eugen Ciurtin. Studia Asiatica 4 (2003)-5 (2004). Bucarest: Centre d'Histoire des Religions, Faculté d'Histoire, Université de Bucarest / Paris: De Boccard 2004. 832 pp. ISSN 1582-9111. € 55.–.

This monumental volume of tribute to Arion Roşu, who passed away in 2007,[34] comprises 40 studies – 23 in French, 16 in English and one in Italian. These are preceded by three introductory essays on the man Roşu and his ac-

[34] See his obituary on pp. 1-15 above.

complishments (by Colette Caillat, Priya Vrat Sharma, Eugen Ciurtin), a bibliography (prepared by Eugen Ciurtin) complete up to 2004, a *tabula gratulatoria* of 116 names, abbreviations and an editorial note (again by Eugen Ciurtin), and followed by French and English abstracts of all the studies, alphabetically ordered – with some discrepancies – according to the author's surname. Several English abstracts, as well as a few of the studies in English, would have benefited from language editing.

The studies are arranged in six groups. The first, 'Plantes', contains five essays. Suzanne Amigues examines anew the problem of the Homeric Lotophagi and the identification of *lōtós*, and suggests looking at the Indian plant *badara-/badarī-*, identified here as *Ziziphus mauritiana* Lam.[35] For further investigation it should be borne in mind, however, that this is not the only identification of *badara-/badarī-* current.[36] André Couture looks at lotus symbolism in the *Puṣkaraprādurbhāva* section of the *Harivaṃśa*.[37] Pierre-Sylvain Filliozat discusses Vedic und Purāṇic passages pertaining to the consciousness and divinity of trees, paying due attention to the relevant commentarial literature too. His presentation is so interesting that it is a pity that he did not decide to look at the subject more systematically on the lines of, or taking into consideration, the studies of Lambert Schmithausen[38] and Albrecht Wezler[39] on other texts.[40]

---

[35] On *caryophyllon*, discussed on pp. 57ff., see now also R.A. Donkin, *Between East and West. The Moluccas and the Traffic in Spices up to the Arrival of Europeans*, Memoirs of the American Philosophical Society 248, Philadelphia (American Philosophical Society) 2003, pp. 111ff.

[36] Cf., e.g., G.J. Meulenbeld, *The Mādhavanidāna and its Chief Commentary. Chapters 1-10*, Orientalia Rheno-Traiectina 19, Leiden (E.J. Brill) 1974, p. 580; Rahul Peter Das, *Das Wissen von der Lebensspanne der Bäume. Surapālas Vṛkṣāyurveda*, Alt- und Neu-Indische Studien 34, Stuttgart (Franz Steiner Verlag Wiesbaden) 1988, p. 102. On the problem of *Ziziphus* nomenclature in general see, e.g., *<http://www.plantnames.unimelb.edu.au/Sorting/Ziziphus.html>* (consulted on 12.2.2008).

[37] Probably because it is quite peripheral to his topic, Couture does not touch upon the exact meaning of *puṣkara-*, which our dictionaries also give as 'blue lotus'. On this see Jürgen Hanneder, 'The Blue Lotus. Oriental Research between Philology, Botany and Poetics?', *Zeitschrift der Deutschen Morgenländischen Gesellschaft* 152 (2002): 295-308.

[38] E.g. his *The Problem of the Sentience of Plants in Earliest Buddhism*, Studia Philologica

Next, Samia Al Azharia Jahn offers us a loose collection of vignettes and data centred around early European descriptions of plants of 'Malabar'. We learn interesting details about persons associated with the study of plants, the nomenclature and usage of individual plants, the various languages and scripts used for the transmission of the relevant data, etc. It is surprising, though, that this loosely structured collection of miscellanea does not mention what Arion Roşu himself has published on the subject.[41] Finally, Georges-Jean Pinault proposes a new etymology of *óṣadhi-*, namely *óṣ-adhi-* 'qui tranche la brûlure'.

In the second group, 'Médecine et alchimie', we have 11 studies. The first is a reprint of Willem B. Bollée's article on Jaina medicine published in issue 7 (2003): 69-110 of this journal. Eugen Ciurtin then discusses the Āyurvedic concept of 'opportune time' (*kāla-* and *kṣaṇa-*) and possible extra-Āyurvedic, particularly Buddhist, connections in detail. Pierre Delaveau argues against the current Western legislation of drug approval, cites 'le grand principe de la polypharmacie que les auteurs du XVII^e siècle en Europe s'efforçaient de cultiver' (pp. 238f.), and lobbies for approval of two *rasāyana-* preparations of Maharishi Ayurved, which will probably raise a few eyebrows. Vijaya J. Deshpande gives an overview on Chinese medical texts attributed to (not necessarily: by) Nāgārjuna, and reverts to an issue already raised by her previously, namely possible Indian influence on Chinese ophthalmology. One hopes that

---

Buddhica Monograph Series 6, Tokyo (The International Institute for Buddhist Studies) 1991.

[39] See his 'Paralipomena zum Sarvasarvātmakatvavāda II: On the Sarvasarvātmakatvavāda and its Relation to the Vṛkṣāyurveda', *Studien zur Indologie und Iranistik* 16 (1992): 287-315, where further literature is also mentioned.

[40] Cf. too Walter Slaje, 'Bewusstsein und Wahrnehmungsvermögen von Pflanzen aus hinduistischer Sicht', in: Bernhard Scholz (ed.), *Der Orientalische Mensch und seine Beziehungen zur Umwelt. Beiträge zum 2. Grazer Morgenländischen Symposion (2.-5. März 1989)*, Graz (RM – Druck- & Verlagsgesellschaft) 1989, pp.149-169.

[41] 'Les missionnaires dans l'histoire des sciences et des techniques indiennes (I). Un inédit jésuite sur la phytothérapie indienne au XVIII^e siècle', *Journal of the European Āyurvedic Society* 3 (1993): 174-228. The second part is less relevant: 'Les missionnaires dans l'histoire des sciences et des techniques indiennes (II). Les jésuites dans l'histoire de la médecine en Asie et dans le Nouveau Monde', *Traditional South Asian Medicine* 7 (2003): 162-185.

someone will undertake a detailed study of the Chinese and Indian data (for instance by looking for specific correspondences between Chinese and Āyurvedic doṣic classifications of glaucoma) to enable us to advance beyond the stage of possibilities. In the next study, Jinadasa Liyanaratne gives an overview of Rasacikitsā in Sri Lanka through an analysis of the Sinhala *Prayogaratnāvaliya*, in the process also tracing the various sources of influence on its matter, as well as its borrowings from Sanskrit medical works, particularly the *Siddhasāra*. G. Jan Meulenbeld then shows how the commentators on the *Kauśikasūtra* 'strive at the incorporation of Āyurvedic practices in the healing traditions of the *Atharvaveda* and *Kauśikasūtra*, while maintaining a dichotomy and recognizing that diseases, not due to a transgression of the *dharma*, belong to the realm of Āyurveda. The authors of the classical medical treatises, on the other hand, try to incorporate the *Atharvaveda* ..., in this, they are not convincing and give the impression that merely lip-service is being paid' (p. 308).

Sandra Smets examines the data on the development of the embryo in the *Jaiminīyasaṃhitā* of the *Brahmāṇḍapurāṇa*, and its relation to that in the *Yājñavalkyasmr̥ti* and its commentary *Mitākṣarā* by Vijñāneśvara. B.V. Subbarayappa speculates on a Chinese origin of both Rasaśāstra and the Siddha system. On slightly over four pages, various apodictic statements with known contents are strung together. Gyula Wojtilla gives a concise, but authoritative, overview on Pākaśāstra, Sūdaśāstra and Sūpaśāstra. He asks, and attempts partially to answer, questions like why 'real cooking i.e. preparing tasty food became an art while making healthy food became science in India in the last three hundred years' (p. 343), and why only texts regarded as medical literature have been preserved. Dominik Wujastyk gives a good overview on the classification based on the polarity of *agni-* and *soma-*. Just prior to the appearance of Wujastyk's study, this reviewer had published a short overview on the opposition of *āgneya-* and *saumya-* in medical works;[42] though the two studies share material, they differ substantially enough to complement each other. Finally, Francis Zimmermann examines metaphors of wellbeing in Sanskrit texts against the backdrop of man's relationship with his natural environment, thus

[42] See pp. 521-527, with further references, of the work mentioned in note 25.

continuing a line of research he started over twenty years ago. Incidentally, it must be pointed out that Zimmermann wrongly writes that the work mentioned in note 36 above misses out the 'distinction between tillage (*kṛṣi*) and gardening (*vṛkṣāyurveda*)' (p. 377, note 6). In fact, this distinction is clearly mentioned in the very first sentence on p. 1 of the work, namely 'daß im alten Indien zwischen Landwirtschaft im engeren Sinne (d.h. Ackerbau und damit Zusammenhängendem) und Gartenbau (d.h. Anlage und Hege von Hainen, Gärten und dergleichen) unterschieden wurde'!

Five studies comprise the third section, 'Littératures et savoirs'. Three deal with theatre (Lyne Bansat-Boudon), Arthaśāstra (Irma Piovano), and poetry/ mathematics (Sreeramula Rajeswara Sarma) respectively. Nalini Balbir examines Middle Indo-Aryan sources on Indian ants, with fascinating details on their nomenclature, classification, behaviour, significance etc. Gérard Colas writes on the *Snānavādavīci* (contained in the *Vādavāridhi*), which describes and analyses the act of bathing from a Navyanyāya perspective.

In 'Histoire des religions en Asie du Sud', the fourth section, there are eight studies. M.L. Gharote opines that among the various versions of Svātmārāma's *Haṭha(yoga)pradīpikā* it is manuscript 6756 of the Rājasthān Oriental Research Institute in Jodhpur with 1553 verses that 'represents original text of *Haṭhapradīpikā*. It was called *Siddhāntamuktāvalī*' (p. 485). Jacqueline Filliozat provides us with a reference tool, an alphabetical index of mystical syllables and formulas from protective Pali literature from South-East Asia. Minoru Hara, taking up a thread spun by Arion Roşu himself, discusses the various meanings of the full jar (*kumbha-*, *ghaṭa-*, *kalaśa-*), on the one hand for producing auspiciousness in various contexts, on the other in connection with Yogic practices of breath control. André Padoux examines the relationship between mantras and the human body. David Gordon White interprets three *Yogasūtras* of Patañjali (3,26 and 3,38f.), against the backdrop of Vedic, epic and tantric texts, as containing elements predating all other Indian teachings on Yoga, elements that have, according to him, unfortunately been obfuscated by the subsequent textual tradition. He castigates in particular Vivekananda's 'diminished, derivative, dilettante revisionist reconstruction of the history of yoga that has held the field in India and the west for over one hundred years' (p.

627). The other studies concern two Nepalese painted scrolls with Buddhist rebirth stories (Siegfried Lienhard), a Buddhist prodigal son parable (Boris Oguibénine) and the iconography of Viṣṇu as a dancing boar (Charlotte Schmid).

The fifth group of four studies is entitled 'Philosophies indiennes'. Problems of *Bhagavadgītā* 4 (Henk W. Bodewitz), of suffering, *karman-* and rebirth (George Chemparathy), of time in Buddhist tantric and Śaiva Kashmirian texts (Jean Naudou) and of Nāgārjuna (Amalia Pezzali) are discussed.

Finally, we have the section 'L'Inde, au-delà de l'Inde' with seven studies. Their subject matter is respectively: Sanskrit epigraphy in Cambodia (Kamaleswar Bhattacharya), data on India in the works of Lucianus of Samosata (Klaus Karttunen), the painter August Schöfft and his Lahore painting of Fezli Azam Joo Court (Jean-Marie Lafont), the founding of the Institut de Civilisation Indienne (Roland Lardinois), Kőrösi Csoma Sándor/Alexander Csoma de Kőrös in the Sikh kingdom (Bernard Le Calloc'h), ancient South Asian maritime routes and sites (I.K. Sarma) and eschatological corporality in Zoroastrian theology (Mihaela Timuş).

Collecting the material for and editing this monumental volume must have been a herculean task. There are a few misprints and glitches in the layout, but these are really minor and cannot in any way impair the overall favourable impression it leaves. The decision to use footnotes instead of endnotes, even though this entails the use of more space, is commendable, as it facilitates consultation of the notes immensely. The only thing that might be criticised is the mode of presentation in the bibliographies: indenting the first line of each entry,[43] while at the same time putting the first name of each author first, makes them a bit difficult to consult.

RAHUL PETER DAS

[43] With the odd inconsistency; cf. e.g. pp. 344ff., 417.

# Other Publications Received

*Anthropology & Medicine. Volume 9, Number 3, December 2002. Speical Issue: Countervailing Creativity: Patient Agency in the Globalisation of Asian Medicines*. Basingstoke, Hants.: Carfax Publishing. ISSN 1364-8470. Pp. 205-363. ⟨Several articles deal particularly with South Asian and Tibetan medical systems.⟩

*Aṣṭāṅgahṛdaya*: Śrimad Vāgbhaṭa. *Aṣṭānga Hṛdayam. Das achtgliedrige Herz. Erstes Buch. Sūtra Sthāna. Die grundsätzlichen Prinzipien.* In der Übersetzung von Hendrik Wiethase. Fachliche Beratung: Markus Ludwig. [Seesen/Ildehausen]: Kalari Kendram / [Untergriesbach]: Wiethase Verlag 2006. ISBN 3-937632-43-4. 335 pp. ⟨This first volume of a proposed many-volume and indexed German translation of the whole text does not satisfy scholarly requirements, but is interesting nevertheless as it derives from a Keralan martial arts-cum-medical tradition, and also utilises a Malayalam translation of the Sanskrit text.⟩

**Bagchi, Asoke**: *Sanskrit and Modern Medical Vocabulary*. Kolkata: The Asiatic Society 2002. Monograph Series 36. ISBN 81-7236-123-8. xiii;132 pp. Rs 240.– / US-$ 24 (!!). ⟨"According to Author", "a Ph.D. in Therapeutic Philosophy from the World University of Phoenix, Arizona, USA", "English lexicographers claim that the overwhelming majority of medical terms originate from Greek, a sizable portion being derived from Latin, but he feels that many of these terms which are supposed to have originated from Greek or Latin in fact did so from Sanskrit" (from dust jacket). This is a publication of the Asiatic Society.⟩

**Bode, Maarten**: *Ayurvedic and Unani Health and Beauty Products: Reworking India's Medical Traditions*. Academisch Proefschrift ter verkrijging van de graad van doctor aan de Universiteit van Amsterdam … . Amsterdam: Faculteit der Maatschappij- en Gedragswetenschappen, Universiteit van Amsterdam 2004. xiii;220 pp.

**Chén, Míng**: *Dūnhuáng chūtǔ húyǔ yīdiǎn "Qípóshū" yánjiū. A Study on Sanskrit Text of* Jīvaka-pustaka *from Dunhuang*. Táiběi: Xīnwénfēng Chūbǎn Gōngsī 1994. Xiānggǎng Dūnhuáng Tǔlǔfān Yánjiū Zhōngxīn Cóngkān 10. ISBN 957-17-2024-0 (hardcover) 957-17-2025-9 (paperback). 4;12;752 pp. ⟨Includes Chinese translation of the Sanskrit text.⟩

**Deshpande, Madhav M.; Hook, Peter E.** (ed.): *Indian Linguistic Studies. Festschrift in Honor of George Cardona*. Delhi: Motilal Banarsidass Publishers 2002. ISBN 81-208-1885-7. xxv;384 pp. Rs 695.–. ⟨Pp. 315-343: Albrecht Wezler, "Some Remarks on the Final Verses of the Kāmasūtra", pp. 344-346: Hartmut Scharfe: "The Language of the Physician".⟩

**Dvivedī, Kapil'dev; Dvivedī, Bhār'tendu**: *Vedoṃ meṃ āyurved (Medical Sciences in the Vedas)*. Jñān'pur (Bhadohī): Viśvabhār'tī Anusaṃdhān Pariṣad· 2001. Vedāmṛtam· 13-16. ISBN 81-85246-36-X. 15;296 pp. Rs 200.– (cloth), Rs 125.– (paper). ⟨Actually first published in 1993; this is not mentioned, though the foreword still bears this date.⟩

**Eichner, Heiner; Nedoma, Robert** (ed.): insprinc haptbandun. *Referate des Kolloquiums zu den* Merseburger Zaubersprüchen *auf der XI. Fachtagung der Indogermanischen Gesellschaft in Halle/Saale (17.-23. September 2000). Teil II = Die Sprache. Zeitschrift für*

*Sprachwissenschaft. Band 42, Heft 1/2. 2000/01.* Wien: Wiener Sprachgesellschaft / Harrassowitz Verlag 2001. ISSN 0376-401X. 242 pp. ⟨Also pays great attention to the medical parallels in the *Atharvavedasaṃhitā.*⟩

**Girke, M.; Hoppe, J.-D.; Matthiessen, P.F.; Willich, S.N.** (ed.): *Medizin und Menschenbild. Das Verständnis des Menschen in Schul- und Komplementärmedizin.* Dargestellt vom Dialogforum Pluralismus in der Medizin. Köln: Deutscher Ärzte-Verlag 2006. ISBN 978-3-7691-0514-8 / 3-7691-0514-1. 114 pp. ⟨Pp. 99-106: Ananda Samir Chopra, "Welches Menschenbild bestimmt das ärztliche Handeln im Āyurveda?"⟩

**Gupta, Brahmananda** (ed.): *Papers on the Āyurvedic Studies.* Kolkata: The Asiatic Society 2006. viii;140 pp. Rs 200.–. ⟨Seventeen essays on diverse aspects both ancient and modern.⟩

**Hook, Peter E.**: see **Deshpande, Madhav M.**

**Hoppe, J.-D.**: see **Girke, M.**

*Indian Journal of History of Science. Volume 41, No. 4, December 2006.* New Delhi: Indian National Science Academy. ISSN 0019-5235. Pp. 345-490;S317-S415;i-iii;i-iv. Annual subscription Rs 700.– / US-$ 180 (institution), Rs 500.– / US-$ 130 (individual), Rs 350.– / US-$ 90 (student/researcher). ⟨Contents: B. Sasisekaran, B. Raghunatha Rao and S. Sundararajan, "Bronze Sieve from Kodumanal – An Archaeo[-]metallurgical Study"; Dominik Wujastyk, "The Questions of King Tukkoji: Medicine at an Eighteenth Century South Indian Court"; Ajoy Shankar Verma, "Ice-making in Late Medieval India: Processes and Principles"; Kaushik Roy, "Technology and Transformation of Sikh Warfare: Dal Khālsā against the Lāl Palṭans, 1800-1849"; Historical Notes; Book Reviews; Obituary of David Edwin Pingree; News; S. Balachandra Rao and S.K. Uma, "Grahalāghavam of Gaṇeśa Daivajña [last part]"; Index.⟩

*Indian Journal of History of Science. Volume 42, No. 1, March 2007.* New Delhi: Indian National Science Academy. ISSN 0019-5235. 115;xv;S41 pp. Annual subscription Rs 700.– / US-$ 180 (institution), Rs 500.– / US-$ 130 (individual), Rs 350.– / US-$ 90 (student/researcher). ⟨Contents: R.K. Dubey, "Sources of Gold in India as Described by Ṭhakkura Pherū – An Assessment"; Job Kozhamthadam, "Jesuit Contribution to the Origin and Development of Modern Science and Mathematics"; Dhruv Raina, "Jesuit Collections of Indian Scientific Manuscripts: Ideologies and Interpretations"; Subhasis Sahoo and Binay Kumar Pattnaik, "Scientist as Interlocutor betweeen Science and Society: Two Biographical Studies from Orissa (India)"; Historical Notes; Book Reviews; S. Balachandra Rao and S.K. Uma, "Karaṇakutūhalam of Bhāskarācārya II [first part]".⟩

*Journal of Indian Philosophy. Volume 32, No. 1, February 2004.* Dordrecht|Boston|London: Kluwer Academic Publishers. ISSN 0022-1791. 111 pp. ⟨Pp. 31-56: Viktoria Lyssenko, "The Human Body Composition in Statics and Dynamics: Āyurveda and the Philosophical Schools of Vaiśeṣika and Sāṃkhya".⟩

**Matthiessen, P.F.**: see **Girke, M.**

*Namah. New Approaches to Medicine and Health. Volume 11 Issue 1, 24th April 2003.* Pondicherry: Sri Aurobindo Society. ISSN 0971-684-X. 56 pp. Rs. 50.–/US-$ 8.– (by air)/

US-$ 6 (by sea). ⟨Selected contents: Michael Miovic, "Non-local studies – implications for health"; K.H. Krishnamurthy, "Mirchi or Chilli (Capsicum, Linn.)"; R.L. Bijlani, "Scientific medicine shows signs of a paradigm shift"; N. Shakuntala Manay and R. Sreelakshmi, "Qualitative vibration of thought energy on the environment"; K.H. Krishnamurthy, "Hospital construction in ancient India".⟩

*Namah. New Approaches to Medicine and Health. Volume 11 Issue 2, 15th July 2003.* Pondicherry: Sri Aurobindo Society. ISSN 0971-684-X. 58 pp. Rs. 50.–/US-$ 8.– (by air)/ US-$ 6 (by sea). ⟨Selected contents: Cromwell Crawford, "The goals of medicine: setting new priorities (a hindu perspective)"; K.H. Krishnamurthy, "Khas or Sugandhimūlaḥ (Vetiveria zizanoides, Linn.)"; Ashok Panagariya, "Science of mind in health and happiness"; N. Loganathan, "Some ethno-medicinal plants".⟩

*Namah. New Approaches to Medicine and Health. Volume 11 Issue 3, 15th October 2003.* Pondicherry: Sri Aurobindo Society. ISSN 0971-684-X. 73 pp. Rs. 50.–/US-$ 8.– (by air)/ US-$6 (by sea). ⟨Selected contents: D.B. Bisht, "A case study on the evolution and strategies of leprosy control and elimination"; K.H. Krishnamurthy, "Methī or Fenugreek (Trigonella foenum-graecum. Linn.)"; NAMAH – Indexing (August 1993 – October 2003).⟩

*Namah. New Approaches to Medicine and Health. Volume 11 Issue 4, 15th January 2004.* Pondicherry: Sri Aurobindo Society. ISSN 0971-684-X. 61 pp. Rs. 50.–/US-$ 8.– (by air)/ US-$ 6 (by sea). ⟨Selected contents: D.B. Bisht, "Health at the crossroads – the Indian scene"; K.H. Krishnamurthy, "Ikṣuḥ or Sugarcane (Saccharum officinarum, Linn.)"; Michael Miovic, "Flower remedies in psychodynamic psychotherapy"; D.E. Mistry, "Treatment of Craniopharyngioma in a 'little Zen master'"; Tinus Smits, "Post-vaccination syndrome".⟩

*Namah. New Approaches to Medicine and Health. Volume 12 Issue 1, 24th April 2004.* Pondicherry: Sri Aurobindo Society. ISSN 0971-684-X. 47 pp. Rs. 50.–/US-$ 8.– (by air)/ US-$ 6 (by sea). ⟨Selected contents: David Johnston, "The individuation process and care of the self"; K.H. Krishnamurthy, "Āmra phala or Mango (Mangifera indica, Linn.)"; D.E. Mistry, "A case of Wilson's disease".⟩

*Namah. New Approaches to Medicine and Health. Volume 12 Issue 2, 15th July 2004.* Pondicherry: Sri Aurobindo Society. ISSN 0971-684-X. 51 pp. Rs. 50.–/US-$ 8.– (by air)/ US-$ 6 (by sea). ⟨Selected contents: D.B. Bisht, "A unified system"; Alok Pandey, "Illness: an integral view"; Arya Maloney, "Alchemy of the soul. The encounter of psychology and spirituality"; Y.V. Chawla, "Disease – the inner disharmony"; K.H. Krishnamurthy, "Amrutaphalam, Guava (Psidium guyava, Linn.)"; R. Ramanan, "Attitudes of approach"; R.L. Bijlani, "Body-mind medicine in action: the Integral Health Clinic of All India Institute of Medical Sciences".⟩

*Namah. New Approaches to Medicine and Health. Volume 12 Issue 3, 15th October 2004.* Pondicherry: Sri Aurobindo Society. ISSN 0971-684-X. 49 pp. Rs. 50.–/US-$ 8.– (by air)/ US-$ 6 (by sea). ⟨Selected contents: David Johnston, "Transference, counter-transference and Jungian depth-therapy"; K.H. Krishnamurthy, "Eraṇḍa, castor (Ricinus communis, Linn.)"; Asit Kumar Panja, V. Sreedhar and B.L. Gaur, "Flowers in ancient classics"; Alok Pandey, "The healer within".⟩

*Namah. New Approaches to Medicine and Health. Volume 12 Issue 4, 15th January 2005.* Pondicherry: Sri Aurobindo Society. ISSN 0971-684-X. 50 pp. Rs. 50.–/US-$ 8.– (by air)/ US-$ 6 (by sea). ⟨Selected contents: Alok Pandey, "The human body: machinistic and consciousness view"; John B. Mulliken, "A sense of wonder"; K.H. Krishnamurthy, "Haridrā, Turmeric (Curcuma longa, Linn.)"; M. Paramkusha Rao, "Herb Thesaurus of Āyurveda".⟩

*Namah. New Approaches to Medicine and Health. Volume 13 Issue 1, 24th April 2005.* Pondicherry: Sri Aurobindo Society. ISSN 0971-684-X. 50 pp. Rs. 50.–/US-$ 8.– (by air)/ US-$ 6 (by sea). ⟨Selected contents: Bhalendu S. Vaishnav, "Integral Health: concepts and clinical practice"; Arya Maloney, "Alchemy of the soul. The body and psycho-spiritual process"; K.H. Krishnamurthy, "Gokṣurah, puncture vine (Tribulus terrestris, and Pedalium murex, Linn.)"; N. Shakuntala Manay and R. Sreelakshmi, "Psycho-physiological concept of health and nutrition: qualitative vibration of food".⟩

*Namah. New Approaches to Medicine and Health. Volume 13 Issue 2, 15th July 2005.* Pondicherry: Sri Aurobindo Society. ISSN 0971-684-X. 51 pp. Rs. 50.–/US-$ 8.– (by air)/ US-$ 6 (by sea). ⟨Selected contents: Arya Maloney, "Alchemy of the soul. A soul-centered psychology"; K.H. Krishnamurthy, "Drākṣā or Grape (Vitex vinifera, Linn.)"; "Interview with a sungazer who doesn't need to eat".⟩

*Namah. New Approaches to Medicine and Health. Volume 13 Issue 3, 15th October 2005.* Pondicherry: Sri Aurobindo Society. ISSN 0971-684-X. 53 pp. Rs. 50.–/US-$ 8.– (by air)/ US-$ 6 (by sea). ⟨Selected contents: Arya Maloney, "Alchemy of the soul. Bridging spiritual practice and psychotherapy"; K.H. Krishnamurthy, "Palāṇḍu, Onion (Allium cepa, Linn.)"; Vandana, "Flower blessings: a glimpse (A note on flower remedies from SAIIIHR)"; Letters on the sungazer – Mr. Hira Ratan Manek.⟩

*Namah. New Approaches to Medicine and Health. Volume 13 Issue 4, 15th January 2006.* Pondicherry: Sri Aurobindo Society. ISSN 0971-684-X. 59 pp. Rs. 50.–/US-$ 8.– (by air)/ US-$ 6 (by sea). ⟨Selected contents: Alok Pandey, "Psychotherapy and Indian thought – I"; Arya Maloney, "Alchemy of the soul. The process of integral psychology"; K.H. Krishnamurthy, "Madhu, Honey"; R.L. Bijlani, "What is death?".⟩

*Namah. New Approaches to Medicine and Health. Volume 14 Issue 1, 24th April 2006.* Pondicherry: Sri Aurobindo Society. ISSN 0971-684-X. 51 pp. Rs. 50.–/US-$ 8.– (by air)/ US-$ 6 (by sea). ⟨Selected contents: Arya Maloney, "Alchemy of the soul. The suffocated soul"; Sampadananda Mishra, "Treatment of Elephantiasis in Suśruta Saṁhitā"; Sanjeev Rastogi, Rajeev Rastogi and R.H. Singh, "What are we losing by ignoring Āyurveda? (Analysis of current Indian medical practice referring to a case of chronic migraine)"; Alok Pandey, "Psychotherapy and Indian thought – II"; K.H. Krishnamurthy, "Lavang, Clove (Myrtus caryophyllus, Linn.)".⟩

*Namah. New Approaches to Medicine and Health. Volume 14 Issue 2, 15th July 2006.* Pondicherry: Sri Aurobindo Society. ISSN 0971-684-X. 55 pp. Rs. 50.–/US-$ 8.– (by air)/ US-$ 6 (by sea). ⟨Selected contents: Arya Maloney, "Alchemy of the soul. Transforming torture"; Sampadananda Mishra, "Treatment of Elephantiasis in Suśruta Saṁhitā – II"; K.H. Krishnamurthy, "Jāmun, Black plum (Eugenia)"; David Johnston, "Shamanism and contemporary depth-therapy".⟩

*Namah. New Approaches to Medicine and Health. Volume 14 Issue 3, 15th October 2006.* Pondicherry: Sri Aurobindo Society. ISSN 0971-684-X. 50 pp. Rs. 50.–/US-$ 8.– (by air)/ US-$ 6 (by sea). ⟨Selected contents: Alok Pandey, "Systems and beyond systems"; Arya Maloney, "Alchemy of the soul. The uninvited guest"; D.B. Bisht, "Hospitals – health or ill-health institutions?"; Vallath Nandini, "Idealistic vision of a Healing Centre".⟩

*Namah. New Approaches to Medicine and Health. Volume 14 Issue 4, 15th January 2007.* Pondicherry: Sri Aurobindo Society. ISSN 0971-684-X. 56 pp. Rs. 50.–/US-$ 8.– (by air)/ US-$ 6 (by sea). ⟨Selected contents: Arya Maloney, "Alchemy of the soul. Spontaneity of soul: an autobiographical glimpse"; K.H. Krishnamurthy, "Kesar, Saffron (Crocus sativus, Linn.)"; Hemant Kapoor, "Mysticism and schizophrenia"; Brenden Skudder, "Are all diseases curable?"; Pamela Siegel and Nelson Barros F. [sic], "Yoga and health: a systematic literature review".⟩

*Namah. New Approaches to Medicine and Health. Volume 15 Issue 1, 24th April 2007.* Pondicherry: Sri Aurobindo Society. ISSN 0971-684-X. 60 pp. Rs. 50.–/US-$ 8.– (by air)/ US-$ 6 (by sea). ⟨Selected contents: Mamta Saxena, B. Sen Gupta and Pranav Pandya, "Yagya vs. Non-Yagya: a case study on indoor microbial environment"; K.H. Krishnamurthy, "Infection and its management in Āyurveda"; Y. Balasubramanian, "Pearls on garlic: the wonder bulb (Allium sativum; Family Liliacea)"; Surendra Pal Singh Jaijania and Archana Verma, "Clinical study on banyan milk and turmeric powder".⟩

*Namah. New Approaches to Medicine and Health. Volume 15 Issue 2, 15th July 2007.* Pondicherry: Sri Aurobindo Society. ISSN 0971-684-X. 63 pp. Rs. 50.–/US-$ 8.– (by air)/ US-$ 6 (by sea). ⟨Selected contents: Alok Pandey, "Search and research"; K.H. Krishnamurthy, "Pāṣāṇabhedī or Indian Borage (Coleus aromaticus, Benth.)"; D.B. Bisht, "Spiritual dimension of health with special reference to traditional healing practices"; "Allopathy and Ayurveda".⟩

*Namah. New Approaches to Medicine and Health. Volume 15 Issue 3, 15th October 2007.* Pondicherry: Sri Aurobindo Society. ISSN 0971-684-X. 77 pp. Rs. 50.–/US-$ 8.– (by air)/ US-$ 6 (by sea). ⟨Selected contents: K.H. Krishnamurthy, "Khadira (Acacia catechu, Willd.)"; NAMAH Index (August 1993 – July 2007).⟩

*Namah. New Approaches to Medicine and Health. Volume 15 Issue 4, 15th January 2008.* Pondicherry: Sri Aurobindo Society. ISSN 0971-684-X. 65 pp. Rs. 50.–/US-$ 8.– (by air)/ US-$ 6 (by sea). ⟨Selected contents: Sanjeev Rastogi, Hem Chandra and Rajiv Rastogi, "Practice of the Āyurvedic system of medicine: a pilot study"; K.H. Krishnamurthy: "Barburah or Indian gum arabic (Acacia arabica, Willd.)".⟩

**Nedoma, Robert**: see **Eichner, Heiner**

*Numen. Volume 50, No. 4, 2003.* Leiden: Koninklijke Brill NV. ISSN 0029-5973. Pp. 357-485. ⟨Pp. 416-463: Steven Engler, "'Science' vs. 'Religion' in Classical Ayurveda".⟩

**Saller, R.** (ed.): *Tibetische Heilmittel bei chronischen Erkrankungen*. Basel etc.: Karger 2006. Forschende Komplementärmedizin, Supplement 1 zu Band 13. ISBN 3-8055-8104-1. 32 pp.

*Studies in History of Medicine and Science. Volume XVIII, No. 2 (New Series), July-Dec. 2002*. New Delhi: Jamia Hamdard. ISSN 0970-5562. 132 pp. Rs 100.– for a single issue, Rs 200.– for the whole volume. ⟨Contents: Altaf Ahmad Azmi, "Academic Pursuit of Mughal Kings With Special Reference to Medicine (Ṭibb)"; A. Khaliq Kaifi, "Unani, The Graeco-Arab Medicine in India"; Altaf Ahmad Azmi, "Shah Fatḥullāh Shīrāzī – An Eminent Scholar of Mughal Period"; Vinod Mishra, "Combinatorics and the (So-Called) Binomial Theorem"; Book Reviews.⟩

*Studies in History of Medicine and Science. Volume XIX, No. 1-2 (New Series), 2003*. New Delhi: Jamia Hamdard. ISSN 0970-5562. 126 pp. Rs 100.– for a single issue, Rs 200.– for the whole volume. ⟨Contents: Altaf Ahmad Azmi, "Unani Medicine during Babur's Reign"; Jaweed Ashraf, "Medico-Social Study of Majmūʿa-i Ziyāʾī: A Medieval Persian Unani Manuscript"; Altaf Ahmad Azmi, "History of Cauterization and its Relevance to the Modern World"; Abdul Bari, "Dastūr Al-Hunūd: A Persian Ṭibbī Manuscript"; S.S. Verma, "Magnetic Therapy: A Supplement to Medicine"; Syed Mahtab Ali, "Contribution of Muslim Physicians to Anatomy"; Vinod Mishra, "Similarity of Plane Figures: A Reflection in Indian Geometry"; Book Reviews; Centre's Report.⟩

**Varmā, Vinod**: *Dainik jīvan meṃ āyurved*. Nayī Dillī: Kitāb'ghar 2001. ISBN 81-7106-362-5. 376 pp. Rs 250.–.

**Willich, S.N.**: see **Girke, M.**

*Addresses of the Contributors*

Prof.Dr. Vincanne ADAMS, Department of Anthropology, History and Social Medicine, University of California, 3333 California Street 485, San Francisco CA 94143, United States of America

Dr. Maarten BODE, Vespuccistraat 82–II hoog, 1056 SP Amsterdam, Netherlands

Prof.Dr. Willem B. BOLLÉE, Don-Bosco-Straße 2, 96047 Bamberg, Germany

Prof.Dr. Mandakranta BOSE, Institute of Asian Research, University of British Columbia, 1855 West Mall, Vancouver B.C. V6T 1Z2, Canada

Ananda Samir CHOPRA, Arzt, Sandbuschweg 5A, 34132 Kassel, Germany

Dr. Eugen CIURTIN, Crisana 20, Apartament 43, 010828 Bucharest – 1, Romania

Prof.Dr. Rahul Peter DAS, Dorotheenring 5, 25451 Quickborn, Germany

Prof. Renchen DHONDUP, Tibetan Medical College, Qinghai University, Xining, People's Republic of China

Prof.Dr. Frances GARRETT, Department and Centre for the Study of Religion, University of Toronto, 123 St. George Street, Toronto ON M5S 2E8, Canada

Prof.Dr. Minoru HARA, 1-19-1-201 Ishikawa-cho, Ota-ku, Tokyo, 145 Japan

Dr. Oliver HELLWIG, Zossener Straße 33, 10961 Berlin, Germany

Prof. Jampa KELSANG, Men-Tsee-Khang, Gangchen Kyishong, Dharamsala 176215, India

Prof.Dr. Catharina KIEHNLE, Blüthnerstraße 5, 04179 Leipzig, Germany

Dr. Makoto KITADA, % Sumiko Kitada, Sashizuki Mansion 102, Nakayamatedori 6-6-5, Chuo-ku, Kobe 650-0004, Japan

Dr. Damodaran Suresh KUMAR, Sami Labs Ltd., 19/1 & 19/2 I Main, II Phase, Peenya Industrial Area, Bangalore 560058, India

Prof.Dr. Mauro MAGGI, Via Castellaccio Carano 30, 00040 Lanuvio (RM), Italy

Dr. Muhammed MAJEED, Sabinsa Corporation, 70 Ethel Road West, Unit 6, Piscataway NJ 08854, United States of America

Dr. Gerrit Jan MEULENBELD, De Zwaan 11, 9781 JX Bedum, Netherlands

Prof.Dr.Dr. Klaus MYLIUS, Bergstraße 13, 79288 Gottenheim, Germany

YUMBA, Mentsikhang, Lhasa, Tibetan Autonomous Region, People's Republic of China